A Different Kind
of AIDS

A Different Kind of AIDS

of AIDS

Folk and Lay Theories in South African Townships

David Dickinson

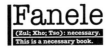

Fanele
(Zul; Xho; Tso): necessary.
This is a necessary book.

First published by Fanele, an imprint of
Jacana Media (Pty) Ltd, in 2014

10 Orange Street
Sunnyside
Auckland Park 2092
South Africa
+2711 628 3200
www.jacana.co.za

This title has been subject to an academic peer review process.

ISBN 978-1-920196-98-1

Cover design by Shawn Paikin
Cover photograph by David Dickinson
Set in Sabon 10.5/15 pt
Printed and bound by Creda Communications
Job No. 002157

See a complete list of Jacana titles at www.jacana.co.za

This book is dedicated to the memory of
Solomon Mveli Nhlapo
(1939 – 2010)
Mosuwe, Motswalle, Ntate

Acknowledgements

Many people assisted, in many ways, in the research and writing of this book. I am grateful to them all.

In addition to placing the book's characters into the fictitious townships of Potlakong and Butleng, I have changed their names and other details in order that they remain anonymous.

I thank: Karen Birdsall, Harold Bokaba, Faniswa Bolawa, Nomsa Bongwe, Dries Burger, Tracey Calmeyer, Pule de Roland Phillips, Charles Deutsch, Zanele Dhladhla, Thandiwe Dhlalisa, Milton Dhlamini, Sibusiso Dhlamini, Madlamini Dlamini, Obed Dlamini, Cecily Falcon, James Goso, Michael Greyling, Siphamandla Gumede, Thapelo 'Touch' Hlahatse/Mosia, Jonathan Klaaren, Mampho Koli, Lefu Kokota, Morongwe Kokota, Nyane Kokota, Thabo Kokota, Jabulani Lekhuleni, Mamosa Lesitha, Masingoaneng Lesitha, Mpuse Lesitha, Nelly Letuka, Seabata Mafaisa, Elliot Mahlalela, Hollyday Maila, David Mailola, Jan Makatees, Thandiwe Malindi, Lehlohonolo Maqwaza, Kate Mashabela, Puleng Mathe, Katse Matsebe, Lucas Mavundane, Rochelle Mawona, Majeki Mbhele, Mamohlolo Mbhele, Maqhawana Mbhele, Masera Mbhele, Sheila Mbele, Sibusiso Mbele, Brad Mears, Mmopiemang Memani, Issa Mofoka, Clement Mncwabe, Themba Mndebele, Ntombi Mnisi, Lefa Mofokeng, Malebohang Mofokeng, Motebang Mofokeng, Motsoso Mofokeng, Palesa Mofokeng, Puleng Mofokeng, Tlala Mofokeng, Maja Mokhutsoane, Modise Mokhutsoane, Kenilwe Molawa, Lolo Molepo, Lesufi 'OJ' Moloi, Tshepiso Moloi, Themba Morajane, Tuane Morakoane, Elias

Motshweni, Napoleon Mpharu, Pamilla Mudhray, Sani Ndaba, Alice Nhlapo, Calestina Nhlapo, Robert Nhlapo, Seiponi Nhlapo, Joel Nkadimeng, Musa Nkambule, Lucky Nkuna, Ellen Nkutha, Emmanuel Ntako, Pumla Ntlabati, Bheki Nonyane, Celia Nonyane, Joe Nonyane, Saki Pheleu, Tankiso Pitso, Susan Preller, Mbozela Radebe, Mpho Radebe, Thulani Radebe, Tsidi Radebe, Violet Radebe, Lekgotla Ralieta, Nkaki Ralieta, Tebza Rasenekal, Charles Rathebe, Nirvana Sandra, Helen Schneider, Mathews Sebeko, Paulos Sebolai, Dudu Serekeho, Mmasibidi Setaka, Mpho Sewela, Matshediso Shoahle, Thulani Shunobe, Krish Sigamoney, Percy Simelane, Courtenay Sprague, Katleho Suping, Maleeto Suping, Motebang Suping, Morena Thulo, Masetjahaba Tlatsa, Andrias Tshabalala, Johannes van Coller, Gregory van Dyk, Sarel van Wyk, Louise Whittaker, Leonard Zungu, Bafana Zwane and Lina Zwane.

Presentations based on this research were made at the Wits Business School, Wits Sociology Department, Wits Society, Work and Development Institute, the South African Sociological Association Congress, 2009, the American Public Health Association Congress 2010, the World Congress of Sociology 2010, and the International Social Science and Humanities Conference on HIV 2011. Two articles on the Digco participatory action research project were published in the *African Journal of AIDS Research* in 2011 and 2013. The manuscript was reviewed by Jonathan Stadler and Suzette Heald. Both provided immensely useful feedback and suggestions.

Funding for the project came from the Wits Faculty of Commerce Law and Management's Research Committee and my Research Incentive Account. The first draft of the book was written while on sabbatical leave at the National University of Lesotho, a visit funded by a grant from the Anderson Cappeli fund.

For much of the time that I was researching and writing this book I was also President of the Academic Staff Association of Wits University (ASAWU). I would like to thank all my colleagues on the ASAWU Executive Committee as well as ASAWU Coordinators Brian Holmes, Vincent Kgosana and Sharon Vergie for their support over this period.

Acknowledgements

This book would have been completed significantly earlier without this responsibility, but for that they are not liable.

Leanne Bell encouraged and improved the book immensely as it took shape, and I am grateful for the faith she showed in the evolving manuscript. At Jacana, Leigh-Ann Harris and Ester Levinrad saw through the book's publication with enthusiasm.

David Dickinson
Johannesburg, April 2014

Contents

Abbreviations

ABC	Abstain, Be faithful or Condomise: HIV-prevention slogan
ANC	African National Congress: Liberation movement and the ruling party since 1994
ASAWU	Academic Staff Association of Wits University
HIV/AIDS	Human Immunodeficiency Virus/Acquired Immune Deficiency Syndrome
KAP	Knowledge, Attitude and Practices: Information sought in survey/questionnaires
KFC	Kentucky Fried Chicken: Fast food
PWA/PLWHA	Person Living (openly) with HIV/AIDS: The PWA abbreviation is most common
RAF	Road Accident Fund: Provides universal insurance for road accidents via a fuel levy
RDP	Reconstruction and Development Programme: Now superseded, but the name remains for the four-room, low-income houses built with government support
TAC	Treatment Action Campaign
TB	Tuberculosis
ZCC	Zion Christian Church

Terms & names

African (race)	South African racial categorisation: People of indigenous African descent
Allopathic medicine	Synonymous with biomedicine, scientific and Western medicine
Biomedicine	Medical diagnosis and treatment based on scientific principles
Bio-moral theories	Theories of disease and affliction linking moral values with physical and social health
Black (race)	South African racial categorisation: Africans, Coloureds and Indians
Butleng	A fictitious Free State township
Coloured (race)	South African racial categorisation: People of mixed racial decent
Digco	Pseudonym for a South African mining company
Emic and etic perspectives	Perspectives from within and from outside a group respectively
Ethnoecological disease	A condition identified or self-identified as particular to one ethnic group
Free State	A South African province: Largely rural with some three million residents

Gauteng	A South African province: Urbanised and industrialised with some 12 million residents
Health-seeking behaviour	The ways in which individuals and families seek help for sickness or other afflictions
Indian (race)	South African racial categorisation: People of Indian descent
Model C School	Formerly, schools which pre-1990 were government schools for Whites only, and post-1990 became semi-private and remained predominantly White. Now indicating, generally, formerly White schools with better academic performance, typically in a traditionally White suburb.
Plaasville	The fictitious Free State town to which Butleng township is attached
Potlakong	A fictitious Gauteng township near Johannesburg
Proximal and distal causes	The way in which sickness is explained through an immediate cause, e.g. infection, and underlying or deeper cause, e.g. witchcraft
Scientific medicine	Synonymous with biomedicine, allopathic and Western medicine
Township	Residential areas previously reserved for Blacks in South Africa
Western medicine	Synonymous with biomedicine, scientific and allopathic medicine
White (race)	South African racial categorisation: People of European descent
Wittenburg	The fictitious regional Free State town some distance from Butleng and Plaasville

Preface

Getting to the point

Why do alternative, non-scientific explanations of HIV/AIDS continue to circulate in South Africa's townships after almost 30 years of AIDS education?

I started to think seriously about AIDS in 1999. I had been commissioned to write a report on a government-sponsored, worker-participation initiative that I researched for my PhD. The Workplace Challenge project was a child of the then still new South Africa; how could management and workers overcome historical differences and increase productivity? I had plunged optimistically and somewhat naively into this project. Having arrived in South Africa in early 1994, just before the first democratic elections, anything and everything seemed possible. Taking on the report meant taking time out from writing my doctoral thesis in the UK, but it was an opportunity to see what had happened in the year that I had been away. One thing that struck me when I re-visited the Workplace Challenge companies was the number of people who had died in what was a relatively short period. Some had died in accidents, some through violence, and others through AIDS-related illnesses.

I returned to South Africa on a permanent basis in late 2000 to take up a post lecturing in industrial relations and resolved to run a short research project on HIV/AIDS. I would use three months or so to research, write a paper and move on with a better understanding of what HIV/AIDS meant for South Africa, particularly the workforce.

I was, of course, a Johnny-come-lately, others had been working on AIDS for well over a decade. However, relatively little had been done on HIV/AIDS within South African companies and I forged ahead enthusiastically with a case study of how Sasol, a large petrochemical company, was responding to the epidemic. The three-month plan had been optimistic; it was mid-2002 by the time I had written up this research.[1]

By then things were in full swing. I collaborated with colleagues to research the responses of other South African companies,[2] organised research symposiums on 'HIV/AIDS in the Workplace',[3] and for a while was seconded from my lecturing, on a part-time basis, to help start Wits University's own response to HIV/AIDS.[4]

By and large, the small group of academics working on HIV/AIDS in the workplace, or other institutional settings, identified with what we saw to be the progressive response to the epidemic. This was dominated by the campaign for antiretroviral drugs that was then under way. Despite our own sphere of interest, we acted, in effect, as auxiliaries to the Treatment Action Campaign (TAC) which skilfully conjoined the new democracy's constitutional emphasis on human rights, political activism and medical solutions to the epidemic. Our workplace studies and reports suggested that companies should respond within a human rights and medical framework. We played down politics, never something business wants to openly identify with. Rather, we used alternative motivations, such as corporate social responsibility and company reputation, to motivate responses.

The TAC succeeded in pushing a recalcitrant government into providing antiretroviral drugs within the public health care system.[5] But their approach was always less convincing on behavioural change. The medico-legal rights approach they took had little purchase here. This weakness was concealed with condoms, the third pillar of the ABC Trinity: Abstain, Be faithful, Condomise, the slogan that has dominated the global response on HIV prevention. Condomise, unlike its A and B partners, offered a quasi-medical response that meshed comfortably with a human rights approach. Or at least it was presented that way with a virtual clampdown on any behavioural questions over condom use.

Condom distribution was an easy thing to run with. In a terribly crude way, installing condom dispensers sorted out who in an institution was *for* the progressive response to AIDS and who was putting their head in the sand over the epidemic. The easiest victory we had in getting the Wits University AIDS programme started was overcoming resistance from one or two Heads of Schools to condom dispensers being installed in their buildings. They were routed when we called in the heavy guns of senior management. It felt as though we were achieving something.

But you can't hunt with the hounds and run with the hares.

My own research was moving on; I was now seeking to understand what was happening within the behavioural change elements of company HIV/AIDS programmes; particularly the role of peer educators, rank-and-file employees drafted in with minimal training, but often great passion, to educate others about HIV and AIDS. I had also stepped outside the workplace environment and was talking to African traditional healers in the townships about AIDS. They were, arguably, the peer educators' strongest opponent and I wanted to see if there could not be harmony rather than conflict. Talking to traditional healers raised eyebrows. There was sometimes concern that I might be on the wrong side of the 'Great AIDS Debate', whether HIV did, or did not, cause AIDS, that lay at the heart of President Mbeki's denialism and the consequent refusal to provide treatment. The question came in different formats, for example, whether I believed that traditional healers could cure AIDS? But it came down to the basic dichotomy: 'HIV causes AIDS? Yes or no?' When I answered, as I had to, that HIV did cause AIDS, there were smiles of relief; I might be engaging with some rum ideas, but it must be in a good cause since I was on the right side of things and on that basis I was invited to present my findings to a range of institutions.[6]

However, what I presented, fascinating as my audiences said it was, wasn't actually what they wanted to hear. I wasn't, I suspect they realised, really on the right side of things. I was suggesting that things were more complicated that we might want to imagine. They wanted me to simplify things and smooth the implementation of their solution to AIDS. This required the population conforming to their prescriptions, whether on sexual behaviour or on adhering to treatment. In short, what was needed from the perspective of clinicians, AIDS activists, programme managers and NGO directors was a translation of African traditional cosmology; a bilingual dictionary of medical and traditional healing terminology. This would allow them to prescribe their solutions in appropriate idiom.

Initially, I weaselled my way through this difficulty. I suggested, compromise-wise, the idea of 'windows of compatibility' between the two systems. The systems were different, but on occasion they happened to be marching in step and, perhaps, we could capitalise on this? [7] This wasn't what the doctors, treatment activists and behavioural change consultants wanted. But what brought my research with traditional healers to a halt was not the clinicians' lukewarm reception to my suggestions, but my own realisation of just how fluid, diverse and idiosyncratic African traditional healing beliefs were. In mid-2008 I had begun a more ambitious inquiry into traditional healers from which I hoped to comprehensively map their cosmology of AIDS. After 12 interviews with Traditional Doctor Mathews Sibeko[8] I had learned a great deal about many things, not least his take on AIDS. But, with this, I could see that his views, laid out in painstaking detail, were different from, and sometimes incompatible with, those of other traditional healers with whom I had started to talk (though I never approached double-digit interview tallies with them). I could weasel this no further; the bilingual medical–traditional dictionary, even in its abridged 'windows of compatibility' form, was not a feasible project. I chucked the idea into the bin of abandoned projects.

I was, however, still left with a problem. If the corpus of healers' knowledge was divided and dispersed, it should be no match for the scientific canon of medical knowledge[9] behind the AIDS programmes that were in full swing. But, on the ground I knew that this was not the case, I had, after all, pursued research into traditional healers' understanding of AIDS because they were the peer educators' most formidable opponent. I had heard plenty of accounts of antiretroviral treatment being abandoned when healers flexed their influence.

My initial research on workplace peer educators, conducted in 2005, was straightforward; a survey, interviews and a few observations squeezed in when opportunity arose. My research was already located at the bottom of the company hierarchy, with its focus on the peer educators who were largely drawn from the ranks of blue-collar workers, most of whom lived in African[10] townships. But I wanted to go deeper. The word in Sesotho is *kakamelo*, it translates as 'curiosity,' but with the not too faint suggestion that you are sticking your nose into other people's business. The next research project that I undertook in 2006 asked peer educators in a mining company to keep a diary of their discussions with peers. I was inquiring into the interactions between peer educators and peers away from the eyes of those who managed the company HIV/AIDS programmes. I wrote up these two research projects with the thesis that what peer educators were doing was multifarious and often difficult, not least because they were operating in contested social spaces when it came to the meaning of AIDS.[11]

A changing approach

Only at this point did I start to question why alternative explanations of HIV/AIDS continued to circulate. I explored this question through two research projects on which this book is based. The first was conducted with a group of 28 African HIV/AIDS peer educators in 'Digco', a South African mining company, between October 2008 and June 2009.[12] The peer educators were asked to identify 'AIDS myths' circulating within their communities. I defined AIDS myths as beliefs about HIV/AIDS that were not medically correct, but which were present in the peer educators' communities. A second, intervention-orientated objective of this project was the development of stories, or parables, that the peer educators could use to counter these AIDS myths.

The Digco project did not go exactly as I had planned. As I describe later, I started to appreciate just how well-constructed, entrenched and legitimate these AIDS myths were within the township settings. Over the course of the project, I began to shift in how I thought of them; not so much AIDS myths but more as alternative, non-scientific explanations or theories of AIDS. This shift in my thinking, and terminology, did not mean that I believed them; rather, I was increasingly acknowledging their power, the benefits they offered, and how they resonated with people's lived experience.

I then planned a second research project that would document 'contextualised illness narratives'. In other words, I wanted to know what township residents infected or affected by HIV/AIDS thought; how they made sense of the disease that they had to live with in their bodies or within their families. This, I reasoned, would complement what the peer educators said other people were saying about AIDS.

I was now less gung-ho about how alternative beliefs about HIV/AIDS could be taken on, or taken out. I was more concerned with grasping how these alternative explanations of AIDS were integrated into individuals' lives. I realised that I needed to take a step back in order to move forward. I attempted to do this with Bafana, Grace, Neo and Paseka between mid-2010 and mid-2011. I sought to understand how these four individuals understood AIDS. None of them were strangers to me, and I have backdated some of the accounts, such as starting Bafana's story with his 2008 health crisis.

I would not have approached this latter project in this way without the previous research. I wanted to establish what alternative accounts of AIDS formed these four individuals' schemas of explanation, and why this was the case, rather than mount a search and destroy operations albeit one using appropriate cultural resources, to neutralise 'AIDS myths'. The Digco peer educators had opened my eyes in this regard. Nevertheless, it would be a simplification of my intellectual journey to say that I was previously unaware of these alternative understandings of AIDS. I had previously spotted alternative accounts, noted how robust these could be, and identified the problem of assuming that people were empty vessels waiting for information on HIV/AIDS,[13] but I had not acted decisively on these insights. I had remained tied to the dominant response to AIDS, even as I argued for a broadening of this from an exclusive reliance on medical interventions and the accessing of human rights. What I now started to see was that we were trying to help people without knowing much about them.

Introduction

Alternative explanations of AIDS in South African townships
HIV/AIDS presents a major problem for South Africa. Some six million people in the country are infected with the virus. Despite three decades of AIDS education and a massive antiretroviral drug programme, in 2012 an estimated 370 000 people became infected and 240 000 died from AIDS.[14]

If we are to grapple with the alternative understandings of AIDS that continue to circulate, we need to challenge some assumptions. The most important of these is that knowledge equals belief. Once we get past that mistaken view, upon which a multi-million dollar AIDS education industry is based, we need to assess how people, really, explain illness. The plurality of health-seeking behaviour indicates that the AIDS epidemic, as well as the illness itself, is being constructed in different ways. Importantly, it is being constructed from below and it is these grassroots constructions that we need to understand.

I start this inquiry, in the following chapter, with an all too common occurrence in South African townships: the funeral of a young man. As the grieving and rituals of burial proceed, the cause of Joseph Sechaba's death becomes increasingly uncertain. Efforts to settle the matter only raise more doubts. We can conclude, though we cannot say with absolute certainty, that Joseph died of AIDS. He hid his illness until the end. But behind the veil of shame, what did Joseph believe? Did he convince himself that there was another explanation, perhaps one of those suggested around the township?

Drawing on the reports of the Digco peer educators, we examine the 'big three' folk theories of AIDS: major constellations of understanding constituted by Christianity, by traditional African beliefs, and by the racial framing of South Africa's social order. Additional to the big three and the medical explanation of AIDS are lay theories of AIDS – hypotheses put forward by individuals that, largely independent of folk cosmologies, model the disease and propose how it can be outsmarted.

These folk and lay theories are coherent, if not mutually compatible, understandings of the disease. The myths that the peer educators and I went hunting for now appeared as formidable opponents. However, even as the Digco peer educators enabled a mapping of township AIDS beliefs, I was also made aware that the peer educators who were providing this information were themselves not separate from it. I was struck by how the peer educators, cleaving to the medical model of AIDS to which they had aligned themselves, often continued to understand diseases and misfortunes other than AIDS within alternative paradigms to that of science.

Although I worked with the peer educators as lay researchers, they were also lay health practitioners with messages to convey. It also became apparent to me that how they engaged with their peers did not always conform to how the Digco peer educator programme was organised – a vertical conduit to deliver medical messages in the idiom of peers. Instead of listening to the peer educators messages, peers would sometimes talk back. This backchat highlights how conversations about AIDS lie outside the control of health professionals.

Beliefs in context

If we are to understand how AIDS is constructed from below, then we must know the context in which these beliefs emerge and endure in the face of constant counter-messages sprayed from above. South African townships are the product of apartheid's regulation of a cheap black labour supply for industry and domestic service, but they continue to endure.

Although the research on which this book is based was conducted in half a dozen townships in the provinces of Gauteng, Mpumalanga and the Free State, to protect the anonymity of participants, and to draw out more clearly what is common rather than different between African townships, we will meet people in this book from two fictitious townships: the huge urban township of Potlakong, situated in Gauteng Province, the economic heartland of South Africa, and Butleng, a small township in the rural Free State.[15] Potlakong, almost 15 square kilometres in size, is a mixture of formal housing, backyard shacks, hostels and informal settlements, close to Johannesburg. Butleng is a small township of perhaps ten thousand residents that lies a kilometre from the small town of Plaasville. Young men and women leave Butleng to find work in Gauteng. They start by renting shacks and rooms in Potlakong. Left behind, Butleng is a township largely of the old, the young, and those unable to work. Left behind, but not forgotten, there is constant traffic between the two townships. Families, relatives, friends and neighbours form networks linking Potlakong and Butleng. These networks are constantly re-woven by long journeys in crowded minibus taxis and overloaded private cars that traverse well-known routes linking the Free State hinterland to the Gauteng metropolis.

My aim when talking to Bafana, Grace, Paseka and Neo and others who appear in their stories about AIDS was twofold. First, I wanted to test that the reported explanations of AIDS were not mere talk. As much as the Digco peer educators provided a source located within, rather than a probe thrust into their communities, it was still possible that what they were reporting was bravado, wishful thinking or simply idle speculation. Or, put another way, rumour and gossip, which might tell us much about how people discussed the disease at a distance, but not beliefs for those who are dealing with the disease at close quarters. Those infected with the virus or responsible for caring for loved ones would, I reasoned, measure their words carefully. At the very least it would be possible to distinguish the flippant from the profound. Indeed, these four individuals opened up complex worlds of meaning around AIDS, framed by their experiences.

The second reason for these discussions was to allow myself, and now the reader, to engage with how understandings of AIDS are constructed within South African townships. What I did not want to do was provide titillating snippets of African belief about AIDS – anecdotal 'ethnobongo' hearsay from deepest, darkest Potlakong and Butleng. I wanted us to understand how these beliefs, different as they may be from the medical explanation of AIDS, are rooted in the lives of township residents and that, within this context, they are not exotic in the slightest.

An unwelcome inquiry, but a necessary labour

An inquiry into why the alternative accounts of HIV/AIDS have proved so tenacious in the face of HIV/AIDS education campaigns that have now stretched over three decades may not be welcomed.

Sympathetic engagement with non-scientific beliefs often provokes disapproval from those attempting to educate people about HIV/AIDS. This is, in part, a legacy of the bitter struggles over Thabo Mbeki's AIDS denialism, but it also comes from a more global concern. Engaging too closely with the emic (or internal) understanding of subordinate populations[16] is viewed as giving succour to the enemies of reason, especially scientific reason, and comfort to charlatans exploiting the vulnerable. This book, in seeking to understand alternative explanations of AIDS, also narrates how I broke with this criticism, and rejected the easy prescription that it suggests. Subordinated and poor populations are vulnerable, but they are not stupid and there are reasons for the persistence of alternative explanations of HIV/AIDS.

There are clear signs that the AIDS epidemic in South Africa is abating, but when it comes to behavioural change it seems this has come about largely despite our efforts and not because of them. The hubris of medical science was exposed when early claims that a cure would be speedily found failed to materialise. Since then there have been intense efforts to change the behaviours responsible for HIV transmission. Measuring the actual success of individual interventions is impossible, but taken together the evidence is stark. Change in behaviour has been so slow that at times it has been hard to detect. Indeed, it's possible that our intervention efforts have achieved little more than an enriched vocabulary of medical terms among the population.

Blaming Mbeki has been an easy response to explain this disappointing outcome, but it is little more than a fig leaf. Unhelpful as Mbeki's stance over HIV and AIDS was, he is not responsible for the dissent from below. Rather than beat the drum that Mbeki's denial set us back, we need to engage the beliefs of South Africans who use alternative paradigms of knowledge, or who simply construct from their own resources more plausible and more attractive explanations of AIDS than that of medical science.

Such an engagement is uncomfortable and it may be tempting to bury this critique of our response to AIDS. After all, if the epidemic is finally being contained, then isn't this jeremiad simply a distraction? Why not continue to maintain our ignorance of dissident discourses around HIV and AIDS? As the epidemic is tamed, will they not become irrelevant to all but social historians?

Yet, the AIDS epidemic is not the first time that expert and popular conceptions have differed. Nor will it be the last. Engaging with this gap between expert and subject may raise uncomfortable questions, but we are better off knowing what people really think. Millions of grassroots dissenters have creatively crafted and woven various accounts of AIDS that draw on diverse resources. This plasticity of explanation is important and we must grasp what underlies the hydra of AIDS belief in the *kasi* (township). It is recognising alternative explanations of AIDS as agency that helps explain why they have endured.

PART I
Alternative Explanations
of AIDS

1

More than one kind of AIDS

When the truth cannot settle

I had arrived in Butleng Township in the early hours of Saturday morning, the day of Joseph's funeral. It had been a difficult drive from Johannesburg. I'd struggled through the Friday afternoon traffic and then spent three hours backed up behind an accident. Amid flashing lights, I had been waved past mangled vehicles and covered corpses. In the township, I could hear hymns from the *moletelo* (night vigil) that was under way *habo* (at the home of) Joseph Sechaba; the house where he had been born, where his parents still lived, and where he would spend one final night. I walked over to join some thirty mourners who sat on plastic chairs in the marquee erected over the small front garden of the house and part of the dirt street in front. Night vigils, a standard part of African funerals, are typically held on a Friday evening before the Saturday burial. Hymns are sung and speeches made for as long as there is energy to continue. It is also a chance for people to assemble, to greet family and friends, and to prepare for the following day.

After I arrived, Joseph's father asked me to briefly address the gathering. I was to reflect later that I did not do exactly what was expected. After introducing myself, for those who might not know me, I should have said something about Joseph whom we were burying in his 35th year, but since I had met him only once there was not much I could say. Instead, acutely aware of the AIDS ribbon on the lapel of the jacket that I kept wrapped tight around me in the cold night, I was as candid as I dared to be. To say, but not really to say, why we were burying Joseph. The truth was that I didn't know, but I believed that he had died of AIDS.

As I left *Ntate* (Mr) Sechaba's side and stood in front of the mourners I realised that I was now standing in the shoes of the braver AIDS peer educators that I have worked with; those who seek to break the silence and talk publicly about AIDS at funerals.[1] Now it was my turn. In a hastily prepared address, delivered in clumsy Sesotho, I said that we suffered in our country, South Africa, because so many people were dying. I said that it was hard for parents to bury their children as *Ntate* Sechaba, Joseph's father and my friend, was doing. Only if we talked to each other could we stop what was happening.

I never mentioned HIV or AIDS. I spoke around the subject as so many others have done. But even this suggestive, cryptic address was sailing as close to the wind as I dared. Indeed, almost immediately, I began to think that I had gone too far. As I sat down, there was the first public explanation of Joseph's death that I was to hear that weekend. It was emotionally delivered by a friend, who, close to tears, described the final weeks of Joseph's life. He explained how each doctor had said Joseph would be *sharp* (fine), but how he had needed masks and tubes as his breathing became increasingly difficult. It felt as though my suggestion was being directly rebuffed; Joseph's illness, we were being told, had been short. It was similar in the printed order of service distributed the next day, the brief *bophelo ba mofu* (life of the deceased) explained that '*Mofu o kutse ka nako e kgutshwane*' (The deceased was ill for a short time [before he died]).

But that was not the truth. When *Ntate* Sechaba had rung me, the previous week, a cold day in the beginning of August, the news of Joseph's death had come as a surprise, but he told me that his son's health had started to deteriorate in March. Initially, he had been kept in the dark about the problem, but had eventually picked up something was wrong. When he confronted Joseph's sisters, they filled him in on how their brother was moving from one treatment to another but always getting worse.

I left the night vigil for a few hours of sleep that were troubled with doubt.

Early in morning the tent was filled with family, friends and neighbours while other mourners stood outside. The sides of the tent were taken down as the sun rose in the sky and *Moruti* (Minister/ Preacher) Radebe started the service. He made a point of telling us that Joseph's life had been *lekker* (good). The Afrikaans expression, a firmly entrenched loan word across South Africa, sent a ripple of light relief around the crowded tent. It was a nod to Joseph's Afrikaans-speaking colleagues who had come from Kimberley in the Northern Cape where he had worked, but it also lent humour to the task that nearly every one of the long list of speakers laboured to achieve; to shore up Joseph's reputation.

But discrepancies between the accounts of his illness undermined attempts to coordinate assessment of his character. Each speaker, referring to his final illness, said something different. At one point, it looked as though we were going to be told what had really happened. Joseph's manager, dressed much more smartly than the other mourners in a light brown suit and yellow silk tie, had arrived in his own car from Kimberley, rather than in the minibus that Joseph's colleagues had hired for the journey. He was on the programme to speak as Joseph's manager. He spoke slowly and clearly in Setswana, easily comprehensible to the Basotho who made up the vast majority of the mourners.

He praised Joseph's work before starting an account of Joseph's illness. In attempting to lay down a definitive account of Joseph's death, he got as far as TB, a new addition to the public list of Joseph's afflictions that already included his heart, asthma and pneumonia. At that point, he was unexpectedly forced from the small front *stoep* (veranda) of the Sechaba house where the speakers addressed the gathering. He was thrust aside by the abrupt emergence of Joseph's coffin, carried by male relatives, from the front door of the house. Joseph's uncle, who led the coffin, shouted that the proceeding could not be held up any longer. Pushed to one side, the manager lost his poise and confidence. By the time Joseph's coffin was resting on the trestles in front of us gathered

5

mourners, Joseph's colleagues, who were next sequenced on the order of service, streamed out to sing *Sweet memories, sweet memories*[2] in English. It was as though anaesthetic was being released over us to numb the unpleasant account that Joseph's manager had started to reveal. Then, to shield Joseph completely from further possible harm, the eldest of the group, a Coloured woman with short cut hair and glasses, spieled forth in Afrikaans a righteous, defiant blessing of God's grace to the good and faithful servant that Joseph had been.

Short of sleep, my mind drifted during the long service. I speculated I had gone too far with what now, the morning after, seemed like reckless words. Words that I could not, if confronted, defend. I had insinuated what I could not prove. I worried whether these defences of Joseph's character were a response to my clumsy speech.

After the funeral, I found *Ntate* Sechaba in his room. We were constantly interrupted by visitors, many of them unobtrusively handing him *matshidiso* (money in remembrance to offset the cost of the funeral) which he wrote down in the pages of an exercise book. Despite distractions, he was at pains to tell me that while much had been said, it was not clear to him what Joseph had died from. He had buried his son, but he still did not know why.

I told him that I thought Joseph was somebody to be proud of, who had helped others, and was loved by many. That so many had travelled from Kimberley testified to that. I told him that I was glad that I had had the opportunity to meet him, if only once. Then I told him that I did not know what Joseph had died from, but when stories about different diseases circle a funeral and cannot settle, the truth is AIDS. *Ntate* Sechaba said nothing for a moment. Then he thanked me for my honesty. It felt that we sat becalmed, the wind stilled around us within a storm of competing explanations. I made my excuses and left.

Whether Joseph died of AIDS cannot be categorically stated. What we know for certain is that young men and women in their twenties, thirties and forties, with access to medical care, should not die of curable diseases without underlying complications. Statistically, the increased burden of mortality in South Africa is the result of AIDS – there is no other explanation. The statistics run into millions and the truth is clear, yet individual deaths can remain surrounded by doubt.

Tshepo Motheo, still a teenager, asked me in a moment of privacy following Joseph's funeral, *o hlokahetse ka baka la lefu lefe?* (What disease did he die from?). I could say no more than I had told Joseph's father. Later, Tshepo's grandmother suggested that Joseph had died of *tswekere* (diabetes). She explained that *tswekere* ran in the Sechaba family. She was validating her choice, at least in this conversation, to stand by the kindest of many explanations that circulated that weekend in the township.

In the Tshabalalas' kitchen two streets away, Florence had held up three fingers. One for 'H,' one for 'I' and one for 'V,' the ubiquitous symbol for the Human Immunodeficiency Virus (HIV), which is as good as saying AIDS (Acquired Immune Deficiency Syndrome), and told me, '*Yena o ne a rata banana hahalo*' (He liked girls a lot). Joseph had left the township more than 15 years ago for work in Kimberley. He had returned only to visit at Christmas, sometimes Easter, and when there were family gatherings. What he got up to away from home, she was suggesting, was the cause of his death. Then she explained that in the Last Days there would be incurable diseases; punishment for breaking God's laws. This was also something I already knew. It was not the first time Florence had pronounced that God punished those who broke the commandment *O se ke wa feba* (Thou shall not commit adultery).

Over Sunday lunch at the Mofokengs, eating in front of the television tuned to Soweto TV, my observation that we are burying so many people nowadays because of AIDS was vigorously assented to. We were not explicitly talking about Joseph, but we all knew we were really talking about him. Then Karabo Mofokeng disrupted the consensus I thought we had when she asked why it was only Africans who died of AIDS. As a family friend I was being excepted, but she was suggesting that this disease was, somehow, being used by Whites against Africans now that they had the right to vote.

On a different tack, Anna, my elderly neighbour, told me that Joseph could have been cured if he had consulted a traditional healer; they had been dealing with this *lefu* (disease) that was now called AIDS, long before Western doctors even knew it existed.

At Joseph's funeral the cause of his death was denied. Around the townships the cause of his death *was* known, but in many different ways. Joseph's funeral tells us about the shame and stigma that cloaks HIV/AIDS in South Africa, but this book is about something else – the circling accounts of Joseph Sechaba's illness.

Knowing about AIDS

It remains a recurring leitmotif in AIDS campaigns and programmes that the major problem is one of knowledge; or, to be more precise, a lack of knowledge about HIV and AIDS. Even if health promotion veterans were not able to convince us that knowledge alone is not enough, those working on the ground have repeatedly re-learnt this lesson. Jonathan Stadler[3] has framed the problem facing HIV/AIDS health promotion efforts, in pointing out that, despite prodigious financial and intellectual resources being employed, people 'are able to recite in parrot fashion the ABCs [Abstain, Be faithful, Condomise] of AIDS prevention ... [Yet,] there is much confusion about AIDS.' Stadler draws our attention to the apparently high levels of knowledge about the biomedical facts of HIV/AIDS, supported by surveys,[4] while alternative explanations continue to circulate. However, rather than explore and understand these alternatives, the most determined reaction is to pursue the idea that people's technical knowledge of AIDS remains inadequate.

Maintaining our own belief that people don't know enough about AIDS can sometimes be difficult. Since people know a lot about AIDS, we may need to ask tricky questions in Knowledge, Attitudes and Practices (KAP) surveys.[5] These can help show that respondents are ignorant of the facts or that their knowledge isn't satisfactory, even if it's sometimes a convoluted process. Karl Peltzer and Supa Promtussanon have to explain to us why the 23 per cent of 3 150 junior secondary school students who answered 'yes' to the question 'People are likely to get HIV by deep kissing if their partner has HIV' are, in fact, wrong. This, they elucidate, is because the statement emphasises the likelihood of transmission and HIV isn't likely to be transmitted by deep kissing.[6] Why it should be a problem that 23 per cent of the surveyed school children think (incorrectly) that they might get HIV from deep kissing isn't clear. Less snogging by school children isn't something we should lose too much sleep over.

What multiple choice-style, tricky-dicky questions do provide is a reassuring sense that people's knowledge about HIV/AIDS is not satisfactory. And if knowledge of HIV/AIDS isn't good enough, then we can carry on educating people until – in some enlightened age to come – they finally score 100 per cent in the trickiest of tests. Only at this point, it is implicitly suggested, will we really be able to evaluate the various behavioural change models that are cut and pasted into our AIDS plans. In the meantime, we can continue repeating facts about AIDS, while remaining immune to criticism that we might be wasting everybody's time and money. Thus, the Metropolitan insurance company,[7] a stalwart partner in the world of corporate AIDS programmes, launched its 'revolutionary new *B the Future* cellbook[8] on HIV and AIDS', with the slogan that 'Education = Prevention'.[9] Or, as spelt out in more detail on their website: 'In order to ensure that South Africans know their HIV status and to ensure that they protect themselves and their partners from infection, they need to be educated on the basics on HIV and AIDS.'[10]

Clearly, people have to have some knowledge about HIV and AIDS if they are going to avoid infection, know their status, or take up treatment, but we have to put knowledge about HIV/AIDS into perspective. It is a necessary, but not sufficient, condition for such change. Joseph Sechaba, as you may have guessed, was a professional nurse. Indeed, he spent several years running a sexual health NGO programme. He knew more than enough to know what he should do, but he chose not to follow the advice that he gave to others.

If Joseph's death illustrates the limits of what knowledge about HIV/AIDS means for behaviour, the varied explanations of his death that circulated in Butleng indicate no shortage of AIDS accounts. I suspect the different residents of the township that indicated to me in one way or another what they thought lay behind Joseph's death, would have all scored reasonably well if tested on the basics of HIV and AIDS, assuming there were not too many tricky-dicky questions slipped in. But nobody that weekend offered me a scientifically compatible account of AIDS as the cause of Joseph's death. AIDS was denied at the funeral and that undoubtedly created confusion. Yet that confusion didn't prevent people saying, away from the public effort made to salvage Joseph's character, that they thought it was AIDS. Still, nobody gave a straightforward biomedical account of the disease – the kind that they could provide if you or I went out to them with a clipboard and politely asked them to answer a few questions.

Illness and explanatory models in the professional, folk and popular sectors

Medical anthropology separates disease, a biomedical condition, from illness or sickness, the lived experience of that disease. The importance of the illness experience has been stressed and there have been attempts to educate medical practitioners to recognise that caring for patients means understanding and responding to their illness, which is more than treating the diseases that they diagnose. An important tool, in this regard, has been to listen to the illness narratives of sick people.[11] Understanding the patients' experience of illness can only improve the effectiveness and experience of health care provision.

One aspect of the patient's illness is their own diagnosis. Cecil Helman illustrated how patients of general practitioners in an English suburban community held complex beliefs about 'colds and fevers' that differed from a biomedical understanding of infection.[12] In the context of the intimate relationship between family doctor and patient, this resulted in compromises over treatment. As Helman puts it, 'Biomedical concepts are tailored to fit in more closely with the patients' model [of illness] …'[13] This, he argued, helps to explain the prescription of vast quantities of scientifically doubtful medication by GPs, since these assist in mediating the different understandings of disease held by doctors and patients. That there are lay beliefs about disease that differ from those of professionals, is not surprising. The vast majority of episodes of illness never get to a health professional, but are responded to at home.[14]

An example is *nyoko*, a widespread condition in African townships that is almost completely unknown to medical science. You'll find no reference to this in a medical textbook and, unless you're African, you'll probably have never heard of it.[15] When I raise this as an example of an ethnoecological disease (an affliction that is uniquely identified by a particular ethnic or cultural group) with first-year health students to whom we give a crash course in the sociology of health and illness, the White and Indian students look puzzled and the African students start giggling. Literally translated, *nyoko* means bile or gall and the condition has some similarities to the European ethnoecological complaint of 'liverishness'. However, within African lay and folk medical knowledge, *nyoko* accumulates as the result of eating and drinking. Particularly problematic are sugary foods and drinks, though alcohol is also sometimes fingered. The accumulated *nyoko* must be regularly purged if it is not to build up with the resulting malaise of feeling off colour and lethargic. Should these warning signs be ignored, the condition becomes more dangerous and can result in an acute attack resulting in collapse, especially if the person is exposed to bright sunlight. There are several ways in which *nyoko* can be removed from the body, including by colonic irrigation or *sepeite* – the reason for the African students' amusement.[16] Such treatments can be carried out in the home on a regular, prophylactic basis, but they also form an integrated part of many traditional healers' and church prophets' healing repertoires.[17] Thus, although *nyoko* is commonly a minor complaint that can be prevented or treated in the home, it is also linked, through belief in bodily pollution, to wider African cosmologies and healing practices.

Similarly to Helman's general practitioners, South African doctors with private township practices engage in compromises with patients' diagnoses. They will, for example, oblige patients who complain of tiredness or feeling off colour with an injection for *nyoko*. Indeed, after the monthly *letsatsi la pae* (pay day; in fact, the day that social grants are paid) in Butleng township, Dr Kasonkola, who runs a surgery there four afternoons a week, has a queue of patients that extends out of the door and into the street. Many of those queuing are there for an injection that will purge them of the *nyoko* they have already self-diagnosed. What is in Dr Kasonkola's injections I do not know, but once the consultation fee has been paid, he never turns down patients' requests for him to *hlaba sepeite* (to clean by injection). Dr Kasonkola is smart enough to put aside what he was taught at the University of Natal Medical School in respect of his patients' explanatory models of health and the health of his bank balance.

In this book, I draw on Arthur Kleinman's model of health care. Kleinman identifies three areas of health care: the popular sector, which I use synonymously with 'lay sector', the folk sector and the professional sector.[18] The professional sector is dominated by biomedicine, alternatively and interchangeably referred to as allopathic or Western medicine. While the diversity of health care in the professional sector should not be underestimated, such practitioners see themselves grouped around the scientific explanation of disease. By contrast, the folk area of health care constitutes alternative systems of healing based on non-scientific bodies of knowledge.[19] However, the boundaries between these three sectors are not absolute and there are areas of overlap.

In seeking to understand how illness is understood across these different sectors, Kleinman (1980) uses the term 'explanatory models' to describe the notions about an episode of sickness employed by those in the clinical process: typically, patients, families and health practitioners.[20] Kleinman's concern is how both practitioner and patient can reach a mutual understanding of illness. Such an understanding can, he argued, have a critical impact on patient satisfaction, compliance with treatment, and the prospect of a successful cure.

Explanatory models of AIDS differ across the three sectors. The professional sector explains disease through the biomedical model, while in the folk sector sickness or, on occasion, disease, is explained through and within particular bodies of knowledge. By contrast, explanations in the popular or lay sector are constructed from individual experience, passed-on explanations, and self-made theories that are not rooted systematically in wider systems of knowledge. Kleinman's hope for a shared understanding of disease across lay, folk and professional sectors is conspicuous by its absence when it comes to HIV/AIDS.

A plural health care system

A vibrant plural health care system, one in which multiple health care options are available, exists in South Africa despite allopathic treatment being freely, if not always effectively, available through the public health care system. Liz Thomas et al. argue that 'strategic, pragmatic and cultural factors interlock with each other in how and why people choose to mix health systems.'[21] These reasons include frustration with the Western medical system's frequent inefficiency, the therapeutic limits of Western medicine, limited access, poor service, a distrust of public institutions, and the value of traditional African and faith-based healing systems that extend beyond responses to specific illnesses.

The relationship between allopathic medicine and alternative healing systems varies. There can be close cooperation; for example, a doctor may refer a patient with a drinking problem to Alcoholics Anonymous, an arrangement that frees the practitioner from the often labour-intensive response to a condition for which medicine has no cure. Such referrals only take place, however, if there is an understanding of the boundaries between the partners. In such cases, allopathic medicine is recognised as the senior partner, and its core area of competence is not to be encroached upon by junior therapeutic partners. Where alternative health care systems, such as African traditional healing, claim competence in areas that biomedical practitioners regard as their domain, such as treating disease, then cooperation between elements of a plural health care system is difficult. Alternative health care systems that are unwilling to play a junior role to the medical professions are regarded as a dangerous nuisance.[22]

Yet, despite the public dominance of allopathic medicine, health-seeking practice is frequently promiscuous with sick individuals, and their families, juggling multiple treatments. Much of this is hidden from competing health care providers. This is especially the case with AIDS, which has become a flashpoint in the conflict between Western and traditional health care systems. HIV-positive patients generally do not tell medical health practitioners about alternative treatments they may be using.[23] Reliance on African traditional healing in South Africa has, taking a long perspective, diminished as access to allopathic health care has increased. Nevertheless, traditional African healing remains firmly present and capable of adaptation to new challenges, including the AIDS epidemic. Moreover, other components of the plural health care system, such as faith healing, may well be increasing, given that the number of people affiliated with Pentecostal and Apostolic churches in South Africa is on the rise.

Whether rival healing systems to Western medicine will perish or persist is an important question. Robin Horton contrasted the 'open' system of scientific medical diagnosis with the 'closed' system of traditional medical 'divination' or inspired diagnosis based on signs, rituals and perceived contact with a supernatural agency, particularly in trance states or in dreams.[24] As specific lines of causality cannot be decisively ruled out when divination means are used, traditional medical beliefs remain, Horton argued, robust in the face of external critique. Unlike scientific medicine, such systems of thought do not allow a hypothesis to be refuted, since confounding factors can always be brought into play. For example, the diagnosis, via divination, that an individual's sickness is the result of ancestral anger is not disproved should the sickness persist after a ceremony to appease the ancestors. It may, for example, be that the ceremony was not correctly conducted, or that witchcraft employed by a jealous neighbour jinxed the process. The result, Horton predicted, was that the struggle between open and closed systems of thought was likely to be protracted and 'inevitably ... painful, violent and partial'.[25] Reaching a similar conclusion, Liv Haram has argued that the adaptability of culture allows traditional systems to selectively integrate or add biomedical elements to their repertoire of knowledge and treatment, thus remaining active competitors in a plural health care system.[26]

Within sub-Saharan Africa, explanations of health and illness are contested between several institutions. The most significant of these, in addition to allopathic medicine, are African traditional beliefs and churches.[27] The relationship between traditional beliefs, with their three key components of ancestors, pollution and witchcraft, and churches is complex. David Macdonald emphasises conflict between the two systems, with Christianity seen as responsible for the erosion of traditional cultural beliefs.[28] Others, however, emphasise the often syncretic nature of Christianity and traditional African beliefs in sub-Saharan Africa.[29] While African traditionalists can argue that Christianity has eroded an earlier public health regime in which sexuality was regulated, for example through the use of initiation schools, both they and Christians can argue that their respective moral orders are being undermined by modern forms of social organisation introduced with colonialism and continued by Western-dominated, secular globalisation.

These narratives of domination are frequently underpinned by understandings of racism that provide a third theory of disease, particularly when it comes to AIDS. Didier Fassin and Helen Schneider stress how South Africa's racial history explains both AIDS denialism and defiance.[30] How far alternative explanations of HIV/AIDS are infused with racial perspectives in South Africa is a matter of degree – it is impossible to separate traditional African beliefs or the beliefs of African Initiated Churches (themselves constituting forms of resistance to White domination) from the racist foundations of South African society.

A vibrant, if hidden, plurality of health beliefs allows individuals to make treatment choices, or to 'window shop' for treatment.[31] This is something that several scholars have identified in relation to AIDS.[32] Murray Last has argued that a plural health care system is based on an ethnoecology of disease, and suggested that individuals working across the range of health care systems on offer are less concerned about looking for the most attractive cure and more about ensuring that they have the right diagnosis, from the right explanatory field, for the illness they are experiencing.[33] This is a significant point regarding AIDS since, as my Butleng neighbour, Anna, was suggesting, traditional healers sometimes argue that what Western doctors label AIDS is the misdiagnosis of a traditional disease which they can cure. Christian faith healers run parallel arguments.

Even in some future modern and homogeneous world, it's unlikely that health care could be completely monopolised by allopathic medicine, however far science had advanced. A plural health care system is the product of both supply and demand. It is not simply that enterprising health care providers promote different explanations and solutions to our ills. The demand is real, and as long as one system cannot solve all problems, alternatives will be sought out. And, short of finding an elixir, ills will be with us till the end of time. Even more so, if we expand what ails us beyond disease, to encompass the varied problems of the human condition. Western medicine limits its considered claims to curing scientifically understood dysfunctions of body and mind. But the human condition throws up problems of love, status, hardship, insecurity, loss, jealousy and much more. Illness is only part of the suffering that we experience and from which we seek relief, and it is across this wide terrain that competing systems of health care operate, putting forward different explanations of suffering and different remedies.

Traditional African beliefs, Christianity and syncretic combinations in the form of African Initiated Churches[34] constitute bio-moral systems of belief. Bio-moral belief ascribes disease, sickness and misfortune to deviations from prescribed, moral codes of behaviour. Suzette Heald describes how the association between AIDS and traditional African conceptions of pollution, resulting from proscribed sexual contact, forms a coherent bio-moral theory.[35] Such theories can operate on a micro or macro level. Thus, a bio-moral theory can explain why an individual is sick. It can also explain epidemics. African traditionalists can attribute AIDS to the breakdown of pre-colonial order, while Christians can cite the breaching of the prohibition on adultery contained in the Ten Commandments. Racial explanations of AIDS also have clear bio-moral components, though the moral infringement is placed on the 'other' and rarely on infected individuals' actions.[36]

Christian faith healing, traditional African beliefs, and racial conspiracy theories constitute the major folk theories of HIV/AIDS circulating in South African townships today. All three of these folk theories of HIV/AIDS have some, albeit different, bio-moral basis.[37] From these bio-moral perspectives, the allopathic or biomedical explanation of HIV/AIDS, which formally eschews moral judgement,[38] constitutes a controversial conversion, or medicalisation,[39] of moral questions into a medical condition.

Understanding the AIDS epidemic

Megan Vaughan argues that illness is socially constructed.[40] By this, she means that illness, despite having a biological basis, can be framed in ways that reflect different social values and positions. Vaughan's study of the 'syphilis' epidemic[41] in Uganda in the early 20th century illustrates how doctors affiliated to the colonial authorities and Christian missionaries drew different conclusions.[42] As she outlines, the problem was first diagnosed by an officer of the Royal Army Medical Corps, as 'the disintegration of their [the Bangandan people's] social and political system brought about ... primarily by the introduction of Christianity'.[43] Not surprisingly, missionary doctors differed, arguing that the epidemic was a result of aspects of traditional Baganda society, such as polygamy, that facilitated the spread of sexually transmitted infections, and this could not be tackled 'other than through a deeper extension of Christian morality'.

The social construction of medical knowledge has, according to Ludmilla Jordanova, 'often [been] caricatured by critics, who impute to it the claim that diseases are not real, and who associate it with a denial that science and medicine really work'.[44] Such caricatures miss the point that agreement over the biological aspects of a disease does not preclude disagreement over why a disease reaches epidemic proportions in some situations. Vaughan's example of syphilis in Uganda illustrates this well, given that the two protagonists were both groups comprising medical doctors. What they differed over was not their perspectives on science and medicine regarding the disease, but the implications of different social orders and values for the disease.

Once a disease reaches epidemic proportions, it's not only medical doctors who compete to define which factors, including social relationships and values, account for the severity of the situation. Elizabeth Fee[45] explores how the pre-antibiotic response to syphilis in Baltimore was an ideological struggle between 'social hygienists', who regarded the fight against venereal disease as a battle for sexual morality, and public health officials, epidemiologists and scientists, who saw syphilis as another bacteriological infection. Following Thomas Parran's influential approach,[46] this latter group argued that syphilis should be addressed by education, testing and treatment, despite this being, at the time, a long and demanding process. In other words, public health officials, in contrast to the social hygienists, were engaged, as Fee put it, in 'a campaign *against* the disease, not a campaign *for* sexual morality'.[47] The health officials and social hygienists did not dispute the biology of syphilis; rather, they differed in their emphasis on whether this, or sexual morality, should be the cornerstone of the public response.[48] The availability of penicillin in the 1940s was decisive in shifting the initiative from the social hygienists' campaign for sexual morality to the public health approach. However, for Fee, such victories are never complete. Pointing to AIDS, she has argued that, 'social and cultural meanings of disease reassert themselves ... whenever biomedical science fails to completely cure or solve the problem'.[49]

Twenty-five years after Elizabeth Fee made this point, medical science, despite advances, does not have an answer for AIDS – at least nothing remotely equivalent to the five-day course of pills that eliminates syphilis. One outcome is the range of explanations of AIDS that are at play or, as Paula Treichler has put it, an epidemic of meaning.[50] I have already questioned the notion that the problem lies in people's ignorance – that they do not know enough about the disease; a perspective easily aligned with the medical approach. Other perspectives on the epidemic have also aligned with relative ease to that of medical science. These include concerns over AIDS stigmatisation, gender inequality and access to testing and treatment.[51] Over the course of the AIDS epidemic, an alliance between medical science and human rights advocates has been forged. This medical–human rights approach to HIV/AIDS has authorised other perspectives only when framed as human rights or medical issues. An AIDS establishment of scientists, doctors, social scientists, health departments, international and national NGOs and activists has coalesced around the medical–human rights framing of the epidemic.

Other constructions or framings of the epidemic have more ambiguous relationships with medical science over HIV/AIDS than that of human rights. The idea of poverty being a cause of the disease has endured a mixed reception. There is an extensive literature on the social determinants of disease, arguing that living conditions influence disease transmission and its impact. For HIV, the connection with poverty is more complex than, say, cholera and its link to inadequate sanitation. Rather, it involves recognising how poverty, along with the migrant labour system, results in extensive sexual networks whose dangers as the transmission routes for HIV are fuelled by the use of alcohol as an 'escape' from the stress that overwhelms the poor. Poverty also increases individuals' vulnerability to infection and speeds the disease's progression as a result of poor nutrition and substance abuse that weakens immune systems.[52]

The condition of the social body is, of course, far more difficult to address than treating individual bodies. However, such an analysis can be conducted in a scientific manner and, in line with the long history of public health reforms, be part of an integrated response to disease – even if it is often an uphill struggle for these arguments to be heard.[53] What pulled the rug from under the feet of those framing the AIDS epidemic through the lens of poverty was President Mbeki's stance linking poverty as an explanation for the epidemic with a denial of the science of HIV/AIDS. In the controversy that followed, the not particularly loved baby (the social determinants of health) got thrown out with the bathwater, as Mbeki's stance on the science of AIDS was opposed and defeated. Poverty as a factor in the AIDS epidemic nevertheless remains; the epidemiological evidence showing how the disease is far more prevalent among the poor remains a stubbornly resilient fact.

The epidemic can also be understood as a behavioural problem, since the virus is predominantly transmitted through sex. This brings us back to the 1930s social hygienists and the construction of behavioural change as a moral crusade. Such perspectives have come into conflict with the human rights framing of the epidemic and enjoyed, at best, an uneasy working relationship. For example, it is impossible to deny the importance of churches as social institutions in a country like South

Africa, and the need to utilise them for health promotion campaigns is a common refrain. Yet, when church leaders, clerics or lay church members put forward their own interpretation of how HIV is to be avoided, which, for example, does not include the use of condoms, churches, for all their value, have frequently been sidelined from the medical and human rights-led response to AIDS.[54]

However, it is not only those driven by moral codes of sexual restraint that have, seeing the epidemic as rooted in behaviour, attempted to influence sexual practices as a response to the AIDS epidemic. In the absence of a decisive medical response, considerable resources have been thrown at promoting the Abstain, Be faithful or Condomise (ABC) message. The degree of sophistication and relevance of such efforts is a moot point, especially when they have often been linked to the 'ignorance' perspective that people don't have sufficient information about HIV/AIDS.[55] But the enormous difficulty of bringing about change in sexual behaviour is evident, given the grindingly slow changes in behaviour. It is clear that the AIDS establishment has lost patience with what can be achieved through these methods, though this patience only evaporated when there was hope that medical interventions, such as circumcision and treatment-as-prevention, could reduce new HIV infections.

Overall, it is clear that official responses to the epidemic have been constructed from a range of elite and expert perspectives. To different degrees these constructions or frames can be combined and allied, though some remain peripheral – if not skirting pariah status – to the dominant AIDS establishment of medical practitioners and human rights advocates. John-Eudes Kunda and Keyan Tomaselli have argued that we need to appreciate the HIV/AIDS discourse circulating in communities so as to be in a better position to engage with them.[56] That has not happened. Indeed, folk and lay theories of AIDS have remained beyond the pale.

The construction of AIDS from below
If alternative explanations of HIV/AIDS are influencing the grassroots response to the disease, getting to grips with what people believe about

AIDS can only be a good thing; education could be more carefully tuned, barriers to prevention identified, testing better promoted, and treatment take-up and adherence strengthened. But we would be correct in being cautious; such improvements would not necessarily be easy to achieve. Some beliefs about HIV/AIDS might be easily 'put right'. However, many AIDS beliefs are not simple misunderstandings, but carefully constructed theories that draw on deeply held, non-scientific beliefs. These may be easy to challenge, but are difficult to change. Nor can alternative theories of AIDS be seen as running parallel to science. The differences are more than linguistic or conceptual. Learning, for example, how African traditional healers classify and treat illness does not empower us to seamlessly insert HIV/AIDS and antiretroviral drugs into their practice. As they are located in different paradigms of thought, there are fundamental differences that will remain, however good the mutual understanding.

Given the difficulties of applying our minds to several alternative conceptions of AIDS, and the limited value that this will bring by a medical yardstick, it is tempting to ignore the existence of these alternative beliefs. And, with some exceptions, that is largely what has happened to date. While numerous exploratory studies of AIDS beliefs have been conducted, enthusiasm wanes as the methodological, conceptual and practical difficulties of pursuing the research become apparent. Far beyond this shallowly revolving research, a far larger enterprise progresses – that of implementing the medical response to AIDS, which largely ignores the belief systems of those it seeks to help. This approach is boiling down to the simple things that are known to work; 'take your pills' and, if you are a man, 'take off your foreskin'.

The benefit of this approach should be acknowledged. After decades of frustratingly slow changes in sexual behaviour, the 'breakthroughs'[57] of treatment as prevention and circumcision in reducing new infections have generated optimism that the epidemic will be vanquished. Inspired primarily by the preventive potential of antiretroviral therapy, Michel Sidibe, Executive Director of UNAIDS, has written, 'We are on the verge of a significant breakthrough in the AIDS response. The vision of a world with zero new HIV infections, zero discrimination and zero AIDS-related deaths'.[58]

This would be a good thing and behavioural change is discernible in, for example, testing uptake, which in South Africa is becoming increasingly routine. Yet, we remain in the dark as to how these changes have come about. Whatever evidence there is will be buried as the epidemic is choked by prevention methods that do not require changing behaviour – at least beyond popping pills or having your foreskin snipped.

If AIDS were the only behaviour-related challenge we face, we would not need to reflect on how the epidemic is to be defeated. But of course, there are myriad problems that are rooted in, or at least exacerbated by, our behaviour. If this is the case, then, following Elizabeth Fee's argument, the alternative worldviews that have surfaced to challenge the scientific explanation of AIDS will continue to emerge wherever health problems cannot be resolved quickly, cheaply and without too much effort through medical science and health technology. And, perforce, they will remain in play while challenges presented by the human condition, of which illness is only a subset, remain.

2

Hunting myths, finding theories

AIDS myths

How do the residents of South African townships understand AIDS? South Africans have been flooded with public health information on the disease since the 1980s, yet alternative explanations to that of medical science continue to circulate. This chapter draws out the non-scientific beliefs circulating alongside public health information in South African townships and explores why they remain in play. It also records how I changed my mind about these alternative beliefs about AIDS; from seeing them as AIDS myths to be hunted down and destroyed, to realising that they were a much more powerful adversary, in fact theories of AIDS, which needed to be treated with respect.

The term 'myth' can describe very different things and disambiguation is necessary. At its most profound, 'myths of origin' explain how the world came about. The biblical book of Genesis, for example, describes the creation of the world in six days, how the Garden of Eden was a paradise, but as a result of Adam and Eve's sin, suffering came into the world. Christian fundamentalists may believe that this is a literal record of what happened, but this is a minority view. Nevertheless, the creation myth contained in Genesis shapes much more broadly held views that God created the world, which is imperfect because of human sin. Excluding fundamental readings of Genesis, such myths of origin are still 'true' – not in the sense that they conform to present-day realities now informed by our knowledge about the origins of our planet and evolution, but that they help many individuals structure their worldview.[1] Myths of origin and the worldviews they support influence social and individual beliefs and behaviour.[2] To continue the example of Christian belief, the creation story, and the subsequent books of the Bible that are contingent to it, influence the behaviour of individuals, congregations, social movements, political parties and entire nations. The influence of this myth of origin is, of course, neither homogeneous, given the fragmentation of Christian thought, nor singular, given the plurality of competing worldviews. However, irrespective of our views on these competing ideas, it is clear that such myths of origin are powerful influences on society and frequently have a strong hold on individuals, who may well see them as self-evidently true.

By contrast, the idea of a myth, when invoked in ordinary, day-to-day language, often implies, in a straightforward way, that a belief is incorrect; a misunderstanding or error. As such, the behaviour that such a misunderstanding may support is misguided, but it is not loaded with values and meaning. Such misunderstandings, although labelled myths, can be easily corrected by providing information that is correct and intelligible to the recipient.

Any examination of beliefs about HIV/AIDS needs to distinguish between deeply held beliefs – AIDS myths in the deeper sense in which these beliefs are integrated into wider belief systems held by the individual – and misunderstandings over HIV/AIDS – AIDS myths only in the shallow sense of their holder being misinformed on the particular point. Unfortunately, surveys of HIV/AIDS knowledge frequently don't do this, and deeply held AIDS myths and simple misunderstandings are not distinguished. The result is confusion over how the results should be interpreted.[3] To illustrate what is simply a misunderstanding and what is a robust AIDS myth, we can look at two different, erroneous beliefs about condoms: the misunderstanding that two condoms are better than one and the AIDS myth that condoms are infected with HIV. Somebody who thinks that 'doubling up' with two condoms will provide extra protection from HIV infection misunderstands how condoms provide protection. It may be a widespread misunderstanding, but it's not one linked to significant beliefs. Should you explain that two latex surfaces may, when rubbed together, 'blast' (rupture) the condoms, your account is likely to be believed. Or, at any rate, any disagreement will be about the properties of latex. [4] But if someone thinks that there are 'worms' in condoms and it is these worms that cause AIDS, you've got a more difficult task on your hands to change their minds. The belief is not really whether or not there are worms in condoms, but about why some people are motivated to use condoms to spread AIDS. As we will see later in the chapter, such beliefs are often linked to racial conspiracy theories in which Whites are infecting condoms to control the African population.

What should concern us are not misunderstandings, since these are factual issues which health promotion education can address with relative ease. Rather, we are concerned with non-scientific beliefs about AIDS that are deeply held. A myth's collective nature is critical in distinguishing it from a misunderstanding. A misunderstanding about AIDS may be common, but unless it is worked into a larger explanation, such as the belief that condoms are infected with HIV because Whites are seeking to control the Black population, it remains a simple error of knowledge that can be corrected with relative ease. By contrast, an AIDS myth is collectively maintained and sincerely believed even if it does not have the scope of a myth of origin. [5] We define AIDS myths, therefore, as a belief about HIV/AIDS that does not correspond to current scientific consensus, but which some people believe is true, and which is collectively constructed, transmitted and adapted. [6]

The term 'AIDS myth' is sometimes used to refer to the macro-level analysis and AIDS policy rather than the grassroots beliefs that we are concerned with. Peter Piot, a former Executive Director of UNAIDS, compiled a list of six policy myths about AIDS, such as the belief that there is a 'silver bullet' (rather than a mix of interventions) that will stop the epidemic. [7] In *Global AIDS: Myths and Facts*, Irwin, Millen and Fallows cover similar ground, arguing against mistaken national policy directions over AIDS. [8] Their work engages with a metropolitan, and implicitly modern, audience – those responsible for shaping the global response to HIV/AIDS – with a range of arguments underpinned by science, political economy and human rights. In the introduction to *Global AIDS*, Paul Farmer clarifies that 'we [the book's authors] do not refer to beliefs about AIDS in so-called traditional societies, whose ignorance of Western science has sometimes been decried by health experts as a reason for the failure of AIDS control efforts'.[9]

Farmer's relegation of non-scientific AIDS beliefs to 'so-called traditional societies' is problematic.[10] South Africa is far from being a traditional society, but it still retains much traditional belief which a number of AIDS myths clearly draw upon. Moreover, as we shall see, there is extensive belief in non-scientific ideas about HIV/AIDS within distinctly non-traditional countries such as the United States. Whether such beliefs are a reason for the failure of AIDS control efforts is a problem with which this book wrestles. The focus here is *not* on those who are responsible for AIDS policies, but on those who, while subjected to modern, scientific and secular explanations of AIDS, are *not* steeped in them or fully convinced by them.

Explanations of AIDS: from north to south

At the risk of simplification, beliefs about HIV/AIDS become increasingly complex in moving from North America to South Africa. Part of this increasing complexity may be an ongoing process of discovery by researchers, and the difference between America and Africa may not be quite as large as the current state of research suggests. Nevertheless, the plural worldviews in many African communities, highlighted by the vibrant plural health care system outlined previously, suggest that there are grounds for proposing an increased complexity of AIDS beliefs running from North to South.

Levine and Siegel explain how gay men in American cities utilised components of the public health model of HIV/AIDS to construct 'pseudo-epidemiological models' that justified unprotected sex;[11] for example, by partner selection in which 'safe' sexual partners are chosen on characteristics such as their physical appearance. Lowy and Ross conclude similarly as to the undesirability of such lay theories since they 'provide a false sense of security and lead to risk of HIV transmission'.[12] Early in the epidemic Steven Epstein outlined how there was a 'genocide frame' put forward as a rallying cry for gay men's response to AIDS, but with their incorporation into AIDS policy-making, these genocidal AIDS myths all but disappeared, leaving the relatively uncomplicated, pseudo-epidemiological models among gay men.[13]

Diane Goldstein, as a folklorist, studied what she calls 'AIDS legends' in Newfoundland, Canada, where prevalence rates, in comparison to either the gay communities of American cities or the general population of many African countries, are low.[14] These legends frequently speak to lay assessments of risk and, Goldstein suggests, sometimes constitute a rejection of public health messages into the public's bedrooms, with a series of AIDS legends placing risk in public rather than private spaces, such as contaminated needles left on cinema seats, phone booths and other public locations. Despite the extensive and rich collection of legends in Goldstein's study, what she did not find was an outright challenge to the medical understanding of AIDS, something found among Afro-Americans and South Africans.

Research among Afro-Americans and other US minorities indicates widespread belief in AIDS conspiracy theories. Sonja Mackenzie identified three types of conspiracy theories over AIDS within the Afro-American population, namely, the implication of government in the creation of the virus, inaction of government agencies that allows genocide, and the mechanism of the conspiracy, such as testing and medication being used to spread the virus.[15] Mackenzie argues that we should move away from seeing these conspiracy theories as individual, and delusional, views, and, rather, recognise that such theories provide a counter-narrative to the dominant public discourse. These counter-narratives help defend the identities of individuals stigmatised by association with high rates of HIV infection among their peers.

It is, however, in Africa that AIDS myths present in a substantially increased plurality. In addition to racial conspiracy theories (constructed with different local detail from those of Afro-Americans) and lay theories of how to avoid infection (also constructed with specific local content), there are African traditional beliefs – witchcraft, pollution and the ancestors, as well as religious-based AIDS myths – all of which provide a range of explanations of AIDS.[16]

To different degrees, researchers and writers recognise that there is a complex mixture of belief over AIDS extending beyond their own particular focus. Additionally, the relationship between these alternative explanations of AIDS and biomedicine is an area that most researchers attempt to grapple with. Edward Green's formulation of proximal and distal understanding of illness is one way in which the integration of biomedical and other beliefs can be achieved; biomedicine provides a proximal (or immediate) explanation of the disease while, for example, witchcraft explains why it is that the individual, and not others, is a victim; the distal or ultimate reason.[17] Helpful as this duel aetiology of disease is, some writers point to an unstable shuttling between the allopathic and witchcraft explanations of AIDS[18] or note that there are two types of AIDS: one resulting from sex and the other from witchcraft.[19] Approaching the range of explanations of AIDS in circulation, Izak Niehaus and Gunvor Jonsson,[20] Jonathan Stadler[21] and Fraser McNeill[22] have all argued that there is a gendered dimension to AIDS beliefs, with women more willing to accept the allopathic explanations and men more inclined to concur with racial conspiracy theories. If nothing else, what we can conclude is that there is a complex plurality of beliefs about AIDS at play within communities, and that we still have only a partial grasp of how and why these emic, or internal, explanations are generated, communicated and believed.

Much of this analysis of AIDS myths critiques conventional health communication strategies which are frequently unaware of (or prefer to remain untroubled by) these competing explanations of AIDS. Some researchers attempt to read beyond the significance of AIDS myths for public health. Izak Niehaus illustrates how HIV/AIDS can be 'a vehicle for talking about moral and political decay ... including the erosion of patriarchy, political corruption, the high incidence of murder and of rape and the legislation of abortion and gay marriage'.[23] Jonny Steinberg's account of a young man's refusal to test for HIV, for which several AIDS myths are mobilised, is linked finally to the undermining of African patriarchy and a crisis of masculinity.[24]

Diddier Fassin argues that in South Africa, race is a reservoir of resentment resulting in mistrust of authority and a belief in racial conspiracy theories, with which Mbeki's denialism resonated.[25] However, for Fassin, what really explains the epidemic in South Africa is racism's real, and not its psychological, legacies. Fassin's fundamental argument is that the epidemic is the result of the impoverishment of Africans in South Africa. Race may be the explanation that is put forward to justify AIDS myths, but it is, he argues, poverty that is the cause.

Thus, we see that in the existing literature, the expert understandings of AIDS myths range from being nothing more than false consciousness concealing the causes of the epidemic, being ciphers for wider concerns, to being structures of belief that shape responses to AIDS. They are all these things and they are also irritating and embarrassing to the legions of HIV/AIDS educationalists. We need to get over the embarrassment of their continued existence and focus on them as a structure of belief. In an epidemic as complicated as AIDS in sub-Saharan Africa, we should recognise that there is not one ultimate cause, just as there will be no magic bullet to bring the epidemic to an end. Clearly, poverty does fuel the epidemic in a number of ways. Yet, there is a danger that in boiling matters down to the social determinants of health, we squeeze agency out of view and erroneously conclude that beliefs are merely the product of social conditions. We need to grasp why and how AIDS myths are produced within communities and how this, in turn, shapes the epidemic.

Collecting AIDS myths

If we are to take AIDS myths seriously, then we need to know which are circulating. Moreover, we need to understand these myths, beyond simply seeing them as 'wrong' when judged against scientific criteria. Surveys can, albeit with considerable uncertainty as to fidelity, identify reported discrepancies from a medical understanding of HIV/AIDS. However, attempts to probe these discrepancies are inherently blunt since they interrogate respondents over individual pieces of information, rather than seek to understand the emic construction of alternative explanations of HIV/AIDS to that of biomedicine. What is being assessed by survey techniques is not the explanations of AIDS known to respondents, but particular concerns of the researchers. From this starting point, all too often we get back to the trope that the population needs yet more AIDS education.

Without checking, we do not really know, when using a questionnaire to ask about AIDS, what responses are based on – which could include AIDS as a biomedicine disease, AIDS as a genocidal weapon, AIDS as a misdiagnosed traditional disease, AIDS as a curse sent through witchcraft, AIDS as a punishment for sin, AIDS as demonic possession, or some other belief. Respondents may assess the source of the research intervention and do their best to answer in line with their biomedical knowledge of AIDS, or they may answer in line with alternative understandings of the disease, or some combination. At best, surveys may point us towards the presence of doubt, but they do so unreliably since there is no way of checking the exact basis of responses.[26]

The AIDS myths identified in this chapter were collected by 28 African peer educators,[27] acting as lay researchers, during a research project I conducted at 'Digco', a South African mining company between October 2008 and July 2009. Peer educators are individuals drawn from their peers, in this case company employees, given some training on HIV and AIDS along with communication skills and asked to engage with peers over HIV/AIDS. The peer educators were asked to record 'AIDS myths' that they heard in their communities, overwhelmingly African townships. These were defined as a belief about HIV/AIDS that is not true (by current scientific consensus) but which some people believe is true, and which is collectively constructed, transmitted and adapted. This latter aspect, an AIDS myth's collective nature, was something that emerged during workshop discussions with the peer educators.

Each peer educator was issued with a digital recorder and asked to provide reports in the language of their choice.[28] A series of six workshops provided an opportunity to discuss the AIDS myths that had been recorded. It also allowed a rough gauge of how common some of the reported myths were, using a 'vox pop' technique in which the peer educators present were asked if they had heard a particular myth within the last two years, though excluding a 'friend of a friend', newspaper or television as sources. While 'rough-and-ready', this vox pop technique provided a useful pointer as to how common these were in their communities.

Many of the workshops were taken up with the development of stories or parables that could be told in response to some of the more common AIDS myths.[29] Towards the end of the project I conducted interviews with 23 of the participating peer educators. The interviews, between one and three hours in length, were structured around AIDS myths that had emerged during the project and the peer educators' own understandings of these.

Using peer educators to collect AIDS myths has advantages over survey methods. While working at the coalface of HIV/AIDS education, they are in conversation with neighbours, colleagues and friends.[30] However, even with the opportunity to discuss these AIDS myths with the peer educators, the capturing and categorising of AIDS myths presented problems. Take, for example, the following five-paragraph monologue by a Zulu man speaking originally in isiZulu, recorded by one of the project peer educators:[31]

1. AIDS is caused by not living in the right way. I mean going around engaging in sex with any woman you meet and you don't know where that person comes from, where she was sleeping.
2. You will penetrate that person and some other blood/semen[32] goes into her body and when you have to go, another person goes into her again, this woman is mixing a lot of blood/semen into her body. This thing when it goes and goes, these people's blood/semen, and you also put your blood/semen in there as well, it affects the body and builds up into a disease.
3. We must not believe that [Dr Wouter] Basson [an Apartheid scientist, see below] injected people and so on and so on.
4. We must just take it like, if you live in the right way and you have only one relationship and one sleeping partner and not doing things which are out of the way, you can live a longer life than if you are unfaithful.

5. Even your wife can infect you with this disease because at this present moment you are at work, you are at work for ten hours, you are not at home, and she is far away from you, and she goes and becomes promiscuous, sleeping around with other men while you are not there, when you come back home, you find that she has bathed, she is clean, sitting at home, cooking and eating and when you get there in the afternoon, you engage in sex with her while during the day she was with other men, what does that thing do? It infects you with this disease.

Several points can be drawn from this monologue. There is a bio-moral theory, of unspecified origin, being suggested as to 'living in the right way' (Paragraphs 1 and 4), safe sex messages of faithfulness (Paragraph 4) and caution over sexual partners' fidelity (Paragraph 5). There is the idea that disease is generated from the mixing of blood/semen within a woman, which appears to draw on traditional conceptions of pollution (Paragraph 2), and there is a *rejection* of the racial conspiracy theories based on Dr Basson, described later in this chapter (Paragraph 3).

When coding this recording, I captured it as a myth of AIDS being generated through bodily pollution, but alternative categorisations could also be argued. Whether accurate or not, coding strips the myth from its context. This is inevitable if we want to collect, categorise and analyse AIDS myths, but we should be mindful of the processing and packaging that has taken place.

The following taxonomy of AIDS myths that I have constructed no doubt remains flawed. What it does illustrate, however, is that the vast majority of recorded AIDS myths can be identified as auxiliary theories to a smaller number of core ideas. As this dawned on me, I realised that while I had set off, with the help of the peer educators, to hunt AIDS myths, we had found an array of theories.

Alternative theories of AIDS

From the peer educator recorded reports, workshop discussions and interviews, some 80 different myths or variants of myths emerged during the action research project. Some of these myths were recorded on multiple occasions and via different channels: recordings, discussions and interviews; others appeared only once or twice. Combining the variants reduces the number of distinct AIDS myths to 40. This section organises the vast majority of these AIDS myths into three folk and three lay theories of AIDS.[33] In doing this, we will see that there is order and coherence to many of the AIDS myths that might otherwise be dismissed as ignorance, idle speculation or simple misunderstandings. That AIDS myths can be linked to a core idea identifies them as auxiliary theories that draw on and develop these core ideas in specific ways.[34]

Organised in this way, core ideas lie at the heart of each folk or lay theory and are surrounded by AIDS myths or auxiliary hypotheses. These auxiliary hypotheses can be nested into several levels, resulting in a layered belt of hypotheses around the core idea. To illustrate, the idea that the HIV virus is being placed in condoms frequently constitutes an auxiliary hypothesis to that of (White) scientists having deliberately created HIV/AIDS, which, in turn, forms an auxiliary hypothesis to that of AIDS being a weapon of racial genocide. Such racial conspiracy theories and their auxiliary hypotheses are not easy to discredit. A belief that condoms are infected with HIV lies not in the scientific robustness of such a proposition, but in its plausibility and palatability to an audience with little scientific schooling and even less commitment to scientific methods.

We also need to think about AIDS beliefs over time. Clearly, although it is hard to capture, such beliefs change. Paul Farmer has presented one model as to how this occurred in Haiti,[35] and Steven Epstein documents shifts in how AIDS was framed by the gay community in the early stages of the epidemic.[36] Core ideas are likely to remain stable, while auxiliary hypotheses are more prone to churn. In South Africa, and elsewhere, oranges have been cited as a mechanism by which HIV is transmitted – frequently this is linked to racial narratives in which Whites inject HIV into oranges eaten by Blacks. In interviews with peer educators, it was clear that this particular AIDS myth had been prevalent in the 1980s and early 90s. Several peer educators recalled having avoided oranges for a spell during this period, believing that there might be some truth to these accounts. Now, however, this AIDS myth, while still remembered, seems to have run out of steam. The two contemporary recordings of this myth collected during the project came across as relics of the past, rather than a current concern. However, the racial beliefs that constitute the core idea to which contaminated oranges was an auxiliary hypothesis are far from exhausted; the belt of auxiliary hypotheses supporting the idea of AIDS as a genocidal weapon retains vigour.

Overly focusing on individual AIDS myths is potentially misleading. We can spend a lot of time working on a particular myth, and even longer on trying to discredit it, but we would have failed to see the wood for the trees. What we need to understand is not each myth, but the core ideas that lie behind these. Individual AIDS myths are usually but one of several auxiliary hypotheses linked to these core ideas.

Folk theories of HIV/AIDS

Folk theories constitute bodies of knowledge or beliefs that differ from science. As outlined, there are a number of core ideas or principles at the heart of these theories from which auxiliary theories are generated. Encountered individually, these auxiliary theories are perceived as AIDS myths. When folk theories are viewed in totality, as a body of knowledge, it can be seen that they are used to interpret the AIDS epidemic and individuals' illness consistently with core principles – principles that are often bio-moral in that they link biological phenomena, such as sickness, to moral codes and their breaching.[37] In Robin Horton's conception these folk theories constitute 'closed' systems not readily subject to falsification and therefore difficult to disprove within their own terms of reference.[38] One implication of this is that while presented as a unitary cosmology, there may be variations of interpretation by custodians or those speaking from within the folk theory. Nevertheless, these cosmologies provide the core idea, or ideas, at the centre of folk theories of AIDS. Three such theories were present in the collected myths: ideas about racism and to a lesser extent political authority, traditional African beliefs, and religious (in this case, a range of Christian) beliefs.

Racism and authority

The core idea of the racial folk theory of HIV/AIDS is that Whites are using the disease to kill, or in other ways control, Africans. The timing of the epidemic, at the very moment that the African majority was able to vote, provides a plausible context for such beliefs in South Africa. The transition to a Black majority government in 1994, however, also negates components of this theory since it breaks the previous alignment of power and race. Box 1 below lists the AIDS myths identified in the project that form auxiliary theories to this folk theory of HIV/AIDS.

Box 1: Racism (and authority) as explanations of AIDS

Core idea: HIV/AIDS is used to kill or control Africans (working class or poor)
Auxiliary theories/AIDS myths 1. Dr Basson created HIV 2. Whites/Americans created HIV 3. AIDS comes from Whites sleeping with animals or African women being forced to sleep with animals 4. AIDS only affects Africans (i.e. designed in this way) 5. A cure is known, but is being withheld (by the South African government or by White scientists) 6. African traditional medicines can cure AIDS, but they are not licensed because Whites want to control the number of Africans 7. Government-supplied condoms are rubbish (i.e. will blast or burst) 8. HIV is put in oranges/other fruit by e.g. White farmers 9. HIV is put in condoms/condom lubricant 10. Doctors inject patients with HIV 11. Condoms are to control the African population (AIDS does not exist)

That racist beliefs might be extended to genocidal policies has been given credence by Dr Wouter Basson (Myth 1), an Apartheid-era government scientist who provides a parallel symbolism to the United States Tuskegee syphilis experiment.[39] Basson investigated the use of biological weapons that would target Blacks.[40] In hearings of the Truth and Reconciliation Commission,[41] it was established that while the front companies used by Basson developed a wide range of chemical and biological weapons, these did not include using HIV. That he did, however, is widely entrenched in popular imagination. In one of the project workshops, 20 out of 20 peer educators reported having heard the myth of Basson developing HIV. Additionally, longstanding attempts to control African fertility by the Apartheid government contribute to racial conspiracy theories on reducing the African population.[42] One recorded AIDS myth (Myth 11) argued that AIDS doesn't exist, but that the insistence that people use condoms to prevent infection was part of a conspiracy to control the number of Africans.

The AIDS myths linked to racial theories generally fit well into Mackenzie's three-part breakdown of 'AIDS counter-narratives' – the creation of the virus (Myths 1–4), a negligent response from those in authority (Myths 5–7), and the various mechanisms by which the virus is transmitted (Myths 8–10).[43] Most of these are located in the South African context in contrast to the work done on racial conspiracy theories in the United States: Dr Basson, White farmers or Boers, the backbone of Apartheid, and White and sometimes Indian doctors[44] in government hospitals make appearances as originators and propagators of the disease.

There is some indication of a transitioning of these conspiracy myths from being purely race-based, to being based on authority, in particular the current ANC government (variations of Myths 5–7 and 10). Where this is the case, such myths cease to be linked solely to a racial folk theory and transform into AIDS counter-narratives rooted in a critique of political power in which class also becomes salient. At what point these two social stratifications might become the basis of two distinctly separated explanations of AIDS is difficult to say (arguably one could split the current data into two different folk theories). However, given the enduring racial legacy in South Africa, racial folk theories will most likely remain strong for some time.

Traditional African beliefs on pollution, witchcraft and ancestors
Christine Liddell et al. have used the term 'indigenous representation
of illness' to explore how Africans have traditionally understood
the ultimate causes of illness – pollution, witchcraft, and ancestral
displeasure – that explain individual sickness and also 'comprise a
powerful mechanism for ensuring social cohesion and stability'.[45]
Box 2 below lists the AIDS myths identified in the project that form
auxiliary theories to this folk theory of HIV/AIDS.

Box 2: Traditional African beliefs on pollution, witchcraft and
ancestors

Core idea: Traditional ideas of ancestors, pollution and witchcraft explain HIV/AIDS
Auxiliary theories/AIDS myths 12. Ancestors can protect you from/warn you about HIV 13. Ancestral calling to be a traditional healer is misdiagnosed as AIDS 14. AIDS is mistaken for traditional disease resulting from taboo sexual contact (e.g. with a widow, with a woman who has had an abortion or miscarriage, etc.) 15. Traditional healers can cure these traditional diseases that are misdiagnosed as AIDS (ARVs are harmful) 16. AIDS and what is misdiagnosed as AIDS can be cured though sex with a stranger/virgin 17. People cleansing for diseases misdiagnosed as AIDS may pass this disease to sexual partners (link to previous myth) through sex 18. Correct cleansing procedures will prevent traditional diseases that are misdiagnosed as AIDS 19. AIDS or disease misdiagnosed as AIDS results from the mixing of bodily fluids (typically within a woman) 20. AIDS or something mimicking AIDS is sent by witches or their familiars 21. AIDS can be cured with patent medicine (stressing herbal/traditional content)

Ancestral belief, that there is a spirit world which ancestors inhabit and from which they can influence the world of the living, is arguably the core component of traditional African belief. However, despite widespread belief in the ancestors, this provides only limited material for AIDS myths, with few being recorded (Myth 12 and, arguably, 13). For many Africans, ancestral displeasure, as a result of being neglected, opens individuals to misfortune including sickness. Generally, however, a line appears to be drawn at the idea of ancestors being malicious enough to send AIDS, given their predominantly protective and benevolent role.

Much more common were myths on AIDS resulting from the breaching of traditional prescriptions on sexual conduct, particularly when this resulted in pollution as a result of contact with death.[46] These myths (14–18) included sex with widows/widowers, sex with a woman who has had an abortion or miscarried without cleansing having taken place.[47] Pollution beliefs, in which taboo activities are believed to contaminate or 'dirty' the blood, extend beyond contact with death to the danger of widespread multiple sexual partnerships which transgress (idealised) traditional value systems. An important AIDS myth that works alongside a number of traditional beliefs is that the indiscriminate mixing of bodily fluids (which may or may not be contaminated with disease) can produce or create different diseases (Myth 19). Importantly, such theories may refer to the generation of AIDS or to traditional diseases that are misdiagnosed as AIDS. The idea of AIDS being a disease resulting from pollution leads to the myth that traditional healers can cure AIDS or its traditional *doppelgänger*, based either on the efficacy of traditional healers' pharmacopoeia or other aspects of their treatment portfolio.

Cures based on traditional healers' pharmacopoeia frequently overlap with myths on patent medicines as a cure for AIDS (Myth 21). In South Africa, such medicines are widely advertised and used to 'clean the blood' (in Sesotho, *ho hlatswa madi*) and users stress their herbal content and traditionally based formulae. That they are aimed at people with HIV/AIDS is frequently indicated with the code that they boost the immune system (often using the metaphor, taken from public health campaigns, of 'soldiers of the body'.)

The ability of traditional healers to cure AIDS or other diseases is generally conceptualised not as the termination of the disease agent (as germ theory postulates), but as the relocation of the disease/affliction elsewhere. Much traditional treatment, which extends beyond curing illness, involves dumping the problem at a distance from the client: out in the *veld* (bush) or at a crossroads (where it will be picked up and taken elsewhere by a passerby), sent back to the originating witch, or directly transferred to another person. This conception of AIDS (or, more likely, its traditional *doppelgänger*) as a problem that can be relocated is linked to some of the AIDS myths around cure – sex with a stranger, virgin, old woman or baby (Myth 16 and, arguably, 17). These are categories that are likely to be selected because the recipients are assumed to be themselves free of AIDS.

Nevertheless, there is a danger that more lurid AIDS myths, such as that of the baby rape cure, become more real in their recounting.[48] There has been considerable media attention to the rape of babies as a cure for AIDS. None of the peer educators reported hearing this myth during the project, but a few reported in interviews that they had heard it. However, when questioned, in all but one case[49] the peer educator was referring to a media report and not to firsthand experience. Thus, although the myth of baby rape as a cure for HIV/AIDS is present within African communities, there is a need to distinguish between myths that are widely repeated in media communication and myths that are circulating within the population through word-of-mouth channels. The former are the material of high-profile moral panics,[50] the latter constitute beliefs away from the headlines that may be underestimated, despite their stronger hold on a population.

The third major component of African traditional beliefs, witchcraft, provides an explanation for infection, often linked to existing social tensions. Many writers have highlighted witchcraft as a significant non-scientific explanation of AIDS,[51] including how it allows people to blame others for misfortune, including HIV/AIDS.[52] Recorded witchcraft AIDS myths focused on AIDS, or a *doppelgänger* of AIDS, being sent by witchcraft/magic or via witches' familiars (Myth 20).

A number of the recorded witchcraft myths formed part of a binary perspective of good and evil, with witches sending AIDS which prayer/ God could heal (see the next section). Such constructions demonstrate how belief in witchcraft, a key component of traditional African belief, can be incorporated into other bio-moral theories.

Christian religion beliefs

At the core of religious folk theory of AIDS, which in the context of this research is focused on Christian denominations, is a bio-moral theory that draws on interpretations of biblical texts that link sickness to sin and offers healing. Box 3 below lists the AIDS myths identified in the project that form auxiliary theories to this folk theory of HIV/AIDS.

Box 3: Christian religious belief in sin as the cause of AIDS and the possibility of a cure for AIDS

Core idea: God's biblical law explains AIDS and that God is capable of miracles
Auxiliary theories/AIDS myths 22. AIDS is the result of sex outside marriage/biblically prescribed relationships 23. AIDS is a disease of the 'Last Days' 24. God can cure AIDS[53]

At the social level, religious interpretations of HIV/AIDS (Myth 22) allow perceived moral decay to be blamed on deviations from an interpretation of God's law, linked to biblical prophecy of incurable diseases in the Last Days (Myth 23), while at the individual level it draws attention to individuals' infringements of biblical laws governing sexual conduct. While this theory places blame on those who transgress these laws, some Christian denominations offer a cure for HIV/AIDS (Myth 24) through a process of salvation achieved through God's grace, provided that a range of conditions are met by the supplicant. One of these conditions is faith in God's ability to do anything. Demonstrating such faith may involve discontinuing other forms of treatment, such as antiretrovirals.

It can be seen that AIDS myths that are derived from religious beliefs are heavily focused on these linked ideas of AIDS as the result of sin, and God's ability to cure AIDS for those who believe. In general, the favoured message in religious discourses is no sex before marriage and to be faithful in marriages, and the hope for a cure of HIV/AIDS is reserved, essentially, for repentant sinners or those who were infected through no fault of their own.

Lay theories of HIV/AIDS

Lay theories can be distinguished from folk theories in that they are put together from observations that lie outside an established canon of knowledge or belief. Although they may borrow from, and overlap with, folk theories (as well as scientific explanations), they utilise only selected ideas and do not indicate a wholesale subscription to the bio-moral content of any folk theory. Most of the AIDS myths linked to the lay theories concern ways in which HIV infection can be avoided. At their centre are either lay observations or lay physiologies.

Partner selection to avoid HIV infection

We have long been aware of HIV/AIDS myths regarding who is and who is not infected with HIV/AIDS. Eleanor Maticka-Tyndale has explained how 'judging [sexual] partners by appearance or reputation' is used to avoid infection, or at least fear of infection.[54] Box 4 below lists the AIDS myths identified in the project that form auxiliary theories to this lay theory of HIV/AIDS.

Box 4: Partners can be selected to avoid HIV infection

Core idea: HIV-positive individuals can be identified by distinguishing features or attributes
Auxiliary theories/AIDS myths
25. Beautiful people are not infected
26. Young people are not infected
27. Fat people are not infected

28. Healthy-looking people are not infected
29. Old people are not infected
30. Educated people are not infected
31. People who are not sex workers are not infected
32. Those you know well/trust are not infected
33. If there is no blood on a person's genitals, then it is safe to have sex

Cues for identification of who is likely to be infected with HIV can take different forms (Myths 25–33), but all are based on the same idea: selection of partners by visual clues or character evaluation allows you to identify who is HIV negative and who HIV positive.

Friction theory of HIV transmission

Two further lay theories on avoiding HIV infection focus not on partner selection but on seeking to exploit loopholes in the understood transmission mechanism of HIV during sex. Through the interviews with the peer educators I established that, away from the scientific understanding of the HIV virus being able to cross mucous membranes, two lay theories of transmission during vaginal sex exist. The first is the 'friction' theory and the second the 'penis sucks' theory.

In interviews it became clear that the peer educators were taught the 'friction' theory of transmission, in which there is always some damage to capillaries in the sexual organs of both men and women during penetrative sex. This meant that the two people's blood would mix and HIV could be transmitted. In some cases it was put forward that this damage was too small to see with the naked eye, i.e. there was no visible blood, but in a supporting auxiliary theory the tingling sensation reported when washing after sex was put down to this slight but invisible damage. Box 5 below lists the AIDS myths identified in the project that form auxiliary theories to this lay theory of HIV transmission.

Box 5: The friction theory of HIV transmission

Core Idea: Friction during sex damages blood vessels and results in the mixing of blood
Auxiliary theories/AIDS myths 34. Sex without a condom on the second and subsequent 'rounds' is safe 35. Sex with an old woman is safe 36. Shallow penetration is safe

A practical advantage of this theory for peer educators was to be able to argue against the AIDS myth that no blood on the genitals meant it was safe to have sex (Myth 33). More significantly, however, the theory allowed trainers to avoid the difficult explanation of how HIV can cross mucous membranes, a concept which the peer educators were not familiar with.[55] Friction theory was, by contrast, a convincing explanation of disease transmission that paralleled the dangers of the virus being transmitted during an accident; a mechanical explanation of infection which peer educators were extremely comfortable in describing. It also resonated with pollution beliefs within the African traditional beliefs paradigm, though this was not the intention of the training.

Friction theory is able to explain the AIDS myths of the second and subsequent rounds of sex being safe without a condom (Myth 34); the woman's vagina has now lubricated/opened and friction reduced. The same reasoning underlies the AIDS myths of the safety of sex with an older woman (Myth 35) whose vagina is now 'loose' and shallow penetration being safe (Myth 36) since it involves less friction.

The 'penis sucks' lay theory of HIV transmission

In the interviews it emerged that there is an alternative lay physiological explanation of HIV transmission from women to men (which was not taught to peer educators, but was present in their communities), based on the penis 'sucking'. This theory posits that during ejaculation the penis sucks in fluids.[56] Box 6 lists the AIDS myths identified in the project that form auxiliary theories to this lay theory of HIV/AIDS.

Box 6: The 'penis sucks' lay theory of HIV transmission

Core idea: The penis sucks during ejaculation, drawing in fluids

Auxiliary theories/AIDS myths
37. Sex without a condom is safe on the first 'round' of sex
38. It is safe if the man ejaculates before a woman reaches an orgasm
39. *Coitus interruptus* protects the man
40. A man can't be infected with HIV because the penis doesn't suck
    (a denial of this lay theory that engages with the idea of the penis
    sucking)

Friction theory (or an explanation based on mucous membranes) can't account for AIDS Myths 37–40, including that sex is safe on the first round (when friction is most likely) but condoms should be worn for subsequent rounds (Myth 37). Indeed, Myth 37 directly contradicts Myth 34 – that condoms should be worn on the first round but are not subsequently necessary. However, belief in the 'penis sucks' theory provides an explanation for this Myth 37, based on the idea that the woman has not yet reached orgasm and released dangerous/polluted fluids into her vagina that the penis will suck up when the man ejaculates, an idea more explicitly indicated by Myth 38. It also explains otherwise perplexing AIDS myths that a man can protect himself (and not the woman) from infection by practising *coitus interruptus* (Myth 39).

This lay theory is contested. This is not surprising given rival lay explanations of HIV transmission during sex. One of the recorded myths is based on the idea that the penis *doesn't* suck and, therefore, that a man can't be infected with HIV when having vaginal sex (Myth 40). This denial of the 'penis sucks' lay theory does not, however, conform to the medical explanation or friction theory of HIV transmission, as it denies male vulnerability to infection completely.

The plausibility and palatability of AIDS myths
Myriad AIDS myths can be located within a smaller number of folk or lay theories, and it then becomes clear that they are not the random products of 'ignorance' of the facts, but components of a wider body of ideas that has internal coherence. This may be a worldview in the

case of folk theories or a central key idea in the case of lay theories. As such, any individual AIDS myth is not a stand-alone concept, but one of several auxiliary theories that are generated from, and support, a particular core idea. This helps to explain their continued resilience in the face of public health messaging. We now examine the power of these core theories in terms of their plausibility and their palatability in comparison to medical science.

The core idea of the medical model of AIDS is scientific knowledge, specifically germ theory and our understanding of viruses, combined with an agreement over scientific method that allows reappraisal and change without threatening the core idea itself.[57] This theory of HIV/AIDS is generally, though not always, supported and propagated by government, academia, NGOs, business, and the leadership of most mainline religions. While to those with an understanding of science, the medical explanations provide a credible account, this is less likely to be the case for those with limited scientific education.

The peer educators who participated in this project had been trained with a manual that introduced HIV as:

> Belonging to the retroviral family that shares one important quality – they carry their genetic material in the form of a single-stranded RNA, instead of the usual DNA. In addition, they all possess an enzyme called 'reverse transcriptase'. This enzyme allows a retroviral to change its genetic material from a single stranded RNA-type to a double stranded DNA-type – reversing the normal process of DNA usually producing RNA.[58]

Such scientific jargon was meaningless to the peer educators and equally so to their peers. The vitality of a core idea starts with its plausibility. Bawa Yamba points out that, where traditional beliefs are in play, it is naive to think that science will trump all in an open contest, as 'biomedical discourse is perceived [by those holding to traditional ideas and perceived traditions] as reverting to concepts such as chance and accident to explain what all people know to be due to infractions of traditional norms, inevitably resulting in evil through sorcery or witchcraft'.[59] Here, our belief in the rationality of science is turned on its head. Seen through others' eyes, it is the explanation of science that becomes vague, flimsy, unsatisfactory or just plain nonsense. Measured against this unsatisfactory explanation, alternatives, such as bodily pollution causing disease or Whites conspiring to kill Africans, can be more easily grasped and provide a more plausible explanation.

If a core theory and the auxiliary theories that are generated from it are not only plausibile but also palatable, then it may well be a truly attractive alternative. The palatability of an AIDS myth may come from the pleasure it allows. Key to this is the pleasure of unprotected sex and the lifting of restrictions on abstinence and faithfulness – the ABC of public health HIV-prevention messaging. Once an individual is HIV positive, key aspects of palatability are: first, denial that it is really HIV/AIDS as defined by medical science; and second, that there is hope of a cure – particularly the hope for a complete cure that rids the person of the burden and stigma of HIV/AIDS.

Care needs to be taken in assigning the underpinning strength of a myth to either its plausibility or palatability. There is clearly an interaction between these two principles. A plausible explanation will be strengthened if its recommendations legitimise, rather than deny, pleasure or hope; consequently a myth that is *less* attractive than medical science is unlikely to endure. Alternatively, somebody seeking pleasure or hope may well be attracted to, and be more willing to believe in the plausibility of, alternative explanations of HIV/AIDS.

Additionally to alternative prevention and cure scenarios, blaming others allows people to maintain existing behaviour in the face of continual barrages of health information. Yamba again: 'Anthropologists ... soon discover that an important first step towards behavioural change lies in whether people accept that the illness they have contracted results from their own behaviour or whether they believe it is due to some agent(s) outside of themselves.'[60]

Thus, AIDS myths, drawing on underlying theories, promote three areas of palatability: first, a way of preventing infection; second, a cure for AIDS; and, third, the shifting of responsibility for illness onto a third party. In comparison, the attractiveness of the scientific explanation of

HIV/AIDS is often limited. Prevention typically requires one of the three strategies of abstinence, being faithful or using condoms, all of which have drawbacks and limitations. While antiretroviral drugs contain the disease, this is not a cure and, even without side-effects, the prospect of a lifetime on pills is far from attractive.[61] Finally, rather than allowing individuals to transfer blame onto others, the explanations provided by Western medicine generally link infection to personal sexual behaviour.

The table below summarises how the different folk and lay theories of HIV/AIDS explored in this chapter compare with the biomedical explanation of HIV/AIDS with regard to plausibility and the three identified components of palatability: prevention, cure and the shifting of responsibility.

Table 1 provides a summarised comparison of the plausibility and palatability of the rival theories of HIV/AIDS. There are many possible nuances that such a simplified presentation cannot capture, but it is clear that different theories offer different benefits. Thus, for example, racial conspiracy theories offer a mechanism for shifting blame along with a range of alternative prevention strategies. Religious folk theories do not, by and large, offer alternative protection strategies, but do put forward a cure and, while responsibility is not shifted from the individual within this paradigm, forgiveness is offered.

While Table 1 indicates the palatability of different theories in the shifting of responsibility for infection, it doesn't distinguish the extent to which this is a collective or individual mechanism. Racial folk or conspiracy theories can be seen as demonstrating (collective) racial defence mechanisms in which HIV is constructed as a White invention, as well as providing an explanation for why an individual has become infected, for example that they were injected by a White doctor. In South Africa, that Whites created the AIDS epidemic as part of a continued racial war is, for some, credible. However, not all theories provide both collective and individual mechanisms for shifting responsibility. The idea of an epidemic of witchcraft, as suggested by Adam Ashforth,[63] has been criticised on the grounds that there is no reason for a proliferation of witchcraft comparable to the scale of an epidemic.[64] Rather, it seems that witchcraft remains a potential

Table 1: The plausibility and palatability of competing explanations of AIDS

Theory	Plausibility	Palatability: Prevention without ABC	Palatability: Cure	Palatability: Shifting of personal/responsibility
Racial and authority	Racial power relationships	✓	✗[62]	✓ Externalises to Whites or to those in authority
Pollution		✓	✓	✗ Responsibility lies with self, but ✓ as failure to comply generally carries limited stigma
Witchcraft	African traditional worldview	✓ (limited)	✓	✓ Externalises to personal enemies
Ancestors		✓ (limited)	✗	✗
Religion	Religious belief and Bible texts	✗	✓	✗ Responsibility lies with self, but ✓ since redemption is possible
Popular or lay theories to avoid infection	Observation and lay physiology	✓	✗	✗ Largely amoral, based on individual being smart enough to avoid infection
Western medicine	Science and support from allied institutions	Only via ABC	Management as a chronic disease	Responsibility for infection largely lies with own sexual behaviour

✓ Indicates a greater palatability than Western medical science ✗ Indicates no greater palatability than Western medical science mechanism for explaining an individual's infection, but, unlike racism, is generally not seen as a credible explanation for the epidemic as a whole, given the implausiblity of an increase in witchcraft that the AIDS-epidemic-as-witchcraft would indicate.

Table 1 does not indicate whether theories of AIDS have a gendered dimension. Isak Niehaus and Gunvor Jonsson sharply divide explanations of AIDS, with women blaming men's careless and unscrupulous sexual conduct for infecting them, while men 'invoked conspiracy theories, blaming trans-local agents ... for the pandemic'.[65] Both sets of gendered narratives allow blame to be shifted from personal responsibility onto others. However, Niehaus and Jonsson see much more externalisation by men than women. While the AIDS myths reported by the peer educators in the research project often demonstrated a gender dimension, this was in the form of blaming the opposite sex and came from both men and women. This appeared to be a reflection of gender tensions and not a fundamentally different way of appointing blame between men and women, as suggested by Niehaus and Jonsson.

Finally, Table 1 cannot distinguish between genuine and sham protagonists of the different folk and lay theories presented. As with all attractive offers, there is room for frauds or quacks to offer hope to desperate people. When it comes to curing HIV/AIDS, there are opportunities to make money. This is particularly true for Christianity and African traditional beliefs, where practitioners stand to gain from providing services of one sort or another. It is also true, of course, for the allopathic paradigm. There are many doctors selling inappropriate but profitable procedures or failing to conduct procedures because they are not profitable. Further, there are 'quacks' who imitate medical professionals or appropriate the profession's language, signs and symbols in order to make money from selling everything from vitamins to cures for AIDS – sometimes the two things are one and the same thing. For those committed to the allopathic paradigm, it may be tempting to believe that there are good and bad doctors, but that anybody claiming prevention or cure outside the allopathic paradigm is a charlatan. Such a view will close off our ability to understand what is being said and done about AIDS. Rather, this book takes the approach that there are, irrespective of what we think about efficacy, genuine and fake practitioners operating within all health care systems. We will see in later chapters of this book how people are attempting to establish which healers are genuine within these competing explanations of HIV/AIDS.

What Table 1 does, however, illustrate is that alternative theories of HIV/AIDS are based on foundations that are plausible to some sections of the population and are able, through the AIDS myths that are their auxiliary hypotheses, to offer more palatable implications than those of allopathic medicine.

Myths as credible explanations

AIDS myths, while seemingly bizarre when viewed from the outside, provide, from the inside, credible explanations of HIV/AIDS for many people. AIDS myths are neither simple misunderstandings nor are they plucked out of the air at random. Rather, they draw on different, if not always discrete, or compatible, bodies of knowledge that provide the underlying core ideas to which AIDS myths are linked. What they offer, and what keeps them circulating, is both their credibility and palatability.

Ignoring cross-fertilisation between biomedical, folk and lay theories, we see that this is a multi-faceted competition between ideas. It is not biomedicine on one side and the rest on the other side. While there can be degrees of alignment between practically any theory, fundamentally all theories are in competition. Moreover, the conflict is asymmetric, different theories draw on different resources, operate across different spectrums of human concern, and, regarding HIV/AIDS, offer different configurations of assistance.

It should now be clear why AIDS myths have proved to be so hard to dislodge despite extensive health-promotion endeavours. Since folk and lay theories are not scientific in nature, attempting to dismantle AIDS myths using scientific information is an inept tool of persuasion. Tackling one myth will leave the core idea from which it was generated untouched and from it new AIDS myths can be developed.[66] And, further, even if we were able to successfully decapitate belief in all auxiliary hypotheses linked to a folk or lay theory, the plurality of theories means that individuals can shift allegiance to another explanation. The hybridisation of folk and lay theories of AIDS makes these transitions easy. We are struggling to defeat a multifarious opponent, which, like the Hydra of Greek mythology, has many heads, and these, if severed by an attacker, will regenerate anew.

3

Managing a mosaic
of beliefs

Elite and popular debates over AIDS

The peer educators participating in the Digco action research project reported back the AIDS myths that they came across in their communities. These turned out to be more coherent and robust than expected – folk and lay theories of AIDS. What we now examine is what the peer educators themselves made of these alternative explanations of AIDS.

Ronald Bayer was the first of many to describe the policy responses to AIDS in the 1980s as 'HIV exceptionalism',[1] distinguishing it from the conventional public health approach to sexually transmitted disease of education, testing, reporting and notification credited to Thomas Parran's approach to syphilis in the US.[2] Such an approach was not taken with HIV/AIDS. Rather, along with education, there was an emphasis on 'prevention measures that were non-coercive – that respected the privacy and social rights of those who were at risk'.[3] This AIDS exceptionalism came about because public health officials had to come to terms with stakeholder contestation.[4] In developed countries, where the response to HIV/AIDS was first formulated, public health officials had to engage with civil liberties lobbies and the gay community, which constituted a well-organised minority group hard hit by the disease.

By the 1990s many were arguing that the period of HIV exceptionalism had passed and that with advances in antiretroviral drugs[5] and 'innovations in prevention',[6] a process of normalising the response to HIV/AIDS was taking place in the developed world. Kevin De Cock et al. argued that the importation of HIV exceptionalism policy, based on developed countries' experiences, was not appropriate for Africa with its generalised epidemic among the population as a whole and that a traditional public health approach should have been taken from the start.[7]

Thus, two debates intertwined. The first was over the most appropriate public health response to HIV/AIDS in developed countries. The second was over whether such an approach was the best one to be adopted (or imposed) in developing counties where the epidemic has evolved in different, much more devastating, ways. However, the existence of debate does not mean that all voices are heard. These debates were between and among health experts and educated activists who did not dispute the scientific explanation of HIV/AIDS. Within South Africa relatively little attention has been paid to those who hold alternative explanations of AIDS, excepting those of President Mbeki's denialism which, as outlined in Chapter 10, was an elite discourse. The beliefs of the population have remained an intellectual afterthought.[8]

Suzette Heald has put forward that, in Botswana, 'two parallel discourse [have been] operating in the 1990s; discourses that were not allowed to meet ... One [a biomedical response] was government endorsed and public, making the second [based on traditional African beliefs] appear as unofficial and *sub rosa*, though for many it was these truths that appeared self-evident'.[9] In South Africa, with Mbeki's alternative explanation of AIDS publicly neutralised in the early 2000s, this cleared the way for treatment to be rolled out, but it also drove further underground alternative explanations of AIDS. It was a matter of alternative explanations of HIV/AIDS being 'out of sight and out of mind' for those promoting medically focused AIDS responses. Without the proponents of these alternative theories being heard, the ongoing conflict over HIV/AIDS has been largely inaudible to health professionals and their vast and varied camp following: Departments of Health, NGOs, health practitioners, academics, columnists, social marketers and more.

Not as one

Peer educators provide one, interpersonal communication method that can be used to educate people about HIV/AIDS and broadly promote health. It is generally assumed that the peer educators recruited into company HIV/AIDS programmes are 'on board' – the foot soldiers of any campaign who will, to the best of their ability, convey correct information to their peers. In this context, peer educators' beliefs are not seen as something to be concerned about. Yet, as the Digco project unfolded, not entirely in the way that I had planned, it became clear that their beliefs needed to be engaged.

Belief in witchcraft is widespread within South African townships. What was unexpected was the difference of opinions within the peer educators themselves over witches and HIV/AIDS. Getting this into the open, however, took time. Early on in the project I attempted to stimulate a discussion among the peer educators about their varied belief in the agency of their ancestors, a much less sensitive topic than that of witchcraft. Their response to a questionnaire I administered during the first workshop of the project indicated a divergence of views.[10] At the following workshop, I projected this data as a bar graph, hoping to stimulate a conversation. I thought such a discussion would help us engage with beliefs around AIDS and the ancestors. What I stimulated was a long and uncomfortable silence. I had exposed that they were not of one mind on these matters and they did not feel secure enough to openly discuss these differences.

That changed as the project proceeded and they realised that the workshops really were a free space to speak and that I would moderate all discussions and insist that all viewpoints be respected.[11] Two discussions that we held over witchcraft, midway through the project, were energetic and lively. In the ensuing discussions, I had my work cut out ensuring that speaking could say their piece without disruption from others keen to contribute.

The first discussion was stimulated when a peer educator reported to the workshop that he had been told that 'witches can send AIDS'. The reporting back on 'AIDS myths' was a regular slot in the workshop agenda that allowed us to discuss what was being said about AIDS and decide on whether a myth merited developing a counter story. What got things started was when I asked how many of the peer educators believed that there were such things as witches. Thirteen out of the twenty present for the discussion did.[12] When I asked if witches could kill somebody, all thirteen agreed that they could, though they stressed that more commonly witches were responsible for other misfortunes, such as destroying the victim's romantic relationship, possibly at the request of a jealous or jilted lover. For men this would come in the form of impotency, for women it could be their vagina starting to smell or continual bleeding.[13] However, when I then asked if witches could send HIV and therefore cause AIDS, only three of the peer educators present thought they could.[14] One of these three also qualified this belief by arguing that witches could send something that looked like, but was not actually, AIDS.

The discussion brought out a range of opinions on witches. Some of the peer educators simply had no truck with the idea of witches. This refutation was based largely on Christian, typically Pentecostal or Charismatic, faith. Others believed in witches, but with different credence over their power. One female peer educator argued coherently for a social interpretation of witches. 'The witch', she said, 'is me [i.e. I'm jealous of somebody]. The traditional healer just assists [with the attempted bewitchment], but can't do anything more than I can.'[15] She went on to say that those who thought they had been sexually assaulted in their sleep, a method by which witches were often supposed to send sexually related problems, had simply had a wet dream, or were putting the blame for real sexual indiscretions on witchcraft. The majority who did believe in witches put forward varied accounts of their powers, including the sending of sexually transmitted infections, but most ruled out HIV/AIDS.[16]

While voluntary enrolment as company peer educators implied a belief in Western medicine and scientific explanation, this was clearly much more of an ideal than a reality. This is revealing, but what needs also to be engaged with is the paradox of many of the peer educators crediting witches with powers, including being able to kill people, but not being able to send HIV/AIDS. Logically this privileged status conferred on HIV/AIDS by the peer educators doesn't make sense. If witches have the power to harm, why should HIV/AIDS be exempted from their munitions of malevolence? We explore this paradox, one that extends beyond the question of witchcraft and HIV/AIDS.

Credible voices?

When, in the final stage of the Digco research, I interviewed the participating peer educators, many of my questions differed from what I had anticipated asking when designing the project. I still used the interviews to get feedback on the peer educators' experience of the project and to establish the extent to which they had used the stories they had developed.[17] However, I also used the interviews to enquire about their own beliefs about HIV/AIDS.

It is pertinent to ask whether their responses to me in the interviews were credible. I have earlier argued that we should be sceptical of information collected in one-off surveys and interviews. Should we believe what the peer educators told me they believed about HIV and AIDS?

I regard what they, eventually, told me as reliable. To begin with, we were working on the same side. They were peer educators who had thrown their lot in with the company HIV/AIDS programme and I was a researcher seeking to strengthen peer education. This alignment was not, however, immediately obvious. At lunch during the first workshop, one of the peer educators complained that Digco always brought in outsiders to conduct training instead of developing its own employees.[18] I was, she was indicating, a case in point. After lunch I repeated to the group what I had told those at the table: while Digco was covering the costs of the project, including the lunch we'd just eaten, I wasn't being paid by the company. Rather, this was part of my academic work paid for by my university.[19] Uncoupling myself from the company was useful; while they might have thrown their lot in with Digco's peer educator programme, their relationship with the company was often difficult. Indeed, during the project there was an unprotected strike and several of the participating peer educators were suspended.[20] Once it was clear I wasn't on the Digco payroll, I was the recipient of frank criticism of company practices and culture.

By the time interviews were conducted, I had worked with the peer educators for six months and, over this time, had built trust.[21] Our interactions had also allowed me to demonstrate appreciation for honesty and maintaining confidentiality.[22] One result was that the interviews were remarkably frank. Various spontaneous 'confessions' on the part of the peer educators indicated a willingness to move beyond giving a 'correct' set of responses. These disclosures included being HIV positive but unwilling to disclose this publicly (or to other peer educators), having multiple partners, having unprotected sex outside supposedly monogamous relationships, and having cleansed themselves of traditional or ethnoecological disease by having unprotected sex with a stranger.[23] Away from these disclosures, which they knew would detract from their status as a peer educator if publicly disclosed, much of what they told me was not, as we will see, 'on message' and they knew it. Their approach indicates that the interviews went beyond providing only acceptable 'public accounts'[24] of peer education in the interviews.

Taking a stand on unfamiliar ground

Before I questioned the peer educators about their beliefs, I asked them about some things they would be assumed to know about HIV/ AIDS, including what a virus was and how HIV was transmitted. Their biomedical knowledge of HIV and AIDS was drawn from the combination of the formal training they had received, the information they receive informally (e.g. though reading, discussions, television programmes, etc.), and their level of educational achievement that provides relevant foundational knowledge, such as biological concepts.[25]

Despite training, the peer educators' grasp of concepts at the heart of any biomedical explanation of HIV/AIDS was sometimes limited. While identifying viruses as something that causes harm to the body, when requested to explain them within the concept of 'germs', ten peer educators did not or could not comment on how a virus might differ from other germs – of those who did comment, two thought that all disease is caused by viruses, five drew a distinction between a virus and other germs on the basis of whether a disease is serious/curable or not, four on the method of transmission, and two on the invisibility of a virus in comparison to other germs. Some of these responses drew, in part, on information given during training: the ways in which disease can be transmitted, the severity of different diseases (and the non-curability of HIV/AIDS), and the small size of pathogens, with viruses being the smallest.

When asked how people got HIV, many peer educators were noticeably relieved to be moving to more comfortable territory (than viruses and germs) and quickly started to list the ways in which HIV could be transmitted. Sexual transmission was generally listed first and accidental/occupational exposure a close second.[26] Their familiarity with mother-to-child-transmission of HIV was much less strong. Despite a page being devoted to mother-to-child transmission in the Digco *Peer Educator Training Manual*, 15 of the 23 peer educators had to be prompted before they added this as a way in which people become infected, possibly reflecting uncertainty on their part over this transmission mechanism. No other ways of acquiring HIV were given at this stage in any of the interviews.

This suggests that training had given them some facts about HIV/AIDS (along with a familiarity, albeit not always on the tip of their tongues, of the main transmission routes for HIV). Beyond these facts, however, there was little if any evidence of a coherent biomedical framework of understanding of the disease that they would be able to use when in dialogue with peers. Expecting peer educators, with their limited training and practically no scientific grounding, to have such a framework is quite unrealistic. Yet, the central focus of most peer educator programmes is the transmission of scientifically correct information to peers.[27]

Although there are a range of reasons for individuals volunteering to become workplace peer educators (a role with few benefits and potentially onerous responsibilities), many take this step as a result of seeing loved ones die of AIDS and a desire to help others (and themselves) avoid a similar death.[28] The Digco peer educators expressed how, as a result of such experiences, they were attempting to educate people about HIV/AIDS, i.e. people who did not know about HIV/AIDS, did not believe that there was such as thing, or did not want to believe it. As one peer educator explained when asked why he had become a peer educator, 'We, as Blacks [Africans] we never believe that AIDS might be a disease. So I wanted to have that explained [to me], so that whenever I talk to people I will talk of something that I am sure of ... I must be informed so that I can convey something that I know and I'm sure of. So I needed to equip myself in actual facts.'

Thus, becoming a peer educator is often about making a stand, on the still unfamiliar ground of allopathic medicine. The peer educators were clearly attempting to take a firm stand in line with what they had been taught, even if their grasp of the 'actual facts' that they were expected, and wanted, to transmit was sometimes shaky. The result was less a holistic grasp of HIV/AIDS and more a series of points around which they stood firm.

The efficacy of antiretroviral drugs was one such point on which they made a stand. That they were essential for an HIV-positive individual to take, when their immune system had been weakened by HIV, was a central tenet of their belief. In this regard, the scepticism of Thabo Mbeki was alternately mocked and chided as misleading people to their deaths. The value of condoms in preventing infection was similarly upheld. Condoms, despite raising a range of complex issues,[29] were also strongly backed by the peer educators. Despite most of the peer educators being religious,[30] and a number attending churches that condemned the use of condoms,[31] all the peer educators interviewed promoted condoms as part of their activities.

Managing beliefs

Beyond these public accounts of their peer educator work, corresponding to their assigned roles within Digco's HIV/AIDS programme, lay a much more complex mosaic of belief. Thus, for example, a Zulu artisan in his 40s, who had identified himself during workshops as an authority on Zulu tradition, turned out during the interview to be highly sceptical of bio-moral explanations of illness. This belief was founded on a 'Road to Damascus' conversion when, some 15 years earlier, he had been cured of a painful neck condition by a minor operation in the company hospital after six months of ineffective treatment by a *nyanga* (a traditional Zulu medicine man) who had said it was the result of witchcraft and warned him against seeking Western medical assistance. Yet, despite his faith in Western medicine, he continued traditional cultural practices, as openly breaking with them would result in a rupture with his family. During the project he had been wearing a goatskin bracelet. The animal had been slaughtered to bring the spirits of his dead mother's ancestors to the family home. It was felt within the family that this had not previously been done properly and was the reason why 'things are not going well'. He explained, 'I had a lot of debate [doubts] on this before I did this. But I had to do it because I knew if I don't do it then my whole family will [be upset] ... So I couldn't say this is not right, because once I say it, that's when they start to have friction in the family.'[32]

The way in which this peer educator provided an account of how he managed a range of beliefs was, however, unique among the interviewed Digco peer educators. In every other interview, the dynamic was the other way round; it was alternative, non-scientific beliefs that emerged from behind an initial front of allopathic explanation.

Some peer educators were managing a wide range of beliefs. Thus, a process operator in his 40s, who had been an active peer educator for over ten years, had a strong belief in the dangers of (traditional) pollution, regularly cleansed himself by means of induced vomiting, had a traditional healer whom he consulted frequently, made use of church prophets at his African Initiated Church, believed that witches could send *isidliso* (a traditional wasting disease, sometimes translated as TB), and made a yearly sacrifice of a goat in honour of his ancestors who he believed could protect him from harm.

Other peer educators' lives were less complex but still held to some alternative beliefs alongside their affiliation to Western medicine. Thus, a female clerk who had been a peer educator for two years rejected outright pollution beliefs, thought that traditional healers peddled lies to get money, mocked church prophets by stating that 'water is for drinking' (blessed water being a critical healing element used by church prophets), didn't think that there are witches outside people's dreams, and thought that ancestors have no influence in the world of the living. She took a feminist position on gender relations, arguing that men, including her own husband, could not be trusted and felt women should insist on the use of condoms. We were well into the interview before she narrated a long story about a friend who had joined, and attempted to leave, the Universal Church.[33] Her friend's experience led her to conclude that financial and health problems could be solved by joining the church, but this was only the case should you remain a church member – you effectively became a prisoner of the organisation. This temporary nature of relief allowed her to argue that the church could only *apparently* cure HIV/AIDS since 'you can think that if I have HIV, my HIV will be cured. It won't, because it's like you won't be permanent[ly HIV negative] ... So if you start leaving the church, your worries they come back again ... Now maybe you will be even fully blown [AIDS stage].' In this way she was able to reconcile her friend's experience with her peer educator training in which antiretroviral drugs suppressed, but did not cure, HIV/AIDS.

Since the peer educators held a range of beliefs, I attempted to systematically probe bio-moral beliefs and their relationships to illness and misfortune, including AIDS. However, my approach to each of these topics was to start questioning the peer educators, not about their own beliefs, but about the beliefs of their peers. This of course took the pressure off them; they were talking about what other people thought. But, this division, between the beliefs of their peers and their own, always crumbled. There came a point in every interview where the distinction between the beliefs of their peers and their own could not be maintained in the context of an honest discussion. I never prompted this switch, but in every interview we always reached a point where it became necessary to clarify that we were talking about *their* beliefs and not those of other people. When we reached this point I would do some backtracking to clarify responses to earlier questions and to what extent they had reported the views of peers or, in fact, their own.

AIDS exceptionalism at the grassroots

In contrast to their stance over condoms and the value of antiretroviral drugs, peer educators' broader understanding of misfortune, including disease, revealed a complex picture. Many remained convinced of the important role of alternative, bio-moral accounts of disease and misfortune that contrasted with the exceptional category into which they frequently placed AIDS.

The different scope of scientific and alternative theories makes exact comparisons difficult. Medical science seeks to identify the cause and cure of specific disease, bio-moral theories frequently operate with much wider categories. Thus, for example, *madimabe*, the Sesotho term literally meaning 'bad blood' but translated as 'bad luck', can originate, within a traditional perspective, from pollution, neglecting ancestors or from witchcraft. It explains, for those who give it credence, not only illness, but also misfortunes such as car accidents, unemployment, infertility, romantic failure and other troubles.

Table 2 below presents the peer educators' views on a range of non-scientific beliefs, distinguishing between their connection to HIV/AIDS, on the one hand, and 'other problems', on the other[34] (the previously mentioned heterogeneous collection of ills). The non-scientific beliefs probed were: three forms of traditional bodily pollution,[35] bewitchment, the power of traditional healers to resolve problems, the ability of ancestors to protect from harm, and the power of church prophets and prayer to heal. On occasions it was simply not possible to place an individual's views clearly within this tabulation. I could not say (and perhaps they did not know themselves) where they stood on a particular issue. In these cases, their views were reported as 'don't know/not recorded'.

Perhaps initially, the most striking result is that a number of peer educators held beliefs that directly contradicted their training. The earlier discussions on witches had alerted me to this, but across the 23 interviewed peer educators none of them fully matched what might be expected of a Western health professional – a belief in scientific explanation of disease combined with an acceptance that non-scientific belief is limited to (albeit valuable) psychosocial support.

Table 2: Peer educators' perspectives on non-scientific beliefs in relation to HIV/AIDS and 'other problems'

Peer educators' perspectives on aspects of belief	Disagree	Agree	DN/Not recorded
Traditional pollution beliefs			
1. Unprotected sex with a widow(er) who has not been cleansed can result in:			
HIV/AIDS	19	2	2
Other problems (not HIV/AIDS)	5	15	3
2. Unprotected sex with a woman who has had an abortion and not been cleansed can result in:			
HIV/AIDS	19	3	1
Other problem (not HIV/AIDS)	3	16	2
3. Unprotected sex with a menstruating woman can result in:			
HIV/AIDS	18	1	4
Other problems (not HIV/AIDS)	7	12	4
4. Witches can send:			
HIV/AIDS	18	5	0
Other problems (not HIV/AIDS)	6	17	0
5. Traditional healers can cure/resolve:			
HIV/AIDS	20	3	0
Other problems (not HIV/AIDS)	7	16	0
6. Ancestors can protect you from:			
HIV infection	19	4	0
Other problems (not HIV infection)	10	13	0
7. Church prophets can cure/resolve:			
HIV/AIDS	20	2	1
Other problems (not HIV/AIDS)	9	13	1
8. Prayer (and faith) can cure/resolve:			
HIV/AIDS	17	4	1
Other problems (not HIV/AIDS)	7	14	2

Yet, this point noted, the dominant pattern is one of the peer educators agreeing with what had been taught about HIV/AIDS, but not applying this to other concerns. For example, a majority of peer educators (18 out of 23) believe that witches *can't send HIV/AIDS*, but also believe that witches *can send other problems* (17 out of 23), including traditional African ethnoecological illnesses such as *sejeso* and 'Western' diagnosed disease such as TB or sexually transmitted infections, as well as being able to jinx a person.[36]

Thus, the peer educators exhibited a deeply equivocal position. Putting AIDS into a distinct category, with different properties from other diseases and misfortunes, appears to have been a way in which they sought to respond to HIV/AIDS alongside Western medicine while frequently holding contradictory beliefs about disease and misfortune generally.

Just too incredible for some: apes, oranges and the origins of AIDS

Over one issue, the origin of AIDS, the scientific explanation appeared to be very difficult for most peer educators to accept, and only a few, when expressing their views honestly, were able to accept what they had been taught. Officially, and in line with current scientific consensus (which has changed over the course of the epidemic), HIV is the result of a zoonotic (animal to human transfer) process in which the virus crossed from primates to humans, most likely in Central or West Africa. This was the information that was given to Digco peer educators. Their training manual stated that:

> The most likely theory [of the origins of HIV] is that SIV, the Simian Immuno-deficiency Virus carried by chimpanzees in Central Africa forests, caused a zoonotic infection in human beings slaughtering the chimps for meat and as part of ritual practices. Once inside the human hosts, SIV mutated into HIV, which was able to spread from person to person.[37]

This information had only a limited grip on peer educators. Putting aside the off-putting jargon in which the manual was couched, many of them simply found this explanation incredible. In the interviews only seven of 23 peer educators agreed that HIV came from primates; 12 disagreed; five said they didn't know; and one peer educator's views were not recorded. As the following quote indicates, this is probably an overestimation of their belief that HIV comes from primates:

> **David Dickinson (DD):** And in your view, where did this AIDS come from?
>
> **Peer educator (PE):** According to my understanding, they say it came from the baboon. They're doing the experiment, they took the blood of the baboon, put it together like in the laboratory, they put it to someone who's ill and then they started this ... [AIDS].
>
> **DD:** [Finishing sentence] ... started AIDS. I have to say that was the most unconvincing explanation. You started off by saying 'they say' and then you've been looking funny all the time.
>
> **PE:** [Laughs] I'm sorry, Professor.
>
> **DD:** So I'm not sure, is that what you think or what you were told?
>
> **PE:** Okay, I was told. And then in my knowledge ... it came to South Africa from overseas, those people coming with the ship or whatever ... They sleep with the *makgosha* [prostitutes] and then they say we get this ... The way I think, Professor, I think the disease, maybe it came from the diseases that were mixed together.

The peer educator starts off with an explanation of where AIDS comes from involving primates, albeit one based on laboratory experiments, but it's not the explanation to which the peer educator actually subscribes. This is, rather, based on a cocktail of diseases, at least some from overseas, prostitutes' wombs as sites of disease incubation, and the combination of different diseases to create new ones.

Of the seven peer educators who did settle for AIDS originating from primates, six cited sexual contact and one the cutting of bush meat as the transmission route.[38] There was resistance to the demeaning implications of Africans having sex with animals as being responsible for the epidemic, and racial defence mechanisms were employed by some peer educators to shift blame from Africans onto Whites. The Digco training manual vaguely refers to 'ritual practices', but peer educators understood the implications of the zoonotic theory. Of the six peer educators who cited sexual contact between humans and animals in the explanation of AIDS's origins, one argued this was the result of an African woman being coerced into such sex, and two re-located the bestiality to White people in America. One of the twelve peer educators who rejected the idea that AIDS had come from primates, also rejected the story that it had been injected into oranges which had then been given to Africans, but of the two it was the orange explanation that had at least some credibility; 'At least that orange one [has some basis], we Black [African] people, we like to eat oranges. You see? We eat oranges [we don't screw monkeys].'

The twelve peer educators who did not subscribe in any way to the idea of zoonosis, and who put forward alternatives, suggested the mixing and progression of diseases (four peer educators), that it was a re-named traditional disease (one), a combination of traditional disease and mixing (two), that it had been made by the Apartheid-era scientist Dr Basson (two), and one that it was a disease of the Last Days, i.e. as professed in the Book of the Revelation.

This spectrum of responses as to the origin of AIDS illustrates the uneven impact of training on the peer educators, despite their desire to learn about the disease. The plurality of alternative explanations reinforces the idea that they are not, in fact, fully aligned with the medical framework that supposedly guided the Digco peer educator programme.

A mosaic of beliefs

Documenting the beliefs of the 23 interviewed peer educators illustrated how shallow their allegiance to a scientific view of the world could be. It also revealed just how varied their beliefs were. When mapped at the individual level, the range of their beliefs produced a mosaic; no two peer educators held the same configuration regarding HIV/AIDS or other problems.[39]

The diverse beliefs of the peer educators poses a problem; over half of them held beliefs that would make it difficult for them to honestly operate alongside medical practitioners in responding to HIV/AIDS, even if we generously stretched what beliefs were compatible with an HIV/AIDS programme.[40] Yet they were part of the company's peer educator programme, committed, sometimes passionately, to their peer educator role. This necessitated a juggling of different beliefs; how the prevention and treatment of HIV/AIDS taught in their training could be integrated into their existing beliefs. This was done in different ways. While members of the group differed on the value of traditional healers, they found common cause in raising technical shortcomings when it came to HIV/AIDS, for example traditional healers' inability to 'see inside blood' and therefore diagnose HIV. On this basis they collectively denied claims that traditional healers could cure HIV/AIDS and asserted that HIV-positive people needed antiretroviral treatment.[41]

Juggling the contradictions between personal beliefs and their training involved a range of manoeuvres and compromises that allowed the peer educators to maintain an equilibrium between the different systems of thought to which they gave credence. Thus, one peer educator sought to emphasise the importance of Christian faith as a way in which problems could be overcome. He cited the biblical story of Job, whose faith was finally rewarded by God. 'He never lost his faith in God. He kept praying and praying until God helped him. That's what the church[42] believes. If you believe enough that let's say you're diagnosed HIV positive, then you believe ... then you live with this. I cannot say you'll be cured, but you'll live with this thing forever.' This formulation, similar to the earlier story about the Universal Church's keeping HIV at bay as long as the member stayed faithful, allowed the peer educator to acknowledge God's omnipotence, and therefore do anything including curing somebody of HIV/AIDS, *and* avoid saying there is a cure for AIDS.

This need to reconcile alternative theories of HIV/AIDS with a committed stand as peer educators was not only a problem for the peer educators themselves, but also for their peer education. Several recounted how peers had abandoned antiretroviral treatment on the grounds that faith in God would cure them of HIV and that by continuing to take antiretrovirals they were failing to demonstrate the faith necessary for a miraculous cure. In responding to the belief that God can cure HIV/AIDS, discussion among the peer educators led to the adoption of the slogan 'God helps those who help themselves' [i.e. you needed to both pray to God and take antiretroviral drugs if HIV positive]. This formulation allowed them to work with those (including some of their own number) who believed that God could do anything *and* incorporate the message that HIV-positive people needed to take antiretroviral drugs. One story developed by the peer educators to capture this message was a parable about a man who meets a lion and kneels to pray.

> One day, a man walked into a forest and stumbled across a lion. Instead of running, he knelt down and asked God to protect him. However, the lion killed and ate the man! On arrival in heaven (the man was a devout Christian), he angrily asked God why the lion had killed him when he was praying for help. God shook his head and told the man that he had been foolish. Instead of kneeling down, he should have used the intelligence that God had given him and run away from the lion. While he was running he should have prayed for help to run faster. If he had done that he would still be alive.

The story, which resonated with the group, is instructive. It puts forward, in allegoric form, that medical science and alternative healing systems (here, Christian faith) should be complementary rather than in competition. This approach was adopted by the peer educators for tactical reasons; they felt they were more likely to have success in keeping people on treatment with such compromises than attempting to 'win' arguments against preachers (or other protagonists of non-allopathic medicine) in the eyes of their peers. However, the compromise also reflects the peer educators' own composite health beliefs which they needed to synchronise.

Constructing compromises

Alternative explanations of AIDS have a complex relationship with allopathic or medical science. Izak Niehaus[43] and Alexander Rödlach[44] have argued that people move between or combine different discourses over AIDS, while Jonny Steinberg notes how AIDS can be blamed on witchcraft or demons, yet at other times it is denied, by the same person who asserted that 'there is only one way to get HIV [i.e. the biomedical explanation]'.[45]

AIDS sat uncomfortably in the understanding of the Digco peer educators. The disease was differently categorised from other forms of misfortune including other illnesses, but this separation was not stable. What was striking was not the weakness of their biomedical knowledge, stark as that was at times, but that they would reach different conclusions should they proceed from different starting points. If a discussion began within one explanatory model it would reach one conclusion, but if it started within another it could well conclude with something very different. Thus, for example, in exploring the view of several peer educators on how having multiple sexual partners could incubate disease in a woman's womb, they arrived logically, and without qualms, at the possibility that this could create, or incubate, HIV. Such a view was never reached when I asked them to explain, from the biomedical information given to them in training, how people acquired HIV.

The limited and unstable hold that biomedical knowledge of HIV/AIDS had on the peer educators can be viewed in three ways: as a training failure, as partial progress, or as unofficial compromises.

The limitations of the peer educator training are not hard to demonstrate. It had failed to equip them with a sufficient biomedical explanation of HIV/AIDS (never mind other diseases) to hold consistently to such explanations. However, while true, this perspective is not very helpful in grasping what is happening and what could be done – the problem of an AIDS educational strategy that requires everyone to have postgraduate degrees in virology and public health is obvious.

The second perspective is to view their, albeit partial, biomedical knowledge about HIV/AIDS as a step forward. From this perspective they had been partly prised away from alternative explanations of disease, at least in regard to HIV/AIDS, and now operated with a dichotomous set of beliefs. It might not be where we would like them to be, but it would be part of the way there. If peer educators are viewed not simply as a conduit of health education, but as early adapters[46] among the target population, then the peer educators' partial shift could be seen as an advance; a beachhead into the wider population's beliefs. However, such progress suggests that AIDS education has only achieved a dualistic, schizophrenic understanding of health and illness, and this after decades of effort.

A third account of the peer educators' knowledge and its utilisation takes into consideration that those not willing or determined enough to turn away from alternative explanations of sickness and misfortune, yet who wish to access and promote the allopathic response to the HIV/AIDS, are attempting to assemble compromises or accommodations.

Constructing compromises is not simply an attempt to demonstrate intellectual coherence – there are higher stakes at play. To turn your back on belief systems may mean turning your back on your family, friends, community, religious faith and your history. The compromises the peer educators put forward typically attempt to promote a biomedical perspective while maintaining respect for alternative perspectives. This could be viewed as purely tactical; they were aware that frontal attacks on alternative cosmologies did not have any realistic chance of success within their communities. However, a fuller understanding needs also to reflect the peer educators' own embeddedness within these alternative, non-scientific perspectives. This embeddedness is more than tact, politeness or an unwillingness to rock the boat; it reflects genuine belief in these systems of thought.

4

AIDS backchat

The limits of expert power

If peer educators struggle with their own embeddedness within alternative worldviews that explain AIDS differently from medical science, it may well be tempting to bypass any form of lay intermediation in health promotion and, rather, rely on direct, unmediated communication provided by educated health professionals. Such communication takes a 'vertical' format with information being transmitted from professional medical expert to lay person. It can take place individually in the consultation room, delivered to an assembled group, or, if necessary, translated into the vernacular, written in boldly coloured pamphlets, aired as public service messages on TV, radio or internet, or plastered on billboards.

Yet, despite a diversity of formats and attempts to adapt messages to the concerns, language and idiom of different target audiences, these vertical health promotion efforts remain firmly under the control of 'experts'. In general, this control over the message limits scope for participatory and inclusive communication. A medical explanation of AIDS leaves little room for discussion over, for example, whether God can cure AIDS or not.[1] That such views are not aired may give the appearance that they are absent. But, rather, counsel is being held for a more appropriate, safer space and time.[2]

It would, however, be wrong to think that if such conversations did take place openly, science would be the winner or the target audience would be convinced. I realised this one wet afternoon in Potlakong when researching traditional healers' understandings of HIV/AIDS. This research had included a survey of 20 healers belonging to a township-based traditional healer association. In response to my question as to whether AIDS was a new or an old disease, all but two of the 20 said that it was an old disease and had provided me, in a follow-up question, with a range of names for this older disease.

I was spending the afternoon going through the survey results with the group's leader, Traditional Dr Mosia. In particular, he was explaining to me the various diseases that the 18 respondents had identified AIDS to really be. Part way through the afternoon we took a break, I shelled out for cool drinks and we sat at the table on which we'd been working together, as the rain came and went outside. 'So, Professor,' Dr Mosia asked me, 'where do you think this AIDS comes from?' This was, I thought, the moment to nail my colours to the mast. Sitting in a dimly lit room with paint peeling from the walls, I carried with me the authority of my university, but had chosen to patiently engage with this group of healers. Now their leader was asking my opinion. I explained how we believed the disease had crossed from primates to humans at some point, probably in Central or West Africa. I kept it jargon-free and I kept it short. Thinking ahead, I aimed to elaborate only once Dr Mosia had reacted to my initial outline.

His response was nothing short of humiliating, though it was not meant to be so. There was a slight pause after I'd wound down my short explanation. Dr Mosia filled the silence. 'You know what I heard the other day, Professor? Somebody said that AIDS was caused by having fleas inside you, drinking your blood from the inside.' Then he laughed uproariously at the crazy ideas people came up with. My story included. Earnestly, I assumed I'd been asked, '*Really*, Professor, where does AIDS come from?' Actually, we'd just been shooting the breeze as we drank our ginger beer. The origins of AIDS lay, obviously, within the older terms and descriptions of traditional diseases that we'd spent the afternoon discussing. Nine out of ten healers couldn't be wrong.

To understand why science is not automatically privileged over explanations of illness and disease, we need to step away from the idea of there being a correct scientific explanation of AIDS, competing with a farrago of ephemeral misunderstandings. Rather, we need to see science as but one idea competing among many. As Heald has pointed out in the context of Botswana, 'The [official AIDS] message is read not as about a neutral scientific "fact" but as a rejection of morality and of culture. The government AIDS message then is seen as politically loaded; not promulgating a universal truth but a sectional Western (White) one.'[3] For most people, there is nothing that advantages science over other forms of explanation.

To repeat something that has already been said, but not accepted, is a futile exercise, however patient both sides are with each other. There is a (probably) apocryphal story circulating about a group of Western doctors and traditional healers who were brought together to reach an agreement over HIV/AIDS:

> Progress at the gathering was slow since both the medical doctors and traditional healers were sticking to their explanations of AIDS. Eventually, the facilitator hit on a compromise that allowed them to salvage something from the encounter and report that they had started a process of meaningful dialogue. She proposed to the gathering that they could agree that traditional healers do not have a scientifically proven cure for AIDS. The proposal is agreed in a flash! The Western doctors think they've won an important concession. The traditional healers are happy that the doctors are smiling, but can't work out why the agreement is such a big deal.

The healers' puzzlement is not surprising. Viewed from their perspective, their 'concession' was akin to the doctors conceding that Western medical treatment was not revealed to them in dreams.

Talking back

If the disputes over AIDS are multiple, responding to challenges to the medical explanation of AIDS can be difficult. But a response is better than talking over, past or through people. Peer educators, lay people given some AIDS education and asked to share this with workmates, friends and neighbours, are able to respond to these challenges; they're able to get to the point with their peers. There are caveats to this, but these aside, peer educators are on the frontline of AIDS education; they are discussing, chatting, talking and arguing with their peers about AIDS.

However, most peer educator programmes give little attention to the discourses between peers. Within vertically organised programmes of peer education, the peer educators' job is to get close to the target so that it can be hit with the experts' educational messages. The peer educator is a stalking horse behind which the expert hopes to get his or her weapons of education and persuasion close enough to score a direct hit. In this model of peer education, what the peer educator really thinks doesn't matter so long as they bring the experts' weapons into range. It's their socio-cultural proximity, shared language and idiomatic familiarity with the target group that are valuable. It's assumed that at close range the experts' explanations and advice will prevail. It's an assumption that doesn't hold in reality.

Rather, close-quarter encounters between peer educator and peers involve complex and contested dialogues. These discussions move away from the careful scripting conceived by experts. Such communication may well be messy. Indeed, peers may 'talk back' and counter the disseminated health promotion messages. The following example, recorded originally in isiZulu, by an African female peer educator during the Digco peer educator project, illustrates how horizontal communication can quickly move away from the propagation of experts' messages.

Here is something that I discovered … One man said he can see how this thing [HIV/AIDS] goes; it is just that White people don't see it. 'When a woman sleeps with a lot of different men,' [he said], 'it causes this [disease] because their blood is different; the blood groups mix but they are not the same.'

'That [the peer continued] is the reason when you are injured or when you have a blood transfusion, they don't just take any blood and put it in you, they start by checking what [blood] group you are, and then they give you your own blood group. So now [if you are] sleeping with a lot of people with different blood groups, those groups, when they mix, they form this disease, which White people end up saying is AIDS.'

Then I [the female peer educator] responded to him [by saying that] … 'My partner and I have different blood groups, but we've been in a relationship and we have a baby without any sickness involved.' He defended himself, saying, 'When you are with your partner and in love [and make love], even though you can have different [blood] groups, as time goes by your blood will change and become one [blood] group.' … I didn't say to him that I was confused, but I was confused as to how to answer him because whatever I said, he came up with his own opinions.

Understanding this interaction requires recognition that the arguments presented by the male peer synchronise traditional and allopathic understandings of blood. The initial argument put forward is that 'AIDS' is an old disease, belatedly mislabelled by Western doctors, that is generated from the mixing of blood, with semen being one form,[4] and not the transmission of a virus during sex. From here it is a short step to the idea that traditional healers can cure 'AIDS' since it is, in fact, an old disease, such as the isiZulu *uGunsula,* one of those identified by Dr Mosia's colleagues and for which cure falls within the competency of healers.

However, the man's argument does not pursue these details further but draws on an allopathic classification of blood groups which he uses to support the thesis that mixing blood is dangerous. In responding, the peer educator faced a difficult choice. She could have gone along with the peer's reasoning, which had preventive value, but would have been acknowledging an alternative explanation of the disease. Instead she attempts to counter his explanation with an argument drawn from her own life: how come she and her long-term partner are not sick even though they have different blood groups? The man trumps this decisively: sharing body fluids over time results in a couple's blood becoming one. This is, intellectually, a knockout blow given the widespread belief in this conception of blood within African communities.[5] The peer educator is stumped. Her attempts to counter the peer's arguments had quickly taken her away from what her training had equipped her for. It also went beyond what any expert could have anticipated such a discussion would lead to.

Peers don't always, of course, talk back. The information peer educators provide may well be welcomed. As one peer educator at Digco pointed out, 'It's easy when a person asks for help from you … Then you start explaining to them how you must go. Now they're listening because they're asking for help.' In such a situation, the peer elects to join the peer educator within a shared paradigm of biomedicine, at least for the duration of their conversation. Restrictions on communication are limited only to what is known and what can be explained. Such conversations provide a valuable alternative mode of delivery to posters, leaflets, TV and radio, but it's talking to those who choose to listen.

Responding to talk: hit and run, preaching and 'call an expert'

When it comes to HIV/AIDS, a focus on communicating the 'facts about AIDS' rules out the value of participatory communication.[6] The knowledge about HIV/AIDS has already been scientifically generated and now must be instilled in the population. There is no room allowed for adaptation in its adoption.[7]

But those on the ground have their own knowledge about AIDS; different knowledge from that generated by scientific inquiry. Peer educator programmes designed as diffusion models, therefore, become *de facto* participatory models if peer educators get 'stuck in' and do not limit themselves to preaching to the converted. But these are participatory processes that are contested. This is somewhat embarrassing; those who are to be saved disagree with the path of their salvation. Peer educators face resistance when they engage with peers.

Those responsible for managing peer educator programmes soon work out that engagement, beyond providing facts and advice to willing recipients, becomes difficult. However, they face a dilemma as to how they should guide peer educators given the complexity of these contested peer-to-peer discussions. One response attempted is to further train peer educators so that they can tackle anything that is thrown at them by peers regarding the science of HIV and AIDS. But there are limits to what is feasible. Even if training resources were unlimited, the problem cannot be solved this way. The worker with a PhD in peer education would be a reliable health promotion ally, but would no longer be a peer educator.

Peer educators sometimes feel they are expected to 'know it all'. Jo Frankham has noted how student peer educators expressed anxiety over how to maintain control within the interactions they had with peers. A common strategy in this regard was to 'try … to set themselves up as experts'.[8] The holding of formal education sessions limits the degree to which peers can object to the messages given to them by peer educators. Typically, formal HIV/AIDS education sessions within South African companies are held during work hours and within the work environment. Consequently, the peer educator is conferred a position of authority, something that limits challenges to what they say.[9] Informal interactions can be a very different matter; it's peer and peer, face to face, in their own environment.

Accepting the limits to which peer educator knowledge can be built and accepting that pretending to be an expert is not going to hold up outside a classroom-type session, the usual response of those managing peer educator programmes is to shore up weaknesses in the vertical model of peer education through one of three tactics: *hit and run*, *preaching*, and *call an expert*.

Peer educators are sometimes advised to employ hit and run tactics, though this moniker is not used. This approach, in which messages should be delivered as simply as possible and tricky engagement avoided, represents vertical communication at its most straightforward. Some peer educators at Digco concurred in their desire to keep things simple. Thus, one Digco peer educator, while understanding that the presence of sores in the genital area increased the likelihood of HIV infection, thought it best not to raise this: 'most of the time when I educate people I just tell them to use condoms. If I start telling them that if you're making love without a condom and you don't have cuts [sores] you won't get HIV, then people would go around sleeping around without condoms.' However, in general, peer educators acknowledged that if a peer had a question, refusing to respond would compromise meaningful discussion.

Some Digco peer educators modelled their activity on the easily accessible model of the *moruti* (preacher), which meant avoiding having to answer too many questions. The delivery of long, often highly fluent monologues that link together information on HIV/AIDS and values over behaviour, provides neither time nor purchase for any disagreement. Such preaching was most easily resorted to when peer educators were given an opportunity to present formally to peers, or if invited to talk to a youth, church or other group. However, it also takes place during informal peer educator activity.[10] In effect, the peer educator is 'clunking' (linking together) various messages drawn from their training and delivering this in a style that draws on the sermons they listen to and sometimes give in their churches.[11] This behaviour was evident in the Digco project workshops, indicating that it had previously been acceptable in peer educator meetings, presumably because it was an extended and articulate repetition of expert-provided information and messages. Preaching prevents problems from surfacing since the length and fluidity of delivery discourage engagement. When challenged in the project workshops, the peer educators agreed that such an approach did little if anything to engage peers who had doubts, questions or contrary opinions.[12] Once this point had been established, whenever a peer educator started 'preaching' during a workshop, he or she would be challenged by others. This allowed discussion to return to the point under debate. Indeed, on a couple of occasions, the peer educators self-consciously stopped themselves as they started to 'warm up' into preaching mode.

Another procedure suggested by programme coordinators to circumvent the problem of peer challenges was for them to avoid answering if they were unsure of their ground, and rather tell the peer that they would ask a health professional and get back with the answer. This obviously maintains the vertical nature of communication, with the peer educator acting as conduit by passively transferring information. The value of such 'call an expert' tactics depends on context. Where a peer approaches a peer educator and is seeking information, this approach can be valuable.[13] However, if there is contestation, then this approach is effectively admitting defeat. Referring to a health professional is likely to be interpreted as going back for instructions from the proponents of a competing worldview.

In different ways these three approaches contributed to the maintenance of vertically organised peer education. Whether they succeed in challenging the views on the ground is a different matter. This back-pedalling from uncomfortable backchat achieves only one thing: a sweeping of the problem under the carpet.

Not so easy as ABC

Peer educators have to grapple with tricky situations with only a cobbled together understanding of the science of AIDS. The simplified ABC (Abstain, Be faithful, Condomise) messages that are condensed out of this body of science and which they are expected to punt, leaves much unexplained. However, what I did not anticipate was the complexity of addressing these gaps. This became apparent as the project progressed.

On a regular basis, the peer educators would recount things they had heard, along with a request for me to clarify whether it was an AIDS myth or, in fact, true. They wanted to know. Since the project's objectives included building peer educators' capacity, I threw these enquiries open. I started this process confidently, assuming that in clarifying issues, and getting us all onto the same page over what was myth and what was not, would assist us to design stories that would counter AIDS myths, the ultimate objective of the project.

Initially, this was successful. One of the first reported AIDS myths that we discussed was, 'If there is no blood on a person's genitals then it is safe to have sex.'[14] This was quickly clarified as not being true and one of the projects' most popular parables, *Tibbos*, was developed:

> Tibbos cycles to see his girlfriend. He comes off his bike and hits his head. He picks himself up and finds that he is not bleeding and carries on. Later in the evening he starts to get a headache, but ignores this as he is enjoying himself too much. In the morning, he is rushed to hospital unconscious, but dies before he can be helped.

The message of *Tibbos* was easy to grasp: appearances can be dangerously deceptive, including the absence of blood. It addressed the myth of sex being safe if there was no blood present, without the need to resort to a scientific explanation of how HIV can be transmitted by other bodily fluids and/or the different risks associated with these fluids. This was what I hoped the project might achieve. We would be able to cut and cauterise each head of the AIDS hydra, just as Hercules and Iolaus, working together, had finally vanquished the Lernaean Hydra in Greek mythology.

My optimism was short-lived. At the next workshop, a peer educator raised the perennial question of whether it was possible for HIV to be transmitted through kissing. As I stood in front of the whiteboard, marker pen in hand, I assumed we were going to build on our previous success – I would facilitate clarity over risks of kissing and the peer educators would, if we thought it was necessary, come up with a story to get the message across. But, as I started to talk, I realised that we were now moving towards a message that was contradictory to that of *Tibbos*. When it came to kissing it *was* safe, unless there was blood or sores in the mouth. The first message, encapsulated in the *Tibbos* story, now started to become convoluted. No blood on the genitals doesn't mean it's safe, but no blood in the mouth means it is safe. Without greater biological knowledge, this is something that looks and sounds contradictory and a difficult message to convey with clear logic, however clever the packaging.[15]

Other areas of HIV transmission that were tricky and difficult to simplify emerged during the project. These included mother-to-child transmission, discordant couples where one partner remained negative despite regular sex, and seminal fluid containing the HIV virus, but not sperm itself. Within a scientific paradigm, these different messages can be accommodated within a single, coherent framework, but even the best AIDS educationalists would likely find these areas difficult to explain convincingly to an audience with limited scientific knowledge.

Many communication forms used for health promotion separate the message proponents and intended recipients. They do not know each other. It is different with peer educators and the peers with whom they talk. Peer educators, unlike distant educationalists, can be directly challenged. A not infrequent assumption or accusation by peers is that peer educators must themselves be HIV positive.[16] This assumption can lead to accusations over their own behaviour. One of the peer educators described how she became discouraged when Digco peer educators were accused of 'attending the workshop or whatever, but you're sleeping with each other'. This forced her onto the defensive, having to explain that 'real peer educators' were disciplined in their behaviour. Another peer educator who was visibly pregnant explained that she had been challenged and felt she had to explain that she had planned her pregnancy with her partner. In other cases, peer educators had histories of multiple partners and this was well known to peers. Such knowledge affected their ability to convincingly role-model behavioural messages.

In the face of alternative explanations of AIDS, peer educators faced a much more difficult task than simply finding a way of explaining the science of HIV/AIDS in the vernacular. They were in competition with alternative explanations of the disease. Below, a Digco peer educator explains how those who don't want to accept they are HIV-positive, can draw on alternatives explanations to shift concern:

> The person that's giving you some questions. You answer the question, then they start coming with other excuses, they've got lots of excuses. When you talk about this thing [HIV/AIDS] ... [They say,] 'No, it's just that I'm sick, not that I'm HIV-positive. No, not HIV.' ... Then you hear people to say, 'No, I don't believe in this White [i.e. Western] medicine.' ... Sometimes you get confused because there are people who say they don't use it, even injection. Or tablets, they say tablets they don't use in their life, they've never used it. But you see that person is sick, you can see. They say, 'No, I'll see my *nyanga* (traditional healer) or someone else. He'll get rid of it, he knows it.' [So] I don't know [what to do next].

A number of peer educators felt that it was necessary to acknowledge the difficulties of the ABC prevention message. Those who put this forward were arguing that the messages that they were being asked to disseminate, did not correspond to the life experiences of peers. This was particularly noticeable around the experience of sex, which prevention messages tend to mechanicalise. For example, the reduction of sexual pleasure and intimacy with condom use is rarely addressed in health promotion messages. Even well-intentioned activists can struggle to consistently use condoms. The Digco peer educators defended condoms. But some pointed out that if they were to explain why condoms were necessary, it needed to be acknowledged that they can intrude on the spontaneity, creativity and pleasure of sex. To be unwilling to do this undermined their credibility as educators. Similarly, the message of partner reduction did not take into account than many people found other potential partners sexually attractive. While peer educators agreed that partner reduction was necessary, not to acknowledge that men and women were sexually attracted to each other was nonsense.[17] Delivering a message of partner reduction, however correct, would not be credible without acknowledging the challenges this represented, challenges that their peers were well aware of.

Whether we like it or not

Peer education is frequently added to the list of interventions recommended for HIV/AIDS campaigns or programmes. Less common is empirical-based analysis of what peer education involves, despite regular calls for evaluations of its effectiveness. The value of horizontal communication in changing beliefs and behaviour around HIV and AIDS is rarely recognised, and we really understand little of what goes on within such communication between peers around HIV/AIDS.[18]

Drawing on the Digco research project, we can see some of the difficulties that working-class African peer educators face when engaging with their peers about HIV/AIDS. In seeing how messages conveyed to peer educators for onward transmission can become entangled in difficult, incomplete and indecisive discourses, or even downright rejection, it may be tempting to drop peer education and focus on more tractable interventions that engage the target audiences from a greater distance. Doing so, however, would also cut off one of the few ways in which we can gauge just what does happen to health education messages within the audiences that we target. This is a problem because conversations about AIDS will happen within target audiences and away from expert scrutiny, whether we have peer educators to tell us about them or not.

Returning from a funeral in South Park Cemetery[19] with my friend Thabiso and four local *batjha* (youth) crowded in the back seat of the car in early 2009, I was party to one such conversation that was a minute fragment of the constant talk of the townships. Having buried one of Thabiso's cousins, we were heading back *habo* (to the home of) the deceased. Initially, the mood was sombre. There had been a frank conversation in the car during which we had said what nobody had said at the graveside: that the 32-year-old man we had just buried had 'obviously' died of AIDS.

But the mood lightened as we drove from the graveyard back to the township with its bustling familiarity. A woman in the street turned all heads in the crowded car. From the back seat where the *batjha* were crowded, there was a joke about all six of us thinking the same thing. Thabiso light-heartedly suggested that he or I should take first option in striking an acquaintance (in the encounter we were collectively imagining). Although he was not saying it, Thabiso was pointing to our age seniority. We were all laughing. We were having fun. The woman was out of sight and the funeral out of mind.

Thabiso continued, only now he was making a point as he grasped what educationalists term a 'teachable moment' – a situation where a message will strike home if delivered deftly. But his message was hardly what health educationalists in the era of AIDS would approve. He explained how a man needs to 'look outside' on occasions. A wife, he said, can provide many things, but she will not satisfy every need. Men must help themselves to meet these needs. We were still jovial, but there was now a slight tension. The five men in the car with me knew I couldn't agree with what Thabiso was saying; they knew I was writing a book on AIDS and they knew well enough the messages of the AIDS establishment. But Thabiso justified his message: it's 'the African way', he said. I was hardly in a position to challenge him and focused instead on the road.

Later, I realised that this wasn't just an abstract lesson on his take on African culture that I'd been given. When the two of us were alone, he told me that he'd arranged to meet up with a woman he'd met in a taxi the previous week. He took it for granted that I wouldn't tell Mpuse, his wife, but when he saw that I was troubled by the prospect of having to lie, he laid it on thick as to how he didn't want his family hurt. *Ke a bapala* (I'm just playing) he told me, his liaison was to be our *sephiri* (secret). He was inducting me into his 'African way', which he knew was not approved in the world I represented but which I needed to understand if I was to share his world. He went on to tell me about the arrangements that would keep Mpuse unaware. Then he mollified me by telling me he would be careful. He said that he would wear a condom; it was too dangerous to do otherwise nowadays, he told me, 'AIDS is everywhere'.

Whether Thabiso did use condoms with this *nyatsi* (girlfriend) is something only the two of them know. Since the fling didn't last long, it's possible. But condoms don't stay on indefinitely, as Saki had already told me. So did Kabelo and Bernard, residents of Potlakong, when I 'bust' Kabelo over his *dinyatsi* (girlfriends) a couple of years after Thabiso had explained the 'African way' to me.

Three plus one

I bust Kabelo in the sense that I opened up a discussion on how he managed the risk of HIV/AIDS, given that he regularly had more than one *nyatsi* or 'spare' alongside his 'main' girlfriend or *kgarebe*. I did not bust him in the sense of calling him out over the risks that he was taking. When this encounter took place I was more concerned with finding out what people really thought than in diligently relaying public health messages. One afternoon Kabelo was holding court with some of my Potlakong friends in the shade of a tree. Kabelo had stayed in the neighbourhood for a few years, renting a room from his friend Bernard. Kabelo had trained as an industrial electrician and was now employed by Eskom, the government parastatal electricity company in South Africa. He was bringing home more than most Potlakong residents and he was not yet married. When he wasn't working he was busy, either with his girlfriends or with friends whom he helped unite with beers and the prospect of heading over to Zanele's Buy & Braai for *pap 'n vleis* (maize starch and grilled meat). Kabelo and Bernard had known each other since school and they maintained a friendly rivalry over who was top dog.

The week before, I'd mistaken Thandeka, one of Kabelo's *dinyatsi*, for Mafaleng, his *kgarebe*. The incident had been minor, his *nyatsi* was well aware of Mafaleng's status, so my social blunder had revealed nothing that was not already known to those present. But now, a week later and among male company, I was being teased over my mistake. So I hit back, '*Hobaneng o na le basadi ba bang?*' (Why have you got other women?), I asked directly.

My question was received with laughter by the group. It was a legitimate response in this teasing session as we were passing the time. I was entitled to defend myself with a counter-attack and Kabelo had to respond. He also needed to respond in a way that would maintain his status within this group. Kabelo was one of the organic intellectuals of the street, and several times I'd seen him give authoritative accounts of issues ranging from strikes to global warming. He had no problem in responding. My question had put the ball in his court, but he was hardly uncomfortable. In this group, having 'spares' was a status symbol. Kabelo used the opening to explain some things. First he provided context, telling us, after a moment's thought, that, currently, he had three girlfriends as well as Mafaleng.

Bernard jumped in and explained, for my benefit, that Kabelo used condoms with these three, but not with Mafaleng, and then he cracked up laughing. Finally he managed to pull himself together and sum up the contradiction of fidelity and this fluid, modern and urban form of polygamy as 'Three Plus One!'[20] Kabelo was tipsy but on the ball and determined to upstage Bernard. Three Plus One it might be, but the idea of keeping condoms on with the three 'spares' wasn't feasible, he told us.

He began by denouncing AIDS education messages, telling his audience that people can't be expected to keep using a condom. He picked up on the language of the AIDS ads that self-consciously attempt to speak directly, yet are constrained by the need for respectability and correctness. 'No,' he insisted, they have to say 'fuck' when they're talking about people fucking. He dominated the discussion and was speaking with an intensity that took me by surprise. As he waved out into the street, I thought that maybe he was pointing out a billboard that had just been erected, or perhaps an advert on the side of a passing taxi. But he was waving in the general direction of 'out there', beyond the shade and our discussion, to the sea of AIDS education which, despite bright colours and glossy presentation, speaks in unrealistic monotone.

He was not denying AIDS. He told us that he's been tested and from the way he told us about his certificate he was telling us that he was negative. But he was not going to keep wearing condoms. He conducted his own tests with his 'spares'; he 'checked' and after a few days could tell if they were 'clean'. Then the condom came off. He made a flicking motion to show the condom being flung onto the floor.

Bernard now got back into the discussion. He suggested it takes longer than a few days before you know if a woman is clean. Bernard played it safe, waiting a month before ditching condoms. There was laughter at the different quarantine periods recommended by Kabelo and Bernard. The point, Bernard stated, conceding that he wasn't coming out as top dog in this competition, was that one had to take precautions, AIDS is everywhere. You can't see it, but it is everywhere.

Kabelo again seized the floor. He agreed with Bernard that AIDS is everywhere, but not everyone had AIDS. It's about, he said, 'friction'. To avoid infection you need to avoid the friction that can *tabola methapo ya madi* (tear blood vessels or capillaries). He was providing the context to his explanation by using the index finger of his left hand to vigorously and repeatedly insert into a ring created by the thumb and forefinger of his right hand. We got the picture. I clocked immediately what he was saying; this was 'friction theory', which I'd heard before in the Digco project.[21] However, he had to elaborate before everybody got the point. I guessed that he'd picked this up in an HIV/AIDS education talk, probably through a workplace programme. But Kabelo now worked the material further than what would be said in any education session. He must have been thinking about it, because he went on, talking about why foreplay is a good thing – if the woman is aroused, there is less friction.[22] He was outlining a lay theory of AIDS transition and an alternative prevention message: ensure you partner is sexually aroused if you want to avoid infection. The audience was all ears. Kabelo was clearly enjoying himself. Bernard could not match this and I suspected that he was now taking mental notes so that he could hold court at another opportunity and with another audience. What Kabelo was saying made sense. He was not just talking, he was one with three 'spares' and a negative HIV test result.

Peer educators, peer discourse and peer power

Alternative explanations of HIV/AIDS are rooted in widespread beliefs and they are not without benefit. This chapter has drawn out the inevitable conflict with biomedicine's health promotion messages. There are various ways in which this conflict can proceed. However, we cannot expect this conflict to be conducted within any one set of rules, since the competing explanations are drawn from different paradigms. We should also recognise that this conflict isn't taking place in the open. The difficulties faced by peer educators when peers talk back provide us with a window into this conflict.

This conflict can be a source of exasperation when peer educators report defeat and confusion. Peer educators are not infallible sources of information and their limits can be tested when peers answer back with their own ideas about AIDS. To then write off peer education because of this amounts, however, to shooting the messenger.

Kabelo, Bernard and Thabiso are just three of the many organic intellectuals, individuals who influence those around them, in the township. They speak on AIDS, just as they would speak on crime, or getting a job, or why the township is plagued with rats. They are more numerous than any army of trained peer educators we can field. Yet they are not the enemy. They are the target audience we should be trying to reach, yet we know little of what they believe.

Despite the value of seeing AIDS myths conceptualised as auxiliary theories to the core ideas that lie at the heart of folk and lay theories of AIDS, I remained troubled as to whether the AIDS myths that the peer educators collected were really the beliefs that residents of African townships used. I was not in any doubt that peer educators constituted a better way to find out which AIDS myths were present rather than conducting a survey, but there is still a considerable gap between knowing that an idea is circulating in a community and knowing that it is being put into practice. After all, talk is cheap.

In the chapters that follow I describe my conversations with township residents for whom AIDS was salient. Folk and lay theories of AIDS applied to everyday necessities ensure their salience. For somebody who is HIV positive or is close to an HIV-positive person, there is little point in entertaining idle speculation over possible causes and cures. Rather, the competing theories of AIDS will be weighed carefully and used judiciously.

PART II

Constructing AIDS in the Kasi

5

The kasi

South African townships

In South Africa a township is, legally, a proclaimed residential area. So, squatters aside, everybody in South Africa's urban settlements lives in a township. But townships in South Africa were for many years racially segregated by law into the four racial categories of Apartheid: African, Coloured, Indian and White. Black townships – those of Africans, Coloureds and Indians – retained the appellation of township, or location, or *kasi*. Whites lived in 'town' and in larger urban areas in the suburbs. Each town had one or more township, sometimes separated by considerable distances, sometimes by an industrial estate, sometimes by a valley or a river, and sometimes by little more than a road or a railway line or strip of open land. But always separate. They still are.

The people of South African townships are all but invisible. With the exception of Soweto, even the names of most townships are unknown. More often than not, the name of the town serves well enough. Bethlehem, for example, is a small Free State town (through which runs the river Jordan). It features on the nightly TV weather bulletins, often with shudderingly cold winter lows. Asking for directions to Bethlehem is straightforward enough, people have a sense of where it is, if only that it is in the Free State (and that it can get very cold there in winter). But if you asked the best route to Bohlokong, Bethlehem's township separated by only a few industrial buildings and a strip of open land, you'll most likely draw a blank stare, unless you happen to ask somebody who hails from the area.

Yet, the population of Bethlehem, in 2011, was approximately 14 000, and the population of Bohlokong some 60 000. Bohlokong's obscurity is because of who is living there. Ninety-nine per cent of the township's population is African. Sixty-four per cent of the town's population is White.[1] In truth, townships are unknown because their inhabitants are invisible. Other than for statistical purposes or research projects, township residents only become important when they are not in the township but working in the kitchens, gardens, factories and mines of the visible South Africa. Soweto excepted, because of its status in the South African narrative of freedom, townships are necessary only for the labour they house, not the people that live in them.

If the names of the townships are unknown, even more so are the names of their streets. Passing a Free State town, your GPS will show the name of every street of the quiet *dorp* (small town) that is good for petrol, groceries, a couple of national retailers selling clothes or furniture, hardware and a bottlestore. But it will not display one street name in the nearby township. If you had reason to enter a township (though it would not be for petrol, groceries, clothes or hardware), you would have to stop and ask. If you were a first-time visitor, you would probably struggle. It is not the street name that is really important in tracking down an address. What is first required is the name of the township section[2] where your host lives. Once you're in their section, you need to ask again, giving the house number. Hopefully, you will happen upon a local person who is familiar with the way the sequencing of house numbers start, break and *qhoma* (jump) in the section. In fact, you might well be better off abandoning house numbers altogether and using local landmarks, whether a school, *spaza* shop, tavern or church.

Of course, this invisibility and impenetrability apply only to those who live outside the township. Those who live in the location are well aware of where they live. In contrast to those outside the *kasi*, they are also likely to have a fair idea about life in town and even in the suburbs. Somebody in the family is likely to be working *kitjhining* (domestic work), as a 'garden boy'[3] or in a company. And they also go into town to shop for groceries, clothes, furniture, building material ... but not beer.

●

So nobody needs to describe township life for those who live in the township, but it is necessary to describe township life for those who don't live in one. Hence this chapter. By and large, people who live in the *kasi* are not into reading chapters in books. Not much beyond *The Daily Sun* and *Sowetan*[4] newspapers get read in the *kasi*. One of the indignant questions raised in the aftermath of 'service delivery' riots is: 'Why on earth did they torch the library?' Burning down a public building that gives access to knowledge is, for those living outside the *kasi*, particularly senseless destruction and perhaps even greater folly than burning down schools. Such attitudes underscore some of the differences and divisions of South Africa. Other than children, who still dream that things will be different and are willing to put up with having their hands inspected for dirt before they are allowed into the library, most people living in the township don't revere books. Those who did well at school, and who washed their hands before going to the library, mostly leave the location for town or suburb. Children and potential Black Diamonds (marketing speak for the emerging Black middle class) aside, township residents know that books are of no benefit to them.

Apartheid's educational policies systematically undermined learning for Blacks. That is changing, even if with frustrating slowness in the townships. Thirty-five per cent of Bethlehem's population is Black. Twenty per cent is African. African Born Frees (those born after the 1994 advent of democracy) who have attended former Model C (semi-private) schools in towns or suburbs can, irrespective of their race, be as clueless about township life as any White suburban resident who has yet to visit Soweto. As Jane Duncan[5] has argued when critiquing media coverage of social issues, 'South Africa has become a society that is unable to see itself accurately.' The following account of South African townships is based largely on my own experiences and aims to contextualise the accounts that follow for readers who may not know the *kasi*. We begin with a not untypical Saturday afternoon in Potlakong.[6]

Potlakong Township, Gauteng, January 2012

It is quiet as I drive into the *kasi* at midday. It is hot. To the south of the township, thunder clouds are building, but it will not rain till evening. In the shade of a single Syringa tree, half a dozen young men are idling in the dusty front yard of a house. There are two open quart bottles[7] of beer on the ground between them. One of young men is crushing *zol* (cannabis) that will be rolled in paper ripped from a telephone directory. The mood is subdued. They talk without the usual teasing, jipping and blagging. It is not the heat that is pacifying them. It is the second weekend of January and 'Christmas', the month-long, South African mid-summer holiday, is almost over. They are *tjhonne* (broke). Practically everybody in the township is *tjhonne* right now. And if you're not, you certainly aren't going to let on.

I park my car and greet my *tjhonne* friends who hang out together here most Saturday afternoons. Matsoso has returned from the small township of Butleng in the Free State only yesterday. He will be back at work on Monday. Butleng is his *lehae* – his real home where he hails from and where he intends eventually to return. There is no work in Butleng and he came to Potlakong a few years ago. He was able to find work in Rossville, one of several industrial estates close to Potlakong. He is lucky to be employed, but not that lucky, as the factory operates a three-shift system and he is about to kick the year off with a week on nights. Matsoso shrugs his shoulders. There is nothing he can do about it. At least as he is a permanent employee the unions have negotiated a shift allowance. Saki, another of my *tjhonne* friends, is employed by a labour broker. His contract has been renewed annually for the last seven years, but he can never be sure if this will happen and he remains a second-class citizen when it comes to employment. But he's lucky compared to Boithumelo who hasn't worked since he dropped out of school in Grade 11, the penultimate year of schooling, six years ago. He talks about studying tourism at a college in town. It's a new year and he's about to be abandoned to the long, empty weekdays of the *kasi*. He wants to make something happen in his life.

This afternoon, I'm visiting Andries in Section 7 in the south of Potlakong where he now stays with his girlfriend, Busi. When I first

problem is and I initially think that he is asking for advice. We set off as a small party: Andries, Busi, Selina and myself, along the dirt streets and narrow passages of Section 7 to reach a tiny brick house where Selina is staying. A rickety set of armchairs are crammed into one small room, which also serves as a kitchen. There are two bedrooms and an outside toilet. The house is full of women and children. If there are men, they are not present when we visit. I squeeze past a low table to reach one of the chairs and am about to sit down when there are squeals of warning. Suspended over the chair, I realise that it is broken and I'll end up on the floor. I move over and sit in the chair indicated for me.

The child whom we have come to see, Lebohile, is asleep in one of the bedrooms. There are howls as she is awoken and explanations that they need to change her Pampers.[10] Finally, she is brought out. She is three years old, but small, and clearly there is something wrong: her eyes roll and she hardly responds, despite the fuss made over her. Handed over to me, her protests subside as she returns to sleep in my arms. Selina explains how at first she had thought the child was just slow, then realised that something was wrong. The hospital referral letter went straight to the point: the child has cerebral palsy. I say that it's a serious and permanent disability. I'm not sure of what further value I can be, but soon realise that I'm not being asked for help. Selina is on top of the situation. She shows me a list of special schools from which she will choose one that Lebohile will attend. She also shows me her notes from the class where she is being taught how to care for Lebohile who, she explains, is a gift from God whom she loves.

We all praise Selina for being so open about the child's disability and point out that families used to hide disabled children away. It's a warming narrative and I see that the visit is an opportunity for Selina to tell, to a new audience, that her situation is a blessing not a burden, especially since she is receiving the child dependency grant which pays four times the normal child benefit rate of R270 a month.[11] At least for the moment, this small child is an economic asset; it's a happy synergy of love and money. I marvel at how, among the endemic inefficiency and corruption that are the hallmarks of the South African state, the social services system is deftly picking up the unlucky lot that life has dealt Lebohile.

On a string around Lebohile's neck is the almost translucent jaw bone of a small mammal. The sharp milky-white canine tooth indicates that it's from a predator. It's a traditional charm and, as our visit winds down, I ask whether it's from a cat. Selina makes light of the question and says that it's from a wild animal but doesn't know which. She's suggesting that the issue be dropped, but I push a little further and ask for confirmation that it's *ntho ya setso* (a thing of tradition). Selina confirms it is. There is slight tension. I only met Selina half an hour ago and I'm intruding beyond the role that I was invited to play. It is easy for us – with our different backgrounds – to agree that a child with cerebral palsy is a gift from God, but beyond a few cultural tropes, little about *ditsela tsa setso* (traditional ways) is shared between Africans and Whites. I know I've overstepped the mark and that I cannot go further for the moment. I will pick up the conversation next time; there will be much more to this *ntho ya setso* than a feline jaw bone. But now, Selina stands up to take the child from me and tells me in English, even though we have been talking in a mixture of Sesotho and Sepedi, 'I believe in both sides.' By this she means that she uses what Western doctors and social services offer, as well as what is prescribed by a traditional healer.

Andries and I take a stroll back to see his new neighbourhood. He stops to buy 'loose draw', a single cigarette, from a small *spaza* shop[12] for *ponto* or R2.[13] Close to home, he introduces me to a neighbour working on a car in the street. When the man stands up he is huge, his oily blue overalls are open and his chest exposed. He speaks in isiZulu and refuses to switch into Sesotho for me, though he clearly understands me. There is laughter as I have to guess what it is he is saying. It's light-hearted, but illustrates ethnic divisions – Zulus are notorious for refusing to speak other African languages. When we get back to the *mosebetsi,* Saki has finished his beer and is ready to go.

By the time we arrive back, it is almost three and we haven't eaten. The food at the *mosebetsi* was finished. Busi had apologised on behalf of her neighbour. '*Hase bothata,*' (Not a problem), we said, 'next time'.

I park the car in the shade of the Syringa tree and we walk the two blocks to Kally's, one of many outlets selling *dikota*, the ubiquitous fast food of the township: a quarter loaf stuffed with chips, plenty of salt, spices, tomato sauce and, depending on your pocket, slices of processed cheese, fried eggs, fried French (polony), fried Vienna (frankfurter), fried Special (garlic-flavoured polony) or fried Russian sausage. Or, should you be really hungry, all of the above! I buy two at R11, for which we get chips, cheese and half a Russian packed into the bread, along with long-tom Cokes.[14] Siting at the metal table in the shade of a rundown veranda at the front of Kally's, we eat the solid, greasy, filling food passed through metal bars to us.

As we are eating, a burly woman in her 30s arrives. Her belly protrudes from between her jeans and the tight top she is wearing. She puts a loaf of bread on our table while she is waiting for her order of chips. She kills the time by asking me where I'm from. I tell her I'm from Jo'burg. She says she is from Frankfort, a small *dorp* (town) in the Free State, though from her Sekasi-heavy language and her manners, Saki and I later concur that she must have been in Gauteng for some time. She turns to Saki and wants to know how old he is and how many children he has. She is looking for a boyfriend and says as much. Saki never misses a chance to greet single women. But right now he's offended; he doesn't think women should be so direct. He says he's 24 and he's got four children; he wants to get rid of her. But it only makes things worse and the interaction degenerates as she ripostes in ribald language, '*O rata kuku baholo!*' (You like pussy a lot!). Riled, he's equally vulgar: '*Ka baka la basadi ba bulang*' (Because of women who open [their legs]). And he's not finished: '*Ke hobane re a kula*' (It's the reason we are sick). He's as good as told her that she's a slut and HIV positive. I'm relieved when there is a shout that her chips are ready. But Saki's insults are water off a duck's back. She returns to the table with her chips and asks for a drink of Coke. We refuse directly, not even bothering to make an excuse, and she leaves.

In fact, Saki is 27 and has no children. Until recently, he's not had a steady girlfriend, though plenty of women have come and gone. A few months ago, the fact that he never fails to greet women paid off when Thandi, fresh from KwaZulu-Natal, welcomed his attention. Now they're an item, though that doesn't stop Saki 'visiting' here and there when she's away or out of sight. But, he insists, he always uses condoms when he's not with Thandi. Maybe. For years Saki told me he used condoms. He had seen his sister die and he didn't want to go the same way. Then one day he'd told me that sometimes he wakes in the night worrying that he's been infected. He prefaced this new version with, '*Ho bua nnete* ...' (To tell the truth ...). The truth was that after he'd been with a girl a few times and had seen that she keeps herself clean, and after the pillow talk when she told him that she's been careful with previous boyfriends, or that there hadn't been many of them, then the condoms were forgotten. He's sure that he can judge. It's just that sometimes alone in the dark he doubts himself.

Walking back to the car we bump into a friend, Nkosinathi. He tells me that he's doing okay, but not really. He's got a *sekoropo* (piece job) laying pavements, only now the taxi fares take up R40 of the R120 that he earns each day. Nkosinathi works only intermittently. He supplements this income with a lodger in the spare bedroom and two *mokhukhu* in the backyard. The rent for these is R200 a month, including electricity, though that costs Nkosinathi nothing. He was cut off long ago, but soon found somebody to rig an illegal connection. Potlakong is full of such connections and on winter evenings, as cooking starts and heaters are switched on, the overloaded system often trips, plunging sections of the township into darkness.

By half past five I'm on the road and leave the township behind me. I will be home in time to walk the dog. This is how I spend most Saturday afternoons and I've got used to seeing things differently in the two worlds that I move between in a 45-minute drive. In my modest suburban street, in Westdene, Johannesburg, there's a guard keeping watch over the cars parked outside a neighbour's house. They are having a *braai* (barbeque). I can hear the chatter and smell charcoal smoke. The dog jumps enthusiastically into the back of the car and we head to the nearby park with its lake, (almost) litter-free grass slopes and trees. While the dog runs off the lead and the sun starts to set, I reflect on the afternoon in Potlakong.

'Deep hanging out'[15] with people in contexts different from our own, over an extended period of time, helps us to see the complexities of people's lives and avoid fragmenting this into artificially distinct components.[16] Only if we grasp their holistic life experience can we see their 'culture'. The term culture has been interpreted in multiple ways, often controversially. Within the African AIDS epidemic, the role of culture has been particularly touchy. Early writings appeared to lay the blame for rapid HIV transmission on particular 'African cultural practices' (such as polygamy or dry sex). This was not particularly helpful. As Quentin Gausset[17] has outlined, different practices, whether part of African or Western culture, can hasten the spread of AIDS.[18] The point, Gausset argued, is not to take sides in a fight between cultures, but to promote safer sexual practices that are culturally acceptable. At a high level of abstraction, in which we conceive of two competing cultures, African and Western, this is a valuable point, but it is less clear how helpful it is at the local level, such as South African townships. Here there is a kaleidoscope of competing cultural influences that are in plain sight during an afternoon's visit, provided you have been hanging out long enough to know what things mean.

It has been argued that the very idea of culture is unhelpful in explaining HIV. Eirick Saethre and Jonathan Stadler,[19] drawing on the perspectives of township residents in Orange Farm, Gauteng, have suggested that decisions about sexual behaviour are not about cultural values, but individual agency. They cite Orange Farm residents locating 'culture' away from their townships and, rather, in the 'rural areas' and historical past. I have sympathy with Saethre and Stadler, but disagree. Dotted around South Africa are 'cultural villages' that present themselves as the repository of traditional African cultures,[20] and on occasion friends in Potlakong and Butleng have suggested we visit. I respond that we are, as we talk, in a cultural village which we don't have to pay an entrance fee to visit. Rather, if they want to see a culture different from their own, they should visit me in my Jo'burg suburb (even if much of what goes down is hidden behind high walls). The point I'm trying to make is that culture is what we do, not what we try to preserve, whether in assigned 'cultural villages' or in imagined spaces that are far away or happened long ago. What is undeniable is that life in my suburb is different from that in the townships of Potlakong or Butleng, and if we want to understand anything – anything – we need to know the context.

I describe township culture, as a lived experience, in the sections that follow: movement, rhythms, church, tavern and values, wealth and status, living cheek by jowl, relationships, and, finally, my notion of the extended township.

Movement

To talk of a township's population paints only a still-life picture with people frozen into place. Thus, the statement 'The population of Bohlokong is some 60 000' is true enough within the confidence intervals of the census, but people are always on the move. The 2011 Census captures the historical migration of people across provincial boundaries. We know that of Gauteng's population of 12.2 million, more than four million people were born in another South African province, and more than one million came from beyond the borders of South Africa. Almost 380 000 of Gauteng's internal immigrants come from the Free State, which has a population of just less than three million.

People move. But there is much more to people's movement than migrating to a province or country different from one's birth. People are constantly in transit in ways that may not be picked up by census questions. Matsoso, one of my *tjhonne* friends, is one of those 380 000 born in the Free State but now resident in Gauteng. But his regular journeys between Butleng and Potlakong are not captured in statistics. Nor can the statistic tell us whether he will eventually return to Butleng, as he plans, or whether he will settle in Gauteng. How Matsoso came to Potlakong is a story in itself. A story that is far from over and has yet to fully play out ... he has a child in Butleng and a girlfriend in Potlakong.

Work in Butleng is limited to government posts and seasonal work on nearby farms. If there was work in Butleng, Matsoso would have stayed. He looks forward to his visits home. The journey from

Potlakong takes a few hours by car, but by taxi it can take much of the day. Driving into Butleng with Matsoso at the beginning of a long weekend entails spotting what is new and what has changed since our last visit. When the phone company Vodacom[21] changed its corporate colours from blue to red, its public phone outlet in Butleng, housed in a shipping container on the corner of one of the few tarred roads, was rebranded. For years it had been referred to as the 'container *e blue*', a township landmark distinct from the 'container *e tshehla*' (the yellow container). The two rival public phone services had become navigational aids in the location. Now, we laughed over what we were supposed to call the container, *e* blue, which was now *kgubedu* (red).

For those, like Matsoso's girlfriend who stay behind in Butleng, Gauteng is a faraway place about which they know little. Gauteng is the place of gold, the place where people go for money. It is not uncommon to talk to women in Butleng who do not know what work their fathers did there, or what their boyfriends or their husbands now do in Gauteng. They go for work, but it is not the work that is important. It is the money. In Butleng, there is often vagueness about the details of what happens in Gauteng. The connection boils down to the *moputso* (wage) that is paid and the remittances that it allows. From this it can be a small step to seeing distant menfolk staying in Gauteng as *motjhini wa tjhelete* (money machines) or ATMs (Automated Teller Machines) whose purpose shrinks to what they are able and willing to provide and on which their worth is gauged. Of course, it is not only the young men of Butleng who look for work. Women also travel to Gauteng looking for work *kitjhining* or *femeng* (domestic or factory work), but still more men than women uproot in this way.

Butleng provides a reservoir of young men and women who know that there is more opportunity for them elsewhere, and who sooner or later gather up the courage to leave, but who nearly always keep the option of return open. Potlakong absorbs young people looking for work, and spits back to Butleng those who can no longer labour. This skews the profile of those who reside in the large urban townships that ring Johannesburg and those who stay in small provincial townships like Butleng. That profile is further differentiated with parents sending children to live with grandparents and *bala* (study) in Butleng's schools, away from the crime and violence in Gauteng and out from under their feet.

Simplifying, Potlakong accommodates an African proletariat, while Butleng is a reservoir of young workers and a sump for those not needed or wanted in South Africa's fast lane: children, the elderly and the disabled.

Rhythms

The populations of the Potlakong and Butleng are different. So too are the rhythms of the townships.

Potlakong wakes to work in the surrounding factories, town centres and suburbs. Then, as the working day closes, the township breathes back in deeply and people return crowded into taxis, buses, trains and cars that drive past streams of pedestrians hurrying home to different parts of the vast township, to eat an evening meal and watch 'soapies',[22] and perhaps the television news in Sesotho or isiZulu before bed. Between these exhalations and inhalations of morning and evening, there are shallower breaths. Many of the surrounding factories never stop outside the long Christmas break. Machines work 24 hours a day, seven days a week. Shift systems for factory production and South Africa's vast private security industry mean that Potlakong is never really asleep.

Not so Butleng. Butleng sleeps deeply. So deeply that you should not expect help from the police should something happen *lefifing* (in the darkness). Everybody knows that the police are asleep with their *dicheri* (girlfriends). In Butleng you wake not to the honking of taxi horns, but the 'swish, swish, swish' of women sweeping out their *mabala* (dirt yards) and the dull rhythmic sound of *dipatsi* (firewood) being chopped for the stoves. Old men and *badisa* (young shepherds) often hired from Lesotho head out to release cattle from the *masaka* (kraals) where they have been penned overnight. Children in green, yellow or red uniforms make their way to school. A long queue of women has already formed outside the township clinic.

All this changes at the weekends. No school, no work, no clinic.

104

In Butleng, the cattle still need to graze, but otherwise weekends are different. Saturdays are for funerals, Sundays are for church, and the whole weekend is for drinking. There are, of course, permutations of these options. There are other *mesebetsi* (ceremonies) including tombstone unveilings, weddings that are usually scheduled for the summer, and the catch-all *mosebetsi wa badimo* (ancestral ceremony). Some people don't drink; some people don't go to church, but everybody goes to funerals, even if, on religious grounds, you discreetly skip traditional aspects too closely linked to ancestor belief for your comfort.

The drinking peaks at the end of the month, following pay day, but then flags as money runs short. The last weekend of the month sees the many township drinking venues bursting at the seams and spilling out into the streets. There are a range of outlets, from *majabajaba laonj* (a fancy 'lounge') for those with serious money and flashy tastes, to the licensed taverns with pool tables, juke boxes and display fridges secured behind metal bars that cater for solid drinking, to the shifting geography of local *chaf posi* or *shebeens* that you only know about because you live close by. These are little more than a front room of a house or *mokhukhu* and a fridge. They double up as takeaway outlets without closing hours, as well as a place to drink a beer or two out of the house. In Butleng and the informal settlements that make up parts of Potlakong, there are also *dipoto* (spots) selling home-brewed, traditional sorghum beer, or alternative brews fermented from bread and flavoured with pineapple, and sometimes given extra strength with battery acid, eye drops or other innovations. Here men, and a few women, sit around on rough benches or crates, drinking from plastic tubs originally used to sell snuff, or other recycled containers.

Alcohol, particularly beer, is ever present in the townships. How much gets drunk depends on a mix of factors – how much money people have in their pockets, the temperature of the day, and the reasons to *ithabisa* (enjoy oneself). For a full-on township drinking binge, mix together a Saturday at the end of the month (other than January), a hot day and an afternoon football derby between South Africa's two football giants, Pirates and Chiefs.[23] It's a guaranteed formula for drinking to spill out onto the streets, for drunken arguments, and busy hospital casualty wards come evening.

And *ditlamatlama* (hangovers) on a Sunday morning. Then you will be very grateful for the unlicensed outlets nearby. On Sunday morning, after the night before, what is needed is a cold beer to calm the raging headache, the dry mouth, the queasy stomach and the shaking hands that make it hard to even hold a cigarette. A cold beer will *thoba ho thothomela* (calm the trembling), settle the stomach, lubricate the mouth and relieve the pain. The colder the beer the better. You will gladly pay the premium of an extra rand for a really, truly cold, cold beer. *Biri e bata po!* (Icy-cold beer). You will knock on the door of the nearest *chaf posi* without ceremony for a quart, or perhaps two, if that's what it takes. Or three, if the beer is cold and going down well, but then, really, you've started another day of drinking.

The monthly cycle of consumption and subsequent belt-tightening is written in larger font across the township year. Few people are not saving for Christmas, often through *stokvels*, the ubiquitous mutual saving schemes that operate on a yearly cycle, paying out, often through bulk buying of groceries, in December. As the holiday period approaches, the residents of Johannesburg's suburbs routinely ask each other if they are going to the coast or staying in the city. Everybody likes two, three, even four weeks at the sea, but the merits of the city, in which the rush hour has all but vanished and calm has descended, also has its attractions. In Gauteng townships, there is an equivalent question, to stay or to visit, not the coast but *mahae* (home areas) such as Butleng. Whether one stays or travels, the month-long holiday in townships will involve much visiting. Not by appointment or invitation, but by dropping in. Here, another side of the township, one that does not rotate around *jwala* (alcohol), is visible. The cultural norm of *ho tjaka* (to visit) makes township houses at Christmas an open home, where you will be served *dikuku* (scone-like cakes) and k*gemere* (ginger-flavoured cool drink) prepared in bulk for the carousel of visitors that family matriarchs take pride in hosting.

Church, tavern and values

The church and the tavern are like two townships that exist uneasily alongside each other in every *kasi*. There are many more varieties of churches than there are drinking options, but for all the variation, a dividing line is palpable between the two. The broken, scarred and quarrelsome men sitting together in a *sepoto* drinking to forget have little in common with the *nonne* (plump) women in ironed *manyano* (women's guild) uniforms on their way to a church, though they share the same space, perhaps the same house, perhaps the same bed. They proclaim different values.

Men do go to church, but churches are attended mostly by women and children. Women do drink, but it is predominantly a male occupation. The consequences are also an occupational hazard: *monna o na le maqeba* (a man has scars) is a township saying. This division of the township peaks visibly at Christmas. In Butleng, the churches run back-to-back services late into the night while revellers spill out from taverns that pulsate with amplified music. The citadels of God and the centres of mammon go head to head. Churchgoers will tut-tut over the rowdy crowds, bemoan the underage drinking, and take alternative routes to avoid the most boisterous crowds. Drinkers, for their part, will suggest that the churchgoers are too proud to join them, but are not better people; a point that will be illustrated by assertions as to what apparently respectable and upright churchgoers get up to when not under scrutiny.

With some reason. Little is exactly as it seems in the townships. What is said in church on Sundays may not translate into practice on a Monday. Cultures of non-payment are widespread. In November 2012, the state electricity company, Eskom, estimated that Soweto residents collectively owed R3.3bn for electricity and the interest that unpaid bills had accrued. Only 20 per cent of electricity consumed was being paid for.[24] Soweto is, according to Eskom, a particularly bad example of non-payment, but the problem is widespread. The installation of pre-paid meters has been one response, but illegal connections are commonplace and many informal settlements are festooned with a spider's web of wires and cables running power for free from street lighting or other sources of electricity that can be tapped. A few years ago, Eskom ran a short TV advert that highlighted the dangers and anti-social consequences of the *izinyoga* (the snakes that steal electricity). The term caught on in the township, but not in the way Eskom hoped, as a term of abuse. When it came to electricity, the insult of calling somebody a snake dissipated to become a description that held little, if any, disgrace. Practically everybody is an *inyoga*, at least some of the time. Not the menacing *izinyoga* of the Eskom advert with forked tongs, scaly skin and unblinking eyes. But *izinyoga* that look just like your neighbours on their way to church. Back in the house, perhaps the kitchen has been wired past the meter, or perhaps the meter is running on discounted (i.e. fraudulent) electricity coupons obtained through a friend who knows somebody.

Of course this and other *maano* (tricks) or *menyetla* (opportunities) lie below the surface of what causal visits to the township reveal. It's the quiet conversations, the discreet suggestions, the slightly embarrassed smiles and the shifting eyes that reveal this network of everyday fraud – one which any respectable person discreetly covers with a few legally bought electricity coupons, complaints about rising prices, and uplifting, harmonic singing *kerekeng* (in church).

Change

The townships are a changing. They are getting bigger. Even as the Free State's total population remains stable, its townships expand as farms are consolidated and mechanised. Around Butleng, there remain many farms with tied accommodation, sometimes in settlements reaching the size of small villages, but everywhere farmers are ending the housing tenure of labourers. The evidence is rows of crudely build, two-roomed houses sitting empty in isolated fields with doors, window frames and roofs removed. Now, when labour is needed, it is sourced from the townships on a casual basis. In Butleng at harvest time, open trucks arrive at six in the morning to pick up hundreds of women, their faces smeared with white clay to protect their skin from the sun, to labour in the fields.

Immigrants from Lesotho, even less able to absorb labour market entrants than South Africa, also swell the populations of Free State townships. Gauteng's townships, as we have seen, continue to bloat with internal migrants and foreigners: the *batswakantle* (literally: those that come from outside, foreigners) or the commonplace derogatory appellation *makwerekwere*.

Despite this tide of people flooding into the *kasi* with little to offer but their labour, life is for most part improving. A massive programme of social grants for the disabled, children and the old (but not the unemployed) has reduced much of the most desperate poverty in South Africa, while an increasing number of households have electricity, running water and sewerage. In 1996, 58 per cent of households used electricity for lighting; in 2011 that had risen to almost 85 per cent. Over the same period, households with piped water in either house or yard rose from 61 to 73 per cent, and those with flush or chemical toilet from 50 to 63 per cent.[25] That is progress; much of it delivered to townships, though there can be steps back as well as forwards that the statistics do not easily capture. In Butleng the bucket system, by which you must defecate into a bucket that is collected once a week, was replaced with outside flush toilets on every stand in the township a few years ago. For many residents, however, this enthusiastically welcomed development has been eroded as Butleng's water supply has become increasingly erratic. In several parts of the townships it has all but stopped, and water, including that needed to flush the toilets, has to be delivered by tanker and stored in buckets and dustbins.

After the bucket system, the next most resented feature of township life is washing in a *waskom* (plastic wash bowl) for the vast majority who have neither plumbed water nor bathroom. It's a cumbersome and tiring process repeated day after day. In comparison, a shower that you step in and out of when you please, with hot or cold water on tap, is freedom – though that assumes you can afford the plumbing and that your section of the township doesn't *sokola metsi* (lack water), and perhaps that you still have that friend who knows where to buy discounted electricity coupons now that you see just how much electricity the geyser eats.

Becoming middle class in the township is no easy undertaking.

Every step up increases overheads. Every visible sign of success attracts claims from families, neighbours and friends. At least a smart and comfortable house is a nice place to sit in, away from the stream of requests and expectations that have to be negotiated outside. Moving to the once-White suburbs or new 'grey' (mixed) areas resolves some problems, but you need to have well-paying work to make that leap and be prepared to leave *kasi* life behind, other than nostalgic weekend visits.

A visible change in the larger townships of South Africa is the arrival of shopping malls. Previously, any serious shopping took place in town since little more than corner *spaza* shops and bottlestores operated in the townships. Large retail malls, most with the low-end market chainstores and supermarkets, now bring consumer goods closer to where people live. In a consumer-conscious society it is a development that has been welcomed by all but those whose own businesses have been pushed aside by the malls.

Wealth and status

There are new fault lines running through South Africa's townships as the solidarity imposed on Africans by Apartheid and colonialism gives way.

In the workplace, the African proletariat confronts less and less the White managers and their Indian and Coloured subalterns of yesteryear. Now, their supervisor or foreman is also an African, living in a township, perhaps in the same street. He (as is typically the case) is only slightly ahead of those he gives orders to and there is little difference on which to base authority. Indeed, taken in the round, his household income may be less than that of subordinates. It may show in what he can afford. In this changing racial configuration of industrial hierarchy, competition can be intense as social tensions intersect with occupational status. One result is whispered character assassinations, accusations of corruption, and muttering about witchcraft.

Labour-broking and black economic empowerment initiatives have only made this worse. Who better to source and cajole cheap African labour than an African who, while one step ahead, is also vulnerable?

In Potlakong, the municipal collection of household waste has been reorganised into a set of contracts, cascaded down to promote small aspiring Black businesses. Except that the only people who really benefit are those at the top of the pyramid of contracts. On the ground, at the base of this pyramid, the contracts are written so tightly and the penalty clauses so liberal that 'emerging black businessmen' are little more than foremen whose incomes are based on the performance of the men they notionally employ but, in reality, merely supervise.

This places a lot of people in uncomfortable positions. To get ahead, you have to fight the tight corner that you are in. As much as anything, it is the gap between the dreams, the promises of 'A Better Life for All' (an ANC slogan),[26] and the reality of current circumstances in which most people live that drives the incessant conflict of current South African life. It also accounts for widespread xenophobic violence against immigrants who join the competition.[27] The explosion of wildcat strikes in 2012[28] was a challenge to the continued inequality in the country. Changes since 1994 have not ended inequality; any erosion of White people's position at the top of the pile has been matched by an increase in inequality among Blacks.

The impact of this inequality is not just about what you can or cannot afford, but also the status that buying power brings. The imperative of showing success hit home when I bought a new car. A White university professor pottering around the township is judged by a range of criteria. That you are there at all gives you credit, and so does your professional status, even if a university is a remote idea for most township residents. But a car is tangible. When I replaced my visibly ageing VW Golf with a two-year old and still quite smart Toyota Corolla, nobody was shy in telling me how well I had done. Initially, it took me by surprise as people shook my hand, congratulated me and told how nice my new car looked. As this continued, my embarrassment began to evaporate. I began to feel as though I really had done something tremendous about which I should be proud. In a couple of households where I'd helped out with school books or short-term loans, this success was elevated beyond mortal bounds. The blessing of my new car was a just reward from God; those who give shall receive, I was told. If I am honest, I could feel an addictive tug upon me. If I got an even newer or bigger or smarter car, would this adulation continue?

The answer is 'yes', but there is obviously a price. A car represents success: even a two-year old Toyota Corolla does, if you hang out in the right neighbourhoods. Cars carry status in most societies, but it is intense in the *kasi*. They do not say *koloi ke basadi* (a car means [you will have] women) for nothing. Once, in Potlakong, I watched as Saki's persistent (and well-practised) pick-up lines were pointedly ignored by two young women. By chance, as the two women were returning back down the road some ten minutes later, Saki had just moved my car (the Toyota, not the Golf) to be washed by a couple of *loxion managers* (an ironic term for young men hanging around the township). The two young women were parallel with him as he stepped out of the car, stood up and closed the door with the car keys in his hand. Both women swivelled their heads in unison to check out Saki, who, for a moment, had been transformed from a tiresome *loxion manager* into a potential prospect.

The thing about flaunting success embodied in material goods is that it's easy to start competing. The relativity of context means there are many leagues of play. A car that will turn heads wherever you go, say an Audi R8, is beyond the reach of township residents (or university professors). But you can always compete in lower leagues, like letting the neighbours see that you've been shopping at Pick n Pay and not one of Shoprite's U$ave stores[29] as you come out of the taxi flashing your groceries in their branded plastic bags, or that you've eaten at KFC by carefully reserving one piece of chicken from your Streetwise Two meal so that there's a reason to bring the distinctive box back home. But the curse about social competition measured by symbols of consumption is that it never ends. Even in the lower leagues, you've got to keep buying KFC to keep up.

There are limited exits from this competition over status that saturates townships as much as flasher neighbourhoods of South Africa. A working wage isn't ever going to suffice. Winning the Lotto would do and costs only R3.50 a shot, but the odds are long. Then there is the Road Accident Fund (RAF), a national accident insurance scheme paid for by a levy on petrol, which has become a macabre lottery for the poor. Playing requires an accident with disabling consequences, often involves a dodgy lawyer, and can, after several years, see you paid out with what seems, at least initially, more than you could ever spend. If the Lotto and RAF don't deliver, you may end up sidestepping this contest in which the stakes are stacked against you, with the bottle that satisfies for a while or you can choose religion where an afterlife can be banked against current hardships and disappointments.

Living cheek by jowl

Aside from the escape offered by drinking, dreams and devotion, township life is crowded. Privacy is limited and dignity difficult to maintain. Even in death there may be little decorum. On a Saturday morning, South Park Cemetery in Gauteng soon snarls up as funeral cortèges compete to reach funerals in adjacent graves. In the chaos of the graveyard, mourners get mixed up, speeches are drowned out by adjacent services, and grieving families endure the inevitable bottleneck at the cemetery gates as cars, taxis and buses jostle to exit without order or restraint.

Washing in a *waskom* is a daily indignity for the living, before you've even stepped outside the door. *Wa hlapa* (s/he is washing) is the commonplace warning that the closed door of the living room or bedroom of a four-roomed house should not be opened or that the sounds of ablutions coming from behind a curtain in a shack should be subject to civic inattention. Living cheek by jowl means intimate co-operation to provide wafer-thin privacy.

But it is not only bodily privacy that life in the crowded townships makes difficult. There is precious little that is not public. That can be a problem when public claims can be laid on what you'd rather were private resources. Take *kwae* (cigarettes) for example. Many township men prefer to buy *loose draw* (single cigarettes) that are available along with *dos* (a light) at almost every *spaza* and *hukung* (literally 'on the corner': a street-side stall or hawker's stand).[30] It is, of course, cheaper to buy a packet of cigarettes, but only if you smoke them yourself, or expect reciprocal exchange when offering cigarettes to fellow smokers.

But living among people who are unemployed and who can draw on the public morality of sharing means that a box of cigarettes is likely to be rapidly depleted. The standard excuse to deflect requests for money, *Ha e yo* (There isn't any/I don't have), doesn't wash when your cigarette packet has been in full view. The best you can get away with is claiming that the last cigarette in the box has to be saved as your *slapi* (final smoke of the day before sleeping).

If you really did have money to spare, flashing your box of cigarettes would not be a problem. You'd be showing that you had money enough not to worry about keeping the neighbourhood in 'smokes'. But then if that was the case, you'd be driving a Beemer (BMW) and wearing a Breitling watch. The reality is that most people don't, because they can't, and as much as they are competing for status through staged acts of conspicuous consumption, these symbols of success can only be sustained by maintaining a grim front of austerity elsewhere.

Striving to impress while needing to skimp drives some of the psychological dynamics of township life. Showing and hiding at the same time is a toxic recipe for insecurity. When the fragile facade can't be managed, *dihlong* or *skaam* (shame) is the result. *Loxion managers*, sitting out township boredom together every day, get over these feelings and perfect their arts of cajoling, cadging and pleading. But for a worker who is laid off, or who is on strike, the experience is usually one of social isolation in which they become embarrassed about going out without enough money to keep up with friends.

Skaam helps keep the *mashonisa* (locally-based informal lenders), formal loan businesses and hire-purchase credit arms of clothing and furniture shops in business. The rates of interest can be exorbitant, but people get tired of having nothing. Consumption can be flashed today; the bleak struggle of servicing payments can be silently borne over months and years. *Skaam* also feeds into transactional sex, which is far from being for survival only but also a way to obtain luxuries. Most sex has some transactional element, even if it so discreetly managed that the partners do not recognise it, but in the context of the South African *kasi*, and the topic of this book, we should note how escaping from one form of shame can end up with having to bear another.

The flipside of shame is *kwaal,* the pervasive Sekasi term for jealousy, which even has its own hand sign of a hooked index finger protruding above an upright and clenched hand. The sign is often displayed on the back window of taxis; you're reading it from behind and should therefore be jealous of the man in front of you. But *kwaal* goes beyond taunting in South Africa's anarchic traffic; it pervades relationships between neighbours and friends in the townships. That's not unique; around the world people try to 'keep up with the Joneses'. It's the close-quarter competition resulting from *kwaal* in the crowded life of the township that merits attention. *Kwaal* helps explain misfortune, for there will always be somebody who is jealous of you and will seek to bring you down a peg. It takes an extremely confident person to shake off this almost universal sense of danger that comes from those closest to you in the townships. Even those who laugh off the threat on the basis that they are protected by a God are not saying that others are not jealous. And they are not saying that others won't act on that jealousy to bring you down. They are saying that they have more powerful forces at their disposal and shall fear no evil.

Kwaal may explain a broken window or other minor act of petty and anonymous retribution in the location, but it also provides a portal for us to see the parallel metaphysical world of witchcraft that township residents contend with. That world may be scoffed at in the safety of the research interview, but it emerges in everyday conversations and the crises of life. Even if you claim that you do not believe in witchcraft yourself, you know that others, whom you will only suspect, do and will use it to satisfy their jealously. So, it may be circumspect to at least protect yourself with a visit to the traditional healer or church prophet who will know exactly what you are talking about and offer remedies.

But for all the vibrancy of these parallel spirit worlds, everybody still has to survive in the here and now. That takes many forms, but what dominates day-to-day life is a working-class resistance that by and large ignores exhortations from politicians, employers and preachers alike. And it is not only because the African proletariat, in all its diverse forms, sees the hypocrisy of many who urge them to be good citizens, hard workers and moral paragons. It is also because they are constantly reminded that they never have enough and others have more. The default position that results boils down to getting away with as much as one can at work and enjoying oneself as best as one can at home. Work is a necessity generally taken up with a grudge and, if that is so, then it is all the more important to try and *enjoya* back in the *kasi* where at least you are not ordered around like an animal. For all its tensions and irritations the *kasi* is home.

Relationships

The *kasi* may be home to many, but it's a competitive abode where economic necessity impinges on the stability of all relationships. Conversations constantly juggle rands and cents; when money is tight prices are closely watched and cost-benefit calculations are part of every sphere of life.

Need binds people together from necessity and shared lives accumulate betrayals, wrongs and irritations that are laid down like layers of sediment in joint histories along with acts of co-operation, kindness and friendship. One greets every day afresh, but remembers what has happened between you. Again, this is no different from all communities – the striking difference here is that people are in one another's face, every day. Lip service to values of *botho* or *ubuntu* (shared humanity) helps to keep things together, at least for the sake of appearance. Exuberant greetings by young men who have grown up together in the townships mask more critical private evaluations that may well play out with indifference or avoidance in times of difficulties, while neighbours scrutinise one another when witchcraft is suspected.

With money you can make things happen, but you must watch out for those who are jealous of your success. Without money you are nothing. Young, unemployed men in the township might father children, but unless they have work, getting enough money for a marriage, for which *lobola* or bride wealth must be paid, is all but impossible. If you ask them why they do not at least live together, the response is shrugged shoulders. They could not provide for the family and there would only be arguments; better that their girlfriend and child remains with her parents.[31]

For men, only money makes marriage and respectability possible. Money also opens the option of becoming a serious player with *dinyatsi* (mistresses/girlfriends). In an impoverished environment where individuals are hungry to consume and display, money provides bargaining power for sexual partners as well as the basis for social status. As much as preachers and public health proponents may rail against them, macho values and consumerist cultures propel extensive sexual networks within the township – networks that women often play an active part in as they learn how to extract benefit from boyfriends and lovers as well as the notorious 'sugar daddies'. Many people stand apart from these behavioural modes, but certainly not as many as profess monogamy. Multiple partners are part of life that draws together pleasure, desire, money and status, even if there is rarely enough money to keep this whirligig turning smoothly.

The extended township

When I first extended my stays in townships beyond day visits, the thing that struck me most was how I entered a parallel world to the South Africa that I had inhabited till then. My world, since I arrived in South African in 1994, had been populated with Africans, but primarily as domestic workers, as students, as research subjects, as well as politicians on television. With the exception of visits to students' or shop stewards' homes, my interaction with Africans had been in contexts controlled largely by Whites; the suburban home, the university and the factory. I now started to be immersed in an environment where Whites were hardly to be seen, let alone in charge. That did not mean that they were absent completely, either in the historical shaping of these spaces or as *makgowa* (Whites, but also employers) of Africans. But Whites were not on the ground in the townships, and had no say in what happened on a daily basis.

More than a decade on, that observation still holds true, perhaps, if anything, even truer. It is not only Whites who are absent from the townships, but also professionals and upper-middle-class Africans, who live, work and school their children in towns and suburbs away from this parallel and grimmer world.

The township exists as a continuous entity alongside, but separate from, the much smarter and, to most readers of this book, familiar world of town centres, suburbs, shopping malls, holiday resorts, game parks and the connecting roads, freeways and branded service stations. The roads are shared, though only to a point. In reality, there are different ways of travelling on the same roads. My journey to Butleng from Jo'burg involves some four hours in my car with a stop, or two, for coffee in clean, efficient service stations. I can travel when I want and choose which CDs to play. I'm happy to give lifts to Butleng friends if it can be co-ordinated, but will never overload the car. The journey for a resident of Potlakong to Butleng can take much of the day, involves two 'local' trips to and from taxi ranks and one, often two, long-distance taxi journeys, and not infrequently they are stopped at police roadblocks that I'm usually waved through. Their journey needs to start well before noon if they are to be sure of arriving that day and they will have to lug their bags across bustling, dusty taxi ranks and then wait for their taxi to fill before the driver, who will decide what is going to be played in his vehicle, sets off. The journey itself will be cramped, sweaty and uncomfortable. It will also be at the mercy of the taxi driver, who may be impatient to overtake my Corolla, irrespective of double white road lines. The alternative is to pay for space in a private car, but the journey will be not much less uncomfortable in a car packed to the gills.

In provincial Free State towns, there are shops that serve township residents in the rougher end of town, usually next to the taxi rank. In the local idiom these shops are known as *maindia* because they are owned by Indians. They stock cheap food and cosmetics in bulk for those who run *spaza* shops, hawk on the streets, or are buying *groceries tsa selemo* (groceries of the year; i.e. bulk purchases made with the combined savings of mutual savings groups at the end of the year). They also provide a complete service for micro retail outlets in the townships. In *maindia* you can buy cheap *dikwankwara* (hard biscuits) in 4-kg bags, *dipompong* (sweets) in ½-kg or 1-kg packs, or *ghosts* (corn puffs) in enormous pockets, and you can also buy the plastic bags in which you will need to retail them to children, who will pester their parents for change.

It's a tardier, cheaper and poorer world than that of town and suburb. It runs in parallel to this world and forms a continuous, integrated social web connected in multifarious ways that draw the bonds between, say, Potlakong in Gauteng and Butleng in the Free State more tightly than between neighbouring Potlakong and Johannesburg in Gauteng or between Butleng and Plaasville in the Free State.[32] This is despite the physical proximity of town and township and their Apartheid-designed relationship. Townships are linked by social and family networks, shared ways of life, shared beliefs, shared problems, even an emerging common language as Nguni, Sesotho, Afrikaans, English and other tongues meld into Sekasi,[33] the township lingo. This concept of a single South African township spread web-like over the entire country contrasts with other concepts of human geography. While there are many internal divisions within townships, variation between townships and regional influences, not least of ethnicity, imagining one interconnected township helps us overcome other imagined geographies that are unhelpful in understanding the social construction of AIDS.

Particularly unhelpful is a geography of knowledge that imagines a set of concentric circles radiating out from urban centres, and universities in particular, with knowledge decreasing and ignorance increasing the further we travel out from the centres of learning. My students are very quick to utilise such a geography, for which they will receive affirmation in many quarters. Far, far away from the lecture theatre or seminar room where we are discussing AIDS, they tell me of somewhere called the 'rural areas', where ignorance prevails and the people must be enlightened. Between our discussion venue and the rural areas, they suggest there are gradients of ignorance and need. That there are rural areas in South Africa with different characteristics is indisputable, but we should not entertain the static concept of society that this imagined geography of knowledge suggests. People can, and do, circulate between rural areas and townships in both the provinces and urban centres. And since ideas circulate with people, there is much more homogeneity over beliefs than we might imagine. This cuts both ways: ideas generated in the urban centres, including universities, ebb into every corner of the land, and ideas generated in the rural areas flow into urban centres and lap around, sometimes leak into, the centres of learning. These are uneven and incomplete processes which are all but impossible to track, but acknowledging this constant churning of ideas across the extended township is a better starting point than the model of concentric rings of knowledge. Folk and lay theories of AIDS do not increase in credibility the further one moves away from enlightened urban centres. They circulate, just as the HIV virus itself circulates, through this extended township.

Township life & AIDS myths

This chapter has provided a description of life in South African townships. With the exception of a few illustrative statistics, it is drawn from my own experiences. It is therefore partial and it is also particular. Despite my liminal status within the *kasi* as a White, foreign-born university professor that provides some freedom to ignore boundaries of gender and age norms, there are limits to what I can see. But these limits notwithstanding, it is a description of life in the township, not the statistics of the township, which is important in understanding AIDS beliefs.

This chapter has noticeably said little about these alternative understandings of AIDS. That is appropriate: AIDS, and how it is understood, is just one part of the township life and must take its place. As much as the AIDS epidemic is a human tragedy of epic proportions, any account that places AIDS at the centre of township life has lost proportion. There are many problems in township life, and AIDS must jostle with them for prominence. Further, as harsh as township life can be, it is more than a list of problems, but is a home for millions of South Africans – this must also be factored in by any account of AIDS.

The beliefs of Bafana, Paseka and Grace in Potlakong, and Neo in Butleng, that we explore in subsequent chapters are rooted in and moulded by this lived environment of the *kasi*. They make sense in this context. Transported outside, they all too easily become the ethnobongo hearsay that does little but provide giggles and gasps at suburban dinner parties. Within the *kasi* they make sense and we need to take them seriously.

6

The precarious life
of Bafana Radebe

***Hang hang!* (Immediately, without delay!)**

Bafana's health crisis came without warning in September 2008. Two weeks earlier, I had been chatting with him in front of his *mokhukhu* (shack) in the Pheko section of Potlakong. He had been sitting on a plastic crate, leaning back against the zinc sheeting, soaking up the welcome spring sunshine. Later, making my way with a friend and Bafana's neighbour, Tokelo, though the narrow 'double ups' (passages or shortcuts linking parallel streets in the township) of the neighbourhood, I had run across Bafana again. He had left his place in the sun and formed part of a circle of men sharing quart bottles in a backyard *sepoto* or 'spot' where the owner usually has a dozen cold quarts in the fridge and will send out for more if needed.

News of his illness was given to me casually, in passing. Bafana was, I was told by Tokelo, ill and in bed. Unconcerned, I had said I would say hello. Later I knocked, called out loudly '*koko, koko*' ('knock, knock') and pushed open the door to his shack. Bafana lay under a thick mat of blankets on a bed that was half screened from the crowded kitchen-cum-living-space by a faded floral curtain tacked to a wooden roof beam. He was complaining how cold it was. His eyes were prominent and cheeks gaunt. His flesh had shrunk over his bones. It was still Bafana, but it would have been easy to mistake him for someone else.

I sat on a plastic drum that served as a seat in the narrow space between the bed and wardrobe of peeling veneer. There was a clutter on the small cabinet next to him: pill bottles, a glass of water, pieces of paper, some folded bank notes and a doctor's card. Thrust between the padding and the wooden frame of the bedstead was a Bowie knife. Within easy reach. Bafana lived alone.

His account of what was wrong oscillated between his symptoms and how much things cost. He was worried about work. His sick leave was exhausted and his supervisor had suggested unpaid leave. Since Bafana was employed as a casual worker, I guessed that such an arrangement was already in place, but I said nothing. I checked the tablets – antibiotics and mild pain relief. There was also cough medicine. But the cough wasn't what was troubling him now. The problem was the constant hiccups. That, and the swelling on his anus, gave him no rest. He was in constant discomfort, lying twisted awkwardly at his waist to avoid putting pressure on the boil. The doctor's card was for a Dr Mabaso, a graduate of Natal University[1] with a surgery in Naledi Section, some three kilometres away. On a crumpled piece of paper, in shaky handwriting, was the name and cell phone number for a Dr Tshabalala.

Bafana was despondent about the progress he had made with Dr Mabaso. Dr Tshabalala's number had been given to him by a friend. This doctor came highly recommended. Bafana said that for R500,[2] *yena* (he or she[3]) would sort things out. *Yena* would be able to solve everything.

When I returned two hours later, he was up and dressed, almost ready to leave. He had first to go to the toilet. Bafana's friend Ronnie sat waiting – he would accompany us to Dr Tshabalala's surgery. While we waited for Bafana to slowly shuffle to the outside toilet and back, we confirmed to each other how ill he was. How thin he was. That's what everyone was now saying. *O otile haholo* (He's become so thin), sometimes said with a shudder for emphasis.

Ronnie sat in the passenger seat. Bafana sat in the back. We stopped for directions once we were in Phola Section. A landmark we had been told to look out for was the clinic. We found it sitting empty and closed behind a heavy concrete palisade fence. Further down the road, there was a track to the right, and further down that there was Dr Tshabalala, standing, as she had told Ronnie she would be, outside her surgery. She slid open a metal gate and we drove in. The high walls gave privacy to the bare earth yard that we entered.

There were introductions and Bafana was taken to the *rondavel* (traditional round hut) with blue painted walls and a thatched roof that served as Dr Tshabalala's surgery. Ronnie and I sat in the waiting area that consisted of four chairs against the yard wall. I could see through the open door of the main breezeblock-built house, a small kitchen table covered with a clean blue-and-white checked cloth. One of the house windows was broken. Dr Tshabalala made several trips between her surgery and the house. She ignored us. Each time she entered the *rondavel,* her shoes were slipped off. Ronnie explained how important this was – shoes could pick up anything, the surgery needed to be kept clean.

After half an hour she came over to us, pulled over one of the seats and asked us what we knew. As Ronnie later explained, she was checking Bafana's account. Then she went back to Bafana. Then she came back and gave her prognosis. She was going to sort out the problems he had come with: his hiccups and the boil behind. But, she suggested, it might be good for him to check his HIV status. It was left at that.

Now she started to warm towards us as she went backwards and forwards preparing Bafana's *imbiza* (traditional medicine). Not enough to grant my request to watch her at work in the kitchen, but enough to be happy that I'd asked. The value of professional secrets is in people wanting to know them. It took some ten minutes to prepare the *imbiza,* a rough black powder in a plastic snuff box.

With the *imbiza* to her satisfaction, we were invited into the dark of her *rondavel*. The only lighting was a single candle set in a small empty bottle on a dresser surrounded by glass jars of herbs and powders. We sat down on a low couch in the gloom. Slowly, as my eyes adjusted to the dim lighting, I worked out that Bafana was lying on his stomach across a small bed, buttocks exposed. Tessa – that's what I was now instructed to call Dr Tshabalala – put on gloves and opened the box of *imbiza*. She wanted us to know what we were dealing with and Bafana's buttocks were pulled apart, while I held the candle to provide as much light as possible. The boil had been lanced and there was copious thick grey pus around his anus. Tessa told us this was dangerous. Then she threw in a pinch of *imbiza* and tapped it matter-of-factly into the pus. Bafana whimpered. When Tessa was finished, she told Bafana that he could sit up.

He sat shivering on the edge of the bed, while Tessa pulled out a 'two litre' (drink bottle commonly re-used for traditional blood-cleaning *moriana* or medicine) from the dresser and provided precise advice on the manner in which the brown liquid should be drunk: not in gulps, but sips. Bafana was told off for not finishing the *moriana* that she gave him to drink. He dutifully finished it in sips, hands shaking as he held the tin mug in both hands. After he put the mug down, he declared that his hiccups had stopped. Tessa was delighted. '*Bonang!*' (Look!), she exclaimed proudly '*Dr Tshabalala o sebetsa hang hang!*' (Dr Tshabala works without delay!)

By tomorrow, Bafana avowed, he would be fine.

But he wasn't.

A week later, he was much worse. His small kitchen was crowded with relatives, but his sister, Paseka, who had arrived earlier in the morning, was firmly in control. Bafana's blankets had been washed and were hanging over a fence to dry. She had bought nappies for him. On the Monday, with Bafana slipping in and out of consciousness, she asked a relative with a car to get Bafana to hospital. He was too far gone to object.

Di re eng? (What do they say?)

The *batjha* (youth) that Tokelo and I came to the hospital with had *zol* (cannabis) on them. They hurriedly got out of the car to use the pedestrian entrance, when Tokelo pointed out that we might get searched in the car. It felt as though we were entering a prison, not a hospital. I had to get out of the car and was checked by a security guard, who ran a hand-held metal detector over me. I also had to show my driving licence. We were ordered about, told to move the car forward, told to wait. It was Sunday afternoon, and there are far more security guards than nurses in the huge dilapidated building.

We had decided to see Bafana first and then buy him something when we knew what he needed. But as we walked across the car park to the wards, we saw a relative of Bafana carrying fruit. We panicked; shouldn't we, after all, buy fruit? I reminded them of our previous decision and we made a joke of it: *Mohlomong Bafana o tla batla jwala, kapa kwae, kapa basadi!* (Maybe Bafana will want beer, or cigarettes, or women!) We entered the ward laughing.

Actually, he wanted *zol*. But the whispered request was ridiculous and only confirmed to us that he'd lost it. There was a nurse sitting at the entrance to the ward who offered no help when we asked which bed Bafana Radebe was in, but she'd have come running at the first whiff of smoke. Otherwise, he was incoherent with fatigue and it was hard to make out what he was saying.

We crowded around his bed, but there was little to do, other than watch Paseka trying to get him to drink Coke. She gently poured it, little by little, from a bottle into his mouth. Bafana, his head resting on the pillow, indicated with an emaciated hand when he had had enough. Paseka waited with the bottle while he swallowed. Then they'd start again. After around five minutes of this, he'd perhaps managed half-a-dozen mouthfuls. Then there was a palaver to find a bowl to tuck under his chin, as he vomited the fluid back up.

The *batjha* drifted away. Bafana's relatives stayed standing around the bed, occasionally harassed by a deranged man who wandered the wards grinning wildly and asking where visitors were from. People turned their backs on him and he moved on, returning later, once his round of the ward was complete, to irritate them again.

I sat on a metal bench and read Bafana's medical notes which were stuffed into an envelope at the end of the bed. They recorded miliary tuberculosis,[4] severe dehydration, gastroenteritis, and the boil on his anus. He was doubly incontinent. There was a long medication list. Under a section of the notes entitled 'Special Risks' was listed 'terminal cachexia', that is, the wasting of his body that would take him past the point of no return. He looked to me as if he might have already passed that point, but encouragingly we told him '*ho tla loka*' (it'll be OK; a stock Sesotho phrase that can also serve to cheerfully postpone confronting a problem) and left the ward.

As we were leaving, Paseka accompanied me to the exit and said she wanted to talk to me. We stood between the bored nurse at the desk and the sullen guard at the door. '*Di re eng?*' (What do they say?) she asked. I responded to the unarticulated nub of her question. '*Ha di bue ka phamokate*' (They don't say anything about AIDS) – though it all pointed towards AIDS. She told me that Bafana gave permission for an HIV test, but they wouldn't tell her the result.

Later, Tshepo, one of the *batjha* who had accompanied us, was frank: 'We all know it's AIDS. Many people have this disease.' But, though we thought the same thing, we could not say for sure. We were still, however, convinced that Bafana knew. *Monga wa pitsa o ultwa monko pele ho ba bang* (The pot's owner smells what's cooking before others).

Cream soda

Bafana pulled through. When we visited him two weeks later, he was out of the hospital and recuperating at his sister's house in Matala Section. The house was still being built and we had to walk through what was only the shell of a room, with bare plaster walls and hanging wires, that would be the kitchen. The family were already using the space, but it had been cleared for the day, so that Paseka's husband could lay tiles. We traipsed past him as he knelt on the ground, determined to get the floor finished, and found Bafana in one of the bedrooms.

The flesh on his face had returned. He was still thin, but the transformation was astounding. It put everybody in a good mood. He was eating a thick slice of gaudily coloured sponge cake with a fork, while lying on a double bed covered in blankets. He ate sporadically while we chatted, and had got through most of the cake, along with a few mouthfuls of juice, by the time we left.

We asked him what we could get him. What he told us was a long list of things that he couldn't yet digest. He ran through the gamut of common fruit that either made him vomit or upset his stomach. Milk gave him diarrhoea. He could eat *pap* (stiff maize porridge) and *nama* (meat) though only if it had gravy, not if it was dry. He clearly knew how to play the 'sick role'.[5] His major complaint was that he hadn't had a beer, something that Paseka was strictly prohibiting, 'for centuries'. In the end he settled on Cream Soda cool drink.

We came back the following week with Cream Soda. By then the cat was out of the bag – at least within the curious triangle that Paseka, Tokelo and I constituted. Bafana had been tested again, this time at the clinic where he'd been referred for TB treatment, after his discharge from hospital. After that test, he'd asked Tokelo if he would accompany him to visit the clinic's AIDS counsellor.

It's good to know your status, but ...

That was in late 2008 and, with hindsight, it was the highpoint of Bafana's openness. I thought that from there we would move forward along a foreseeable path: a crisis, testing, an acknowledgement of the problem, a healthy (or at least healthier) lifestyle, CD4 tests to monitor the virus,[6] and eventually, when necessary, treatment. An orderly, if unwelcome, response to a situation that could no longer be denied. Bafana would live with his status and take responsibility for his health, unappetising as that might be.

But it was otherwise.

There was a mix-up over the appointment with the AIDS counsellor, and if Bafana did go to the AIDS clinic, it was not with Tokelo. Once he'd completed the nine months of TB treatment, I started to pester Bafana. Did he know what his CD4 count was? He had his excuses for why he'd not gone to the clinic – there were renovations under way, the queues were long. We stalled again and I went back over what we'd achieved so far: he knew his status, it was better to know your status. I was about to go onto the next bit: he should monitor the numbers in his blood, the soldiers of the body, so that the virus didn't catch him by surprise. Only he got in first. 'It's good to know your status,' he confirmed, '*Mara* (but) ...' he paused, 'what if the news is bad?'

I didn't push it further. As we talked, he was looking natty with a trilby hat and an umbrella under his arm. He had come striding out of his *mokhukhu* with a jaunty step, and was heading off to a wedding of a neighbour a couple of streets away. Now our conversation was turning morbid. He didn't say it, but what I was suggesting was perverse. I was proposing to send a well man to hospital so that he might receive bad news.

Over the coming months, he was careful to show me that he was looking after himself. Once, when we had attended a funeral together in a different part of the township, he made a point of collecting his jacket from my car. It was hot and we'd left our jackets, necessary for any funeral, in the car when we had joined the long queue of mourners for a plate of food. Then we had sat in the little shade we could find to eat. Now I was moving on. Bafana and the others were staying behind, where they would club together to buy beer and enjoy the afternoon. I would drop the jackets off as I was heading back to Pheko Section, where they could pick them up later. But Bafana elected to collect his from the car before I left. As we walked together to the car, Bafana explained that the weather might change and he could be exposed to a chill. He was telling me that he was looking after his health.

But there were limits to the front he could project. Drinking wasn't something he could stop – though it was one of the messages he'd been given at the clinic. Once, he tried to hide a bottle of *Zamalek* (an affectionate name for Black Label beer) as he walked past me, but as it was clear I'd seen, he thought better of it, smiled sheepishly, and carried on without the pretence of hiding the bottle. After that, he presented himself as a moderate drinker. Which he usually was, in a modest kind of way. But not always.

One afternoon, I had a distracted discussion with Bafana. He wanted to visit his sister Paseka. We'd driven over together a couple of times since he'd recuperated with her, but I said it wasn't possible today. Before leaving the township, aware I'd turned him down, I went to say goodbye and found him passed out in one of his two armchairs that make up, along with a large TV, the lounge area of his *mokhukhu*. He was slumped back in the chair, his head lolling over, a plate of food on his lap, and a spoon in his hand. The electric heater was between his legs and he was being slowly roasted. Fleetingly, I thought he was dead. After moving the heater back, I managed to get him to stir. He rubbed his face with his hand, still clutching the spoon, but other than issuing a low grunt, he didn't wake.

What bothered me was not the evident limits to a reformed lifestyle, but the sense that his HIV status was slipping from view. Everybody – that is, everybody who knew Bafana – had known he was positive. In the *kasi*, there is no need to specify that somebody is *HIV* positive. In context everybody understands what 'positive' means without the need for three prefatory letters. That Bafana was positive had never been openly discussed, as you might openly talk about, say, somebody being retrenched, or somebody having been in an accident – matters you would talk about frankly, albeit with some tact. But it had only been a short step away from that, I thought. Now his status, never really in the open, was disappearing from sight.

Another time, I found Bafana with a friend, Bongani, when I visited. They were watching television in the shack without much enthusiasm and my visit was welcome. Bafana unnecessarily apologised for not being in two weeks ago when I had called around. He recalled how I had realised that, despite his words *Ke phela hantle, ke sharp* (I'm fine, I'm OK), not all had been well and we had agreed to talk later. He developed this theme with enthusiasm. I was looking out for him. That although he was shy about his troubles, I had picked up that something was amiss. I was like a brother or a father. He wanted to know how was it that when he had been ill, I knew that his favourite drink was Cream Soda. Perhaps, I thought, he didn't remember that I had asked him what he would like. Or perhaps it was convenient for him to put me on this pedestal.

The problem, when we got to the point, had been his *diphio* (kidneys). He didn't bother with the details, since he was now fine, after drinking lots of water. But warming to the topic of health, he got up and took out a packet from the small metal kitchen cabinet where he kept his groceries. It was a packet of vitamin-fortified maize powder, a gift from his sister. He explained how easy it was to make: just add hot water, stir and wait a few minutes, and how much he liked it. He also showed me the back of the packet that listed the dozens of vitamins, minerals and amino acids with which the powder was laced. There was also a list of the product's benefits. These included boosting the immune system of people with AIDS. He pointed to this sentence carefully and specifically with his finger, while saying something innocuous about it being good for him. Bongani, only a few feet away, was unaware of this secret communication between us. Later, I thought that maybe I'd missed an opportunity to force the issue into the open. But, I reflected, he hadn't given me permission to do that. Rather, he had invited me into a conspiratorial silence. Like most invitations, it would not have been easy to spurn. Short of me making a scene, his pointing finger was binding me to his subterfuge.

Hidden truths

When I asked Bafana, in 2010, if I could formally interview him about living with the virus, he was keen and we fixed up a time when I would regularly visit during the week. I explained that I wanted to know more about how HIV-positive people understood their illness, something that the consent letter that he signed for me spelt out.

With the necessary ethical formality out of the way, my strategy with all those I interviewed was to keep away from discussing AIDS for as long as I could. I figured that if I wanted to know what people really believed about AIDS, opening our discussion with a set of direct questions was not the way to get below the answers that everybody in South Africa has been coached, through many and varied health promotion education campaigns, to recite about AIDS.

So, rather, I asked them about their lives, about their families, about their work, and about their neighbours. That I knew each person before the first interview opened made a difference; there were a number of occasions when they told me things that did not correspond with what I already knew. Referring to these inconsistencies would usually result in smiles and sometimes laughter at being caught out, though occasionally annoyance. Invariably, it helped me to better construct my understanding. But even as I pinned them down on occasion, I was more than happy to sidetrack into issues that might have no direct relevance for my research, if it seemed important to them. At times I would be fretting about time and just how many more interviews this was going to go on for, but I did my best to hide these feelings.

Inevitably, these discussions raised issues of health, sickness and treatment, but I strove to keep these interchanges away from direct discussion about AIDS, and confined to other illnesses or misfortunes. Nicodemiously, I hoped to survey the landscape of their beliefs, against which their account of AIDS could be measured. By the time we finally got to the subject of AIDS, my hope was that they would realise that I was indiscriminately interested in anything that they thought was important, and that my curiosity overrode any values or sanctions that might apply elsewhere. Such processes take time.

Of course, the process was not as neatly compartmentalised as this account suggests. There were a lot of mistakes, some embarrassing, along the way. It is in the reviewing of scribbled notes and the careful scrutiny of long interview transcripts, that it dawns on researchers that a particular issue needs to be returned to, a new line of questioning tried, a different framework of understanding employed, or whether, finally, we are done with a topic and can move on. But, in broad brushstrokes, this was how I stalked my eventual objective: what, really, did each individual think about AIDS? I started my quest with Bafana as my first interviewee. He was to demonstrate just how difficult this pursuit could be.

Fragments of a life

Bafana's parents had met in the early 1960s, in what is now Gauteng province. They had come from different corners of South Africa. His father, from the small Basotho homeland[7] of Qwaqwa,[8] jammed up hard into the Drakensberg mountains, where KwaZulu-Natal, the Free State and Lesotho come together. His mother, an Ndebele woman, hailed from the Northern Transvaal, close to the border with the then Rhodesia.[9] Both had come to work in the growing industries of the East Rand.[10] Bafana's father had kept his links to his *mahae* (true ancestral home, in this case Qwaqwa) until his death. They had married (Paseka was later to proudly show me the certificate) and Bafana, their fourth child, was born in 1971. He spent several years at his grandparents' home in Qwaqwa, attending primary school, but after that had rarely returned. Home for Bafana is Potlakong. The Sekasi that he speaks shifts with ease between Nguni- and Sesotho-heavy[11] versions, depending on whom he's talking to, but he is, without having to think about it, a Mosotho (ethnically Sotho). Sometimes, he will pull out a Sesotho *maele* (saying or aphorism) to make a point. Others will not have heard it and you might think he's making it up, but then you'll find it tucked away in Paroz's *Southern Sotho–English Dictionary*,[12] the last published, and long-dated, repository of the Sesotho tongue.

In 1979, his father's throat was slit by *tsotsis* (hoodlums) as he made his way home from work one Friday evening. A few years later, his mother was dragged under the wheels of a bus in the busy streets of Johannesburg. In his final years of school, his older sister was running the household. She had three children. The house was crowded. It wasn't a good space for studying. He failed matric.

It was not a major blow. It was still easy back then to find work, unemployment was rising, but the Group Areas Act[13] was only repealed in 1986 and it took time for the wave of immigration into the urban centres to gather pace. Bafana recalled how he'd be told by a neighbour, or a friend, working in the nearby industrial estates, that a company was looking for hands (casual labourers). After several short stints in different factories, Mpho, an older cousin, had tipped him off about a vacancy in Topshelf, the furniture factory where he worked. Mpho took him to see the supervisor and vouched for Bafana, who started cutting plywood sheets on a band saw. It was noisy and dusty work. In 2002, after ten years working on the same machine, he was clearing just over R3 000 a month. Hanging from his shack wall, above the TV, is a 10-year-long service recognition certificate from the furniture factory. The certificate says, in an italicised font, that Bafana Radebe has given '10 years of loyal service', but that omits the steady pilfering of furniture fittings that he had smuggled out of the factory to supplement his wages.

Refilwe, who grew up in Tembisa Township, and Bafana got to know each other as she was a frequent visitor to her aunt, a dozen doors down from the Radebe house in Potlakong. Bafana had had several girlfriends by then, but Refilwe was around at the time that he was growing up and wanted something more permanent. She was pretty. Unlike him, she had passed matric.[14] He thought she could have got better work than the receptionist job at a tyre and exhaust centre in town.

She all but moved in, and the house was even more crowded. Together, they looked for somewhere of their own. First they rented a backyard room nearby in Potlakong and bought furniture piece by piece on hire purchase. When there was hardly space for the two of them to squeeze in the room, they found a house to rent and married at the local magistrate's office. Two children followed: twins, Dineo and Neo, referred to collectively as 'Bodineo'.

Bafana gave the usual reasons for the various girlfriends he had had while he and Refilwe were together: sexual boredom and the 'home atmosphere'. Their arguments were usually over finances. Even when he showed her his payslip and could account for everything, the arguments didn't stop. There was always food in the house. She, however, was never satisfied, and soon he was resenting her demands for money. He worked the whole month, but there was nothing for him to *ithabisa* (to relax or enjoy himself with).

Although Bafana had started out on a path not dissimilar to his father, his *dinyatsi* (girlfriends on the side) spoke to the growing fragility of the 'patriarchal contract' that Mark Hunter[15] describes in the informal settlements of KwaZulu-Natal. Most of these relationships, fuelled by novelty and excitement, didn't last long. Each *nyatsi* knew he was married and that constrained each liaison to a fling. But each fling took a financial and emotional toll on the marriage.

Bafana and Refilwe's relationship continued to deteriorate. In the end, Refilwe had planned her move. On pay day in March 2005, Bafana had gone to withdraw his wages from the bank, but his bank card was not in his wallet. Inside the bank, the teller had accessed his account and told him there was nothing. He had rushed home to find out what he had feared, she had *thothile jwalo ka Maqhotsa* (left like the Xhosa woman, that is, stripped the marital house empty and gone).

He had then moved into the shack he now currently rented.

At first, he had thought he would be better off without Refilwe. Pulane, a girlfriend, had moved in with him. It was crowded, but fun. Then he was retrenched along with almost half the Topshelf workforce. His retrenchment letter explained that management 'had considered all possible alternatives to your redundancy, but unfortunately are not able to offer you an alternative position'. The letter went on to outline, scrupulously in line with South Africa's labour law, the payments due to him. As well as getting two weeks' pay for each year of service, his company was up to date with contributions to the statutory Unemployment Insurance Fund, ubiquitously referred to by its acronym UIF, and its contributions to an industry-wide provident fund. From the UIF, Bafana received a monthly unemployment payment designed to provide an income for workers between jobs. That lasted for six months. Then the payments stopped. Then Pulane moved out.

Finding a job was not easy. Bafana got by for two years. After Pulane left, he eked out his provident fund payment. He had deliberately delayed applying for it to be paid out, and kept Pulane in the dark about this financial stay. There were also odd jobs that he picked up around the township – clearing somebody's blocked toilet, a few days sweating it out as a *daka boy* (building labourer) mixing cement if someone in the area was building a house extension.

Then, despite his old company's retrenchment letter, they were in contact with him and he was informed that they were able to offer an alternative position. In fact he was back on the band saw. Only this time, they didn't, legally speaking, employ him. Rather he was now employed by the labour-broking company Firstjob, which boasted in its slogan of *People for Productivity*. Bafana now formed one corner of a triangular employment relationship. He worked at Topshelf, but was employed by Firstjob, who provided a labour-broking service to Topshelf. His new contract specified that his employment was contingent on there being an operational need, but this did not concern him; he had previously worked on the band saw for ten years and the work had never stopped. His new casual status was, in reality, ongoing. He had just become a 'permanent-casual'. The real drawback was clearing a lower wage than previously. And he found out the inventory system for the furniture fittings had been overhauled, apparently because of something called 'shrinkage'.

But he took the job. With nothing at home, he was out of options. He stuck it out for three years, until he started to get sick.

But we're not here to learn about AIDS

At the end of our second interview, Bafana pulled out a grubby form from a steel draw in the kitchen 'base' (cabinet). It was the incomplete application form for the provident fund that he had contributed to for the three years he had been employed by Firstjob, while working at Topshelf. As he had done previously, he had delayed drawing down his provident fund. He had figured that it was safe enough where it was and that he should pace his resources. Up till now he had managed with the UIF payments and a few odd jobs here and there. Well over a year later, and still without work, he needed to get hold of the money. Would I help him?

We filled in the form together. He'd been paying R40 a week into the fund. Over three years, that amounted to some R6 000 plus whatever interest had accrued. Bafana was satisfied with this, but would I come with him to the Firstjob offices to hand the form over? What he was really requesting was a lift, which would save him the taxi fare and, though he didn't spell this out, the value I'd be if the matter was not straightforward when we arrived at the Firstjob offices. We arranged to go the following week.

Firstjob is based in a large, brick office building a short distance from Boksburg CBD, one of the seven towns of the East Rand that, along with numerous industrial areas and their historically linked townships, are clustered together as Ekurhuleni, the eastern Gauteng Metropolitan Council.[16] It was a busy 45-minute drive from Bafana's shack to Firstjob's office. Alternatively, it would mean two taxi trips for Bafana, probably an hour and a half door-to-door, and a R40 round-trip fare. After negotiating with the company security guards, we found a large but almost empty waiting room.

The room clearly took a lot of traffic. The lower sections of the yellow-painted walls were dirty. There were around 30 chairs set around the room. At the far end was a sliding, mirrored-glass window labelled as 'Dispatch & Operations'. Beyond the window, which was open, I could see a shelf of flies, each one labelled with a vehicle's registration number and a driver's name.

In one corner, a group of three men, their chairs pulled together to face each other, spoke in Sepedi;[17] one had a ZCC badge[18] on his jacket. There were two other men keeping to themselves. They were waiting, Bafana explained, for casual work. Should somebody not turn up for a shift at one of the companies that Firstjob supplies with labour, one of those waiting would be dispatched in a company vehicle to plug the gap. By comparison, Bafana had been lucky with his three-year 'permanent-casual' placement.

After we handed in Bafana's application, we were told to wait and the mirrored glass of the window was slid closed. We were left to contemplate the yellow walls and a large laminated notice – in English, isiZulu and Setswana – informing us that our stay in the waiting room was entirely voluntary. We could not be considered as job applicants by virtue of merely being there. There was no catching Firstjob out with the small print of the Labour Relations Act! From the moment you walked in, your legal non-status as not-being-an-employee, nor having the rights that this would afford, was firmly established.

There was also a once colourful, but now dog-eared, poster that outlined how AIDS was contracted. It showed a cartoon drawing of a broken bottle with blood dripping from it, illustrating one transmission route. Sex was illustrated with a couple, of indeterminate race, sitting in bed. We were, the poster instructed, to use condoms. Perhaps somebody had thought that this would provide useful education for those in the room waiting for work.

Neither of us commented on the poster. I'm not sure Bafana even saw it. To fill the time, I asked him about Refilwe and whether he regretted that they'd broken up. Bafana took the question seriously, and after thinking for a while he answered, 'Nyala o nyele.' This is not a nice maele; it approximately translates as 'Marriage is like shitting in your pants.'

Then he corrected himself; it wasn't as though one could do without women. They were obviously necessary. The problem, he explained, was that men and women don't understand one another. There was the money. He told me again about how Refilwe refused to accept that he didn't have money to give her, even when he'd run through monthly expenses against his payslip. There was also the way she tried to control him; she had always wanted to know where he was. That was nice at first. It showed that she cared about him, but it became too much. She was jealous if he even looked at another woman. Before you knew it, she'd be accusing him of spending money on a *nyatsi*.

Nowadays, he explained, it was worse. He pulled out his cell phone. 'You've got to be careful. Cell phones make it easy [to arrange a meeting with a girlfriend], but, at the very same time, it makes it easy to split up.' The problem started when your spouse checked your phone to see whom you'd been talking to, and how often. Or perhaps you were too proud of a message to delete it and it got you into hot water. Cell phones were still uncommon when he and Refilwe were living together. Even if there had been a landline in the house, he'd never have used it to 'play around' with girlfriends; it was too risky. Bafana outlined a picture of a much slower epoch, though it was only some ten years earlier. Somehow you would strike up a conversation, perhaps in a minibus taxi going to work. They'd chat and arrange to meet, maybe they'd start to travel back home together regularly. He'd tell her he was married, and she'd tell him if she had a boyfriend. Typically, that was the situation – Bafana preferred younger women. They both had to be careful. He'd arrange to visit her one weekend, but just to be sure there wasn't a problem, he'd *etsa dipatlisiso* (do some research or make enquires) before knocking on the door. If they were both sly enough, they'd prearranged a sign that would signal the all-clear. The next liaison might not be for weeks. Without the convenience of cell phones, things went slower, but it was a pace that Bafana had been quite content with.

'So, did Refilwe ever find out about any of your girlfriends?' I asked. 'No,' was the response. Then he smiled, 'Well, she knew that I'd been outside when I had the *drop* (STI).' Bafana reckoned he had the *drop* five or six times before he and Refilwe moved in together. If he could, he would get pills from friends, rather than face being shouted at in the clinic,[19] and he was always careful to drink *dipitsa* (traditional medicine), which was easy to get at one of the township hostels. The doctor's pills might seem like a cure, but the *dipitsa* would clean you out from the inside, making sure that no dirt remained. The first time we'd talked about STIs, his account had ended pre-Refilwe. Now he explained that he'd been slow about sorting the problem out on one occasion. She had found out when washing his clothes and had found *boladu* (pus) on his underpants. That threw me. My questions dried up as a vision of what Refilwe had pulled from the washing basket, or perhaps picked up from the floor, seized my thoughts. We sat in silence.

When the mirrored-glass parted, Bafana and I were called to the window. We were told that we had filled in the wrong form. I braced myself and, getting ready for an argument, explained that we'd come specially to sort out Bafana's money. My fears of this being a stalling tactic were unfounded. Portia, the receptionist on duty, took a liking to the Radebe–Dickinson team. She got the right form, filled in the company's section, told us what we had to fill in, and send us on our way with detailed directions for getting to the bank so that we could get stamped verification of Bafana's bank account details.

When we arrived back from the bank, the waiting room had filled up. For firms operating a three-shift cycle, the two o'clock changeover between morning and afternoon shifts was approaching. But Portia waved us to the front. She checked that the form was correctly completed and volunteered to provide us with a reference number as soon Old Mutual,[20] the company to which Bafana's deductions had been paid, acknowledged receipt. She'd be faxing the form herself, but, 'just in case', she gave us their number.

The morning had gone well. The matter was as good as sorted. Keen to get back to the office where there was a mountain of work waiting, I dropped Bafana off at the Boksburg taxi rank with money for his fare home. As we arranged for the next interview, he suddenly remembered a piece of news that he'd been meaning to tell me. Ronnie, his friend whom we travelled with to Dr Tshabalala, was ill, *o kula haholo* (he's very ill). 'What the problem?' I asked. 'Same thing,' said Bafana. I hadn't seen Ronnie since the visit to Dr Tshabalala's. I suggested we visit him after our next interview, set for two weeks' time. But I didn't commit myself; I didn't want an extra obligation if my schedule was hectic.

Diagnoses and treatment

I need not have worried about finding time to visit Ronnie. By the time I next saw Bafana, Ronnie had died. Bafana had met me on the dirt road in front of his shack. There was a storm closing in and the sky was dark overhead. He told me the news as I was locking the car. The end had come quickly. Bafana recalled how he had visited Ronnie three days before he died. Ronnie had been sitting on a sofa outside his house where his mother and sister were looking after him. He had been taking in the sun under a blanket and Bafana had chatted to him for a while. He had told Bafana that he had been *docteng* (literally, the place of the doctor; in context, a private medical practitioner's surgery rather than a state facility or traditional healer) in the week, but the doctor had not been able to say what the problem was. Bafana didn't believe Ronnie. Shrugging his shoulders, he told me he had done his best to cheer Ronnie up, *ho tla loka* (it will be OK), he had tried to reassure him. Ronnie used to work as a petrol pump assistant and had suggested to Bafana that inhaling the petrol fumes might be the cause of the problem. Bafana didn't dismiss this out of hand, maybe there was something in it, but he thought Ronnie had been hiding whatever the real problem was.

There were heavy globs of rain starting to fall. Then, without warning, there was an almighty clap of thunder directly overhead and the rain started to bucket down. We both ran for the open door of his shack. Inside it was dark. The lightning strike had knocked out the electricity. It was all but impossible to talk with the noise of the rain on the zinc roof. We sat, in the gloom, waiting for the rain to subside.

Once it was quiet enough to talk, I started to ask Bafana what treatments he had undergone when he was sick. I was still circling the issue of HIV/AIDS and wanted to collect a full inventory of what treatment had been attempted. This was not straightforward. There was the treatment that Bafana had initiated, those which had been recommended and which he'd gone along with, and those which others had initiated and which he'd had no choice but to endure. Then there were a number of discussions about causes and remedies which were considered but didn't get beyond the talking stage.

He'd tried two doctors. The first had been a matter of taking pot luck in Boksburg town centre. He had walked into a doctor's surgery. The doctor had given him some pills and a three-day sick note. He'd charged R120 and said he could do tests, but that would cost more, as would an extended sick note. Bafana had not gone back. The second, Dr Mabaso, came recommended from Oupas, a taxi driver friend. Dr Mabaso had a surgery near one of the Potlakong taxi ranks and his waiting room was always full. Painted neatly on the outside wall were signs advertising '*Udokotela/Ngaka*' (Doctor, in isiZulu and Sesotho) along with his business hours and medical qualification: *MBChB (Natal)*. The first consultation had cost R170 and R30 for the injection. He was given a date to return for another injection. He'd had six in total, each cost R30, but he never found out what his problem was. Rather Dr Mabaso had assured him, 'You'll be fine, this injection will make you strong.'

He'd tried two traditional healers. I, of course, knew about his visit to Dr Tshabalala, but now Bafana filled me in on more details. On the day we'd gone over, she'd told him to bring his test results; she wanted to know if it was TB or HIV. But Bafana had no test results and, in any case, he'd been more concerned about getting directions to her surgery. When he'd gone into the *rondavel,* he'd handed over the R500 he'd been told to bring. This was to treat his hiccups and the boil. But she had told him that if he was HIV positive she could cure him, for R1 000. She'd also told him to tell other people. Bafana appreciated that she'd bother to phone him the next day to enquire if he was still feeling better.

He'd been twice to the second healer. Like Dr Tshabalala, Dr Manyi had come recommended, though this time by a relative rather than a workmate. Dr Manyi had given him a two-litre Coca-Cola plastic bottle filled with her *moriana* (medicine) for which she'd charged him R50. He didn't feel it had helped much and had discontinued the treatment.

Then there was prayer. Lots of it, though Bafana was vague about the details and clearly held little store by it. Various relatives and neighbours had prayed for him in the shack, in the hospital and while he was recuperating at his sister's home. Probably more people had prayed for him than Bafana was able to recount to me. Many Apostolic and Pentecostal church[21] members turn themselves enthusiastically into healers around sick beds. These are more than prayers for God's blessing and peace; they are requests for God to remove the *moya o ditshila* (evil spirit) at the heart of the patient's problems. With somebody like Bafana, this is an uphill struggle; it's no secret that he doubts God and is quite unconcerned about what some might consider his sins. As we'll see in later chapters, banishing *meya e ditshila* (evil spirits) demands fervent belief on the part of the *mokudi* (patient) as well as prayers and the laying on of hands in *Jesu*'s name by preachers, prophets or a patient's visitors.

Bafana did not, however, dismiss the prayers completely – he appreciated them as gestures of concern. It was important, he explained to me, that a sick person was encouraged. Moreover, Apostolic Church prophets were valuable in specific circumstances, such as fighting witchcraft. Bafana recounted how, as a young boy, he'd been ill, and in some kind of trance a church prophet had saved him. Bafana still distinctly remembers that while his body had been lying in his bed, his mind had been kept prisoner in somebody's kitchen which had all the paraphernalia of a witch. It was the prophet's prayers, he was quite certain, that had foiled the witch's scheme of enslavement.

What about witchcraft as a cause of his illness? The hiccups, he conceded, had been suggestive of *boloyi* (witchcraft) and the point had been discussed with him by family members. But neither healer had suggested 'throwing the bones',[22] and had both focused on the physical symptoms for which he had sought relief. If it was witchcraft, the healers would have suggested throwing the bones. He had seen Dr Tshabalala's set in the dim light of her *rondavel* and he was sure that Dr Manyi would have had the same or other means of divination, such as a mirror, to see who was bewitching him. To think otherwise was, Bafana suggested, like saying a doctor didn't have a stethoscope in their office and that they wouldn't have used it if they felt it was the right diagnostic tool. What would have really made the case for witchcraft would be a traditional healer turning up at the door to tell him that their ancestors had given instructions about somebody in the house who was bewitched. Then you would know for sure that witchcraft was afoot.

'So, it wasn't witchcraft?' I asked for final confirmation. But Bafana was demure, he didn't want to rule witchcraft out completely and returned to how *sejeso*, the practice of introducing a small animal to eat away inside you, was consistent with his hiccups. Such bewitchment was easy enough to do; most obviously the necessary *muthi* (traditional medicine, traditional magic) could have been put in his food. That was why, he explained, he was always happier eating at a *lefung* (funeral) rather than a *mokete* (function). At the former you queued up along with the other mourners for your plate of food, which is served from large pots in front of everybody. It would be impossible for somebody to target your meal. But at a *mokete*, when the plates of food were brought out from the kitchen for the guests as they arrived? He raised his eyebrows, indicating that absolutely anything could happen between the time the food was dished out and it was handed to you, as you sat with the men in the yard. Even harder to stop was *sejeso* introduced via a dream. If you dreamed that you were eating, that was a sure sign somebody was bewitching you.

Bafana was warming to the subject now. He was no longer talking about himself, but about *sejeso* in general. Treatment required the expertise of a traditional healer. They would induce vomiting to remove whatever was inside you. It could, he elaborated, be a frog, a snake, or a lizard, or ...

He must have caught the scepticism in my face. I've heard firsthand accounts of people diagnosed with *sejeso* who have vomited out creatures, but these have been described as pieces of meat, too large to have been swallowed whole, which must, therefore, have been a malevolent creature still in a stage of re-constitution or creation. Whole creatures being vomited out are commonly cited, but always as third-hand accounts. Bafana started protesting at my facial slip.

'It's true. I've read it!' Then he started laughing, 'OK, it was in *The Daily Sun*.'[23] But even as he acknowledged the sensational nature of his source, he was only going to retract the more lurid passages of his *sejeso* account. Backtracking prior to the disruption that the menagerie of *sejeso* creatures had introduced, I pursued the slim possibility of witchcraft being responsible for his condition. For the sake of completeness, I asked him, if it had been witchcraft, 'Who might have been responsible?' 'Obviously,' he responded, '[It would be] Refilwe [his ex-wife].' Obvious it might be, but he was still leaving open different possibilities. *Sejeso* can serve two purposes. It can be used to harm an enemy or it can be used to control or bring back a lover: '*Sheba nna feela*' (Look only at me). Sometimes, it is suggested that *sheba nna feela* can go wrong, and the lover ends up ill rather than besotted. I assumed Refilwe would be suspected of using it for the former purpose, but the second was not impossible to imagine; she might want Bafana back, especially if he was working.

'Was anything else talked about when you were ill?' I asked. Bafana paused to think and said that there had been talk of a *kotlo* (blow or punishment) from the *badimo* (ancestors). There had been several problems in his extended family over the last two years, more deaths than usual and a cousin had been stabbed in an argument. His own illness could be added to these problems. Not that the ancestors would kill people, but maybe they had felt neglected, even annoyed. It was also true that the extended family had not gathered together for some time. Younger members didn't even know one another. If so, maybe the ancestors would be less vigilant in protecting you, perhaps they would even allow something to happen. It could be a way of their telling people that they were being neglected. 'It's not', Bafana sought to clarify for me, 'that they'd make you ill, like by sending TB. *Mare* (but) on the other side [also] maybe there is something else.' He was suggesting that the something else constituted a parallel explanation located in a different dimension. 'Like if you're [be]witched.' He illustrated what he was explaining by returning to witchcraft. 'We know you're sick, but on the other side, there is that something else.'

'So,' again, I was trying to get a firmer reply, something that I could clearly capture in my notebook, 'maybe it was a *kotlo*?' He responded by making a face. It wasn't something he thought was important in regard to his illness. Rather, as he had told me, it was an explanation that some people had talked about. We moved on.

We were still in the gloom. I was exhausted from this long narration about the various treatments and possible explanations that Bafana had laid out for me over the last two hours. However, despite being tired, I was intrigued about how Bafana's friends might have contributed to these different diagnoses. All the talk that he had reported to me was about discussions in the family. Yet, Bafana was often with a friend whom he'd introduce to me, usually somebody he'd grown up with, or had been to school with, or worked with. You'd meet one friend and the next time you'd meet another. Other than Ronnie accompanying us to Dr Tshabalala's, and Tokelo's invitation to accompany him to the AIDS counsellor, none of them seemed to have been involved in his illness. So I asked what these many friends had said about his illness.

Bafana was candid. They hadn't talked openly with him. Rather, they had encouraged him: '*ho tla loka*'. But he knew what they were saying *ka thoko* (on the side) – that he had AIDS. He knew that they did it because he'd done the same thing with other people. Ronnie, for example.

'Did you ever talk openly with any of them?' I asked, without myself being completely open about what it was I was asking.

'Only Mosa,' Bafana replied.

I had to ask Bafana who Mosa was. I'd apparently met him, but I couldn't recall him among the many people whom Bafana had introduced me to over the years as his friends.

Bafana continued, 'We went to the clinic together. He had the same thing.' They had found themselves sitting together in the clinic, waiting for the HIV counsellor.

'And now?' I asked.

Mosa was dead.

As I drove out of the township, I felt as though I was fleeing a world saturated in death. I've lived in the same modest, middle-class suburb for ten years and I know my neighbours. I've not yet been to a funeral for somebody from the neighbourhood. In the township, I've long got used to the Saturday morning burials, but now I seemed to be drawing further into a world in which death is everywhere. In which any enquiries could add to the tally. Didier Fassin[24] notes the same grim situation that the AIDS researcher enters in South Africa. After the death of a young woman whom he interviewed, Fassin writes, 'Investigating AIDS is like working on sand. Each time I return, I am informed about those whom I know and who are no more.' Yet, it is not only the researcher who finds that they tread without traction. Those who are dying seek explanations. Which are offered in profusion, but which do not hold – over AIDS, everything is sand.

Penalty shoot-out

The next time I interviewed Bafana, he had a cough and was complaining about a headache. I suggested *setlamatlama* (hangover), but he denied it; despite taking pills, the pain had remained. He thought it was *nyoko*. What he needed was a 'full service'. He would use pills (laxatives) and would also *kapa* (induce vomiting, see Chapter 1). The problem, he volunteered, was that he didn't *kapa* on a regular basis. His mother, when she was alive, used to prepare a bucket of warm water every Monday morning for him. This prevented *nyoko* building up and causing a problem, as it was now doing. Despite feeling under the weather, he assured me he was up for the interview.

What, I asked Bafana after a few follow-up questions on the previous interview, had they told him at the hospital? They had told him he had TB. This had been a surprise to Bafana. Nobody had thought he had TB. But he explained to me now that there were different kinds of TB. Sometimes the symptoms were just like HIV. 'What were these?' I probed. Bafana reeled off a list: losing weight, the skin became dry, the hair dull, then there were the lips, they would become pink. He was talking about Black people. He pulled down his lower lip to show that it was pink on the inside. You'd see this colour on the outside, he explained.

I moved on. 'Did they test for HIV at the hospital?'

'Yes,' he responded.

'And what did they say?'

'No, they said I was *sharp* (good).'

'They said you were *sharp*. Did they say if you were positive or negative?'

Bafana hesitated. '*Ha ke hopole hantle*' (I don't remember well). '*Empa* (but) they said I would be *lekker* (good/fine).'

I asked about the clinic. He'd attended his first appointment there two weeks after being discharged from the hospital. Thereafter, he'd gone every month to collect his TB treatment. Had he been tested for HIV there?

'Yes.'

'And did they tell you the result?'

'They said it was positive.'

'Positive?'

'Positive. The same as Mosa.'

'OK. Thanks. So what happened after they said you were positive?'

He'd had a CD4 test to determine the strength of his immune system. He couldn't remember what it was. Maybe around 200,[25] he suggested. They had told him it was good. Then he'd been sent to see a counsellor who had talked to him about living healthily. After that, there had been home visits from a *mofumahadi* (an older woman) to check that he was taking his TB medication.

I went back to the testing. 'So they said you were *sharp* at the hospital and at the clinic they said you were HIV positive?'

'Yes.'

My turn to pause; I was wondering how to tie this down. Bafana was hedging, but the message he was trying to get across was that he'd had two HIV tests and the results had been different. It was a draw: one all. I needed a penalty decider. 'If you went back to the clinic,' I suggested, 'do you think you'd test positive or negative?'

'*Ha ke tsebe hantle*' (I'm not really sure), he replied and we both burst out laughing. Sometimes in research, it's best to accept defeat, at least for the time being. I would come back to this in a later interview.

Meroho le jwala (Vegetables and beer)

'What did the counsellor tell you?' I asked, moving on to what I assumed would be an easy topic. But whatever the counsellor had told him hadn't made a strong impression. He did recall the need to eat vegetables. He started to list the vegetables he knew. This was not a long list: *kgabetjhe* (cabbage), *cumumberi* (cucumber), *ditamati* (tomatoes). Then he stalled, racking his brains for more vegetables. He knew he was supposed to know more, but Bafana is a *pap* and *nama* (maize starch and meat) man. He doesn't have much time for vegetables other than eating what's on his plate *moketeng* (at a celebration or event). I was about to step in with another question, when he suddenly pulled out a final contribution to his list; '*meroho!*' He was triumphant; *meroho* is a Sesotho word for spinach or other green leaves, but it can also be used as a generic term covering all vegetables. Topping his list with *meroho* meant that he had to delve no further into his limited knowledge, or appetite, for vegetables. From the satisfied look on his face it was clear that he felt he had scored full marks on this question.

'Did the counsellor tell you anything else?' I asked. 'Yes,' he answered, she had told him about the importance of eating regularly. I'd had a long discussion with Bafana on how he always liked to have something to eat in the house. He'd talked about how he'd eke out a *Two KG* (a 2kg bag of frozen chicken pieces) for as long as possible to avoid being reduced to *pap 'n lebese* (maize porridge and milk), a staple meal of poverty. I agreed that he was careful that he always had something to eat. But I also thought about him passed out in front of the electric heater with a half-finished plate of food in his lap, spoon in hand. 'What about *jwala* (beer/alcohol)?' I asked.

Although I'd had to probe on this issue, it seemed *jwala* had been prominent in the advice he'd received from the councillor. Bafana explained, drawing on what he could remember of the sessions, that alcohol was something you had to be very careful about. He illustrated the point with an example. 'Why was Mosa dead while he, Bafana, was alive?' I had to wait for Bafana to explain. The answer was brandy. Mosa drank brandy and brandy was *bohale* (strong). It damaged your lungs. Mosa had died gasping for breath; he hadn't listened to the advice about liquor (i.e. spirits). Bafana raised an eyebrow to emphasise his point. That brandy damages lungs is a common belief in the townships and I let it pass without comment. But I pushed Bafana about his drinking beer. How come he was drinking, if he'd been told it was dangerous? But he countered my query, he had taken the advice. He had not drunk during the nine months of his treatment.

'Then you started again?'

Bafana gave me a look. 'Yes.' Once he felt fine, once he was *sharp*, of course he was going to drink. It was so obvious, that he didn't need to spell it out for me. What would be the point of getting better if you weren't able to drink?

After we'd wrapped up for the day, and I was writing out the receipt for his research honorarium, he made a suggestion. Christmas was only a few months away. When the companies closed, people would have their December pay and annual bonus, and nearly all would be drawing down on some kind of saving that they had been making over the year. *Batho ba tla ithabisa* (People will enjoy themselves). Fully translated, what he was saying was that the men who stayed in the township over the four-week shutdown would have money to buy beer and he wouldn't.

Bafana was pointing to a bleak time ahead. It wasn't just that he wouldn't have money to buy beer. It would mean that he didn't have the money to drink with those who were enjoying themselves. He faced the prospect of sitting in his shack, on his own, watching the TV, while outside, for weeks on end, his friends would be sitting, laughing, joking, drinking and fooling around. There would be music blasted into the streets, there would be sessions that went on into the night, sessions that went on all night and into the next morning. And Bafana would have to hide himself in his shack, making excuses about why he couldn't join them.

So, I agreed to his proposal. I would give him half the honorarium now, and keep half. That way, he would build up savings and be able to hold his own, at least for a while, in the coming festivities. I pledged that, even if he begged me, I would not hand over the savings he would accumulate with each interview before Christmas.

The Two Sisters Tavern

In the months before Christmas, I drove out to Potlakong as often as I could. I was steadily consolidating my understanding of Bafana's world. Sometimes I would have to double back on an issue to be sure. Bafana was happy to repeat himself; the honorarium I paid for each interview, now split 50/50 between *kontane* (cash) and his *seketekete* (piggy bank), as we jokingly referred to as his savings tally, meant his pocket and his future were not completely empty.

My research was progressing, but despite the promises from Portia at Firstjob, progress on Bafana's provident fund had stalled. One morning, he sent me a 'please-call-me'[26] message. When I called back, he told me that Portia had rung earlier in the week, and informed him that his provident fund had been paid out. Except that the money wasn't in his account. He was worried that maybe there was a problem with his bank account number. Since I would be in the township that coming Saturday, I suggested we meet.

When I got to his shack the chain was threaded through the hole in the plywood door and around the frame. It was padlocked closed. Bafana was out and his phone was off, probably the battery was dead. But he was not hard to track down. From the direction and manner of his departure, the consensus was on the Two Sisters Tavern a couple of streets away. Tshepo, one of my *loxion manager* friends, who was particularly sure that we'd find him in the tavern, and was himself fond of a drink, came with me.

The Two Sisters Tavern is a converted residential garage. At the back, there are fridges behind a counter with serving hatches in the metal grille that reaches to the ceiling. There's a pool table, plastic tables and chairs, and posters that blend beer and sport in bright cheerful colours. At night, the roller door comes down and they serve till the customers leave. During the day, and if it's warm, the door is up and people spill out into the front yard, and onto the street. Those inside have to talk loudly over the noise of the two competing television sets. The toilets are out the back, behind the house, where, in a small concrete yard, there are stacks of empty beer crates. When it's busy, they are used as seats out in the front yard.

With some rearrangement of chairs, we sat together at one of the tables. Space was tight and, every now and again, a pool player manoeuvred his cue over our heads as he paced the table, seeking the best position for a shot. Tshepo went to the grille with my money. He elected for a Castle Lite, I stuck to Coke, Bafana declined the offer of a drink, pointing out that his quart of *Zamalek* was still two-thirds full.

The matter of the provident fund was quickly dispatched. We agreed that we'd use my phone to ring Portia after our next interview set for the following week and, if necessary, we'd go to Firstjob again. He agreed to check his bank account once more, just in case the transfer was delayed. We moved on to other topics and he morbidly lamented that he hadn't seen his two children for over a year. After Refilwe departed, she'd demanded maintenance. He'd told her he'd pay it when she returned the things she'd taken. He ended up in police cells when she'd taken the matter to the Maintenance Court. After that, he'd started to pay and she allowed him to visit the children. Then he stopped paying maintenance and visiting when he lost his job. 'But you could ring them?' I suggested. He was nursing his bottle of *Zamalek,* but telling me that he didn't have airtime to say hello to his children.

It would have been rude to point out directly this contradiction to Bafana. Tshepo, however, got straight to the crux of the matter once we had left. In Bafana's presence, I'd instead pointed out the way that he was pacing his drinking. It was in contrast to a common weekend pattern of drinking till you are *tauwe* (really drunk). Over time such practice bestows on drinkers an enormous capacity to consume alcohol during sessions that stretch as long as the money holds out. By comparison, Bafana was drinking responsibly.

He again reiterated that he didn't drink brandy. He told me that for someone like himself who is ill it would be dangerous. We were back into the conversation about his health and how he was looking after himself. He told me there was something that he had forgotten the previous time we spoke; he had had a 'narrow escape' over his drinking. With his TB treatment coming to an end, he'd been contemplating shifting from his long-term tipple of *Zamalek* to Hunter's Dry cider. This was based on an assumption that a drink based on *ditholwana* (fruit), like cider, would be good for him. But no! To his surprise, he had heard from somebody, who had got it from a nurse, that this was far from being the case. To the contrary, the fruit used to make cider had been *senyehile* (spoiled, damaged or rotten). *Ha e loke* (It's not OK). In fact, he continued, it was a dangerous drink for someone who is positive.

I noted that he'd said positive, but didn't interrupt his account. I was fascinated by the lay theory he was outlining. He went on to contrast the 'acidified' fruit in cider with the wholesome ingredients of beer. Conveniently, we had a teaching aid to hand and he lifted up his bottle of *Zamalek*, by now half empty, so that I could read from the label the short but nutritious list of contents: water, barley and hops. Happy that he had made his point, Bafana shrugged and put the bottle back down on the table. He rested his quart and his case – clearly he was much better off having stayed with his original tipple. It had been a close call.

Tshepo had downed his Castle Lite by the time Bafana was approaching the last third of his *Zamalek*. As Tshepo and I got up to go, Bafana reminded me of my previous offer of a drink. I smiled at my naivety in thinking that in pointing to his two-thirds-full bottle he had permanently declined my offer of a drink. I handed over a *tiger* (R10 note).

The window and the chair

It was necessary to go to Firstjob again. Once I got hold of Portia on the phone, she told me I needed to talk to Old Mutual; they, she said, had told her the policy had been paid out a long time ago. I was beginning to wonder if Bafana might be using me in trying to pull off some kind of scam. I rang up Dimpho at Old Mutual. I didn't have a reference number, but Bafana's identity number[27] was good enough for the policy to be traced. Dimpho was helpful and clear. Yes, the policy had been opened in June 2006, the month Bafana started employment with Firstjob, but it had been closed the following month, July 2006.

I made Bafana search high and low for his old payslips. I helped by peering into the very dirty space between the zinc wall of his shack and the two-plate electric stove, in case any of them had fallen behind. The running totals itemised on the payslips that we located established that there had been deductions every month of the three years of employment with Firstjob/Topshelf. I took the payslips, made copies, and had them certified by a commissioner of oaths.[28]

When we went to Firstjob, Thuso, another of Bafana's friends, came along. He happened to be visiting Bafana that day and came for the ride. On the way to Boksburg, Bafana asked me if I thought Firstjob was doing things properly. I said 'no', and went on to say that they had either made a *phoso* (mistake) or *leano* (trick or scam), but in either case we were the ones who were being put to inconvenience and cost – *ba bapala ka batho* (they play with people).

I was trying to keep an open mind over Firstjob, but I was aware that, without me, Bafana would not have got this far, his provident fund contributions would have been written off. Not because a rational calculation would demonstrate that the costs involved in pursuing this had now outstripped the value of his provident fund. It would take many round-trip taxi fares to balance that equation. Rather, it was because, without my car and my support to tip the scales, he would have already gloomily concluded that more effort and more money would achieve nothing; he wasn't going to see whatever had been accumulated in his provident fund. The odds were stacked against him. But today was a different matter; driving out of Potlakong playing Johnny Clegg's *Impi*[29] loudly on the car stereo, we were part outing, part war-party.

As we drove, Bafana pointed out township landmarks to me and explained how on occasions, when he was younger, he had walked long distances through Potlakong at night after drinking in far-flung *shebeens* (unlicensed drinking venues). He would carry a weapon; the township was dangerous if you were walking alone at night. He talked about his Bowie knife as a convenient *thipa* (knife) to carry with such vividness that I wondered if it wasn't under his jacket as we were driving. I was relieved when I checked and he told me he had left it in the shack.

Once we got to Firstjob we handed over the payslips through the hatch and waited. After 20 minutes the response we received, from a woman we hadn't seen before, was that they would make copies and be in touch. We were being fobbed off, but we weren't having it.

I said we had copies, handed them over and stuck insistently to the point that I wanted to speak to the person who would be dealing with the matter. I refused to cede the hatch and leant in on the right-hand side, so that the glass window couldn't be slid shut. Bafana and Thuso stuck with me and also took up positions. Between us we had most of the hatch blockaded. Now Portia, brought from the back office by our persistence, explained to us why Ingrid, who would deal with the matter, was unable to see us that day. We didn't budge. I did the talking. I stayed polite but firm; we had come a long way, this was the second time we had come, the matter was straightforward, and we wanted to speak to the person who would sort it out. Eventually, Portia, who had been turned into something of a shuttle diplomat between us and Ingrid in the back room, came with the message that Ingrid would see us shortly.

We held our positions, though allowed those in the queue that had formed behind us to squeeze between us with their requests. If we didn't already suspect it, their inquiries confirmed that Bafana wasn't the only person having problems with his provident payment. Our stand, inconvenient as it might be, was clearly welcomed by those in the waiting room.

Ingrid finally came out, a White woman still in her twenties; she was nervous and clearly unused to dealing with plaintiffs in the waiting room. I carefully explained the situation. She immediately undertook to sort the matter out. I raised a few details: would they pay Bafana the interest that the fund would have accumulated if his contributions had been paid over to Old Mutual? Ingrid replied that she had to sort out what had happened; even if the policy had been closed, the deductions might still have been paid to Old Mutual. Once she had established the facts she would be in a position to respond. I saw her point; clearly she had only just been made aware of the situation. Her request for time was reasonable. I asked for a commitment to resolve the matter by the end of the week and she agreed. Winding down the encounter, I thanked her, cheerily said goodbye to Portia, and turned to Bafana, telling him that we had done what we could for the day, but Bafana wasn't ready to leave.

To my surprise, he started to have a go at Ingrid. Emboldened by our small victory in getting the White *madam*[30] out from the back office, Bafana's anger was bubbling to the surface. I was taken aback that my careful de-escalation of the situation, allowing us to part on cordial terms, had completely passed him by. His voice was rising to wrath. While we had jointly held the hatch, he had told me and those within earshot that he would never work for a labour broker again. They played with people and cheated them. Everybody knows that, but to say that out loud here in Firstjob's offices had been an act of social rebellion. I had not seen the significance at the time. Now, his anger was boiling and in a rising tone he vented not about his provident fund, but how Firstjob treated people badly and that labour brokers exploited people. His anger was resonating with those in the waiting room who had the same experiences. Ingrid had backed away from the hatch as far as she could without fleeing into the back office. Portia was getting ready to slam the window shut, but she hesitated; the mirrored glass might separate the two sides, but it wasn't a solid barrier. Closing the window would be an act of moral defeat and could well further escalate the situation. I could see a chair would end up being hurled through the glass. I spoke directly to Bafana in Sesotho, hosing him down, telling him that it was reasonable that Ingrid have some time to sort his payment out. Ingrid had no idea what I was saying, but she nodded furiously in support. In South Africa, when the chips are down, race trumps pretty much everything. Bafana subsided and we walked out together.

Despite the complex finale to our excursion, we were on a high by the time we got to the car. Perhaps my intervention had allowed Bafana to speak his mind without having to follow through in action. There was much more talk about how contractors were ripping people off and we went for KFC in Boksburg on the strength of our victory. I bought Streetwise Three-piece meals all round. We were hungry. Bafana carefully saved one piece of chicken to take home in the brightly coloured red-and-white box.

Condoms

On my next visit, Bafana reported that Ingrid had rung him. She needed the start and end dates of his employment. Bafana hadn't had these to hand and said he would ring her back, for which he used my phone. With that done, we got back to my research. I returned to his views on condoms. Previously, he'd impressed on me that he used condoms. In fact, to emphasise the point, he explain how with *Mzanzi Fosho* (the government's *Choice* free condoms[31]), he would 'double up' (use two condoms at once) to be sure since he didn't fully trust them. I started by asking him again about doubling up.

He did, this conversation confirmed, double up with *Mzanzi Fosho*, but only on the first time he had sex with a woman, especially if he didn't know if she was 'clean'. This was different from previous conversations, especially the 'first time' bit. With this slight nuance, a crack in his account appeared. And once a fault opens it will often widen. Increasing trust in a partner, Bafana outlined, ends up with the condom being discarded. Bafana illustrated this with a rapid flick of his hand, just as Kabelo had done when we had talked about his Three Plus One in the shade of the Syringa tree, to illustrate the condom being thrown onto the floor, as though it had now become a dirty thing that could not be cast away too quickly. But he was ahead of his story of mutual trust. Told step by step, it starts with doubling up because you're afraid. You're attracted and you're fearful at the same time, especially with AIDS, because it's everywhere. But as you get to know her, two condoms become one and soon you're hoping that she'll say *'entshe!'* (take it off!). Then there will be none.

'So you don't really like them?' I suggested supportively. Pushing into this private territory, I know I'm flouting public health messages. I was in tricky terrain. It felt as though I were stalking a bird, trying to get close. It will fly if I move too quickly or clumsily, but equally it will startle if I stop. I must calibrate my moves carefully even as I'm making them.

'Because of the feelings,' Bafana replied.

He used English, referring to the pleasure of flesh-on-flesh sex, though emotional feelings are wrapped up with this pleasure. With the plastic in place he sometimes struggled to come. Sex is like eating; you might be ravenous and the food might be *masutsa* (delicious), but there comes a time to finish. If you tell her that you're struggling to come, it's a cue for her love – *entshe!*

'So women want to get the condom off as well?' I asked, now more confidently pursuing the topic.

Bafana considered my question. 'Some,' he says. But it's not all of them. He told me about Nthabiseng. She had insisted on condoms and had once pushed him out to check.

'That you were wearing a condom?'

'No, she thought the condom might have blasted [burst].'

'Had it?'

Bafana grinned bashfully. 'I knew it had.' Nthabiseng had suspected as much and stormed off. That was the last time they'd slept together.

Other than with Nthabiseng, however, a burst condom was a good reason for leaving them *thoko* (on the side) for good – as long as this didn't happen too early, when you still didn't really know much about each other – before you'd had chance to reassure each other that you always used condoms with people you didn't know well.

'The other thing', Bafana continued unprompted, 'is *jwala* (alcohol). If you *tauwe* (drunk) they [condoms] take away the enjoyment.'

'For men and women?'

'For both. If she's *tauwe*, she'll want it off just like the man.'

'But, you think people would use them again if they're sober?'

Bafana looked at me. It was the same look he had given me when I'd asked about him starting to drink again when he'd completed his TB treatment. 'What would the point be?' he asked rhetorically and shrugged his shoulders as if to say that there was no point in going back to them. 'If they blast, it's the same thing,' he added.

'Unless you're with Nthabiseng,' I thought, but kept quiet.

Undisturbed by my silent deviancy, he gave the example of Thandeka. The condom had blasted on the fourth time, if he remembered correctly. After that, they hadn't bothered with them.

Back home, going over my notes, I concluded that this was as far as it goes with condoms. Bafana had not held back and I could take his explanation at face value. On the topic of condoms, we had reached what he really felt about them. There were no more layers to uncover.

He didn't like condoms. However well they were promoted, branded or marketed, nobody could tell him they didn't reduce the pleasure of sex. He could feel that for himself. You could talk yourself blue in the face saying otherwise, but you'd be wasting your time.

To use Bafana alone to make this point would, it struck me, be to hide behind him. Sometime previously, I myself had had a condom burst during sex. The surge of pleasure had been intense. It had been a hurried tryst and I thought perhaps the change was a late surge of fluids that had heightened the pleasure. More likely, I reasoned with sober hindsight, I'd wanted to believe that this was the case. When I had withdrawn, the condom was ripped open.

It's not easy to accept something that is obvious, but that you've long refused to confront. There are plenty of people, outside the heat of sex, that proclaim condoms make no difference. I was humbled to realise that, despite my own experience, it took Bafana to bring me around to the fact that this is disingenuous. I thought about the oft-repeated and indignant accounts from well-meaning educationalists about men refusing to use a condom because they were scornfully reported to say that wearing a condom was like 'eating sweets with the wrapper on'. But, I had to admit to myself, that was exactly what it is like. It may be an inconvenient truth, but it's a very good description of a key limitation of condoms; the dulling of pleasure, barrier to intimacy and damper of spontaneity. Not of a mundane, take-it-leave-it pleasure, but a deeply intense and primordial pleasure, one that can be only offset by the fear and tensions of initial encounters.

Pleasure is easy to dismiss with words, much harder to discount in the flesh. Which is why condoms have failed to stop the epidemic. Moreover, they will continue to fail whenever concurrent partners are more than one-night stands. The ABC slogan tells people to condomise if they can't abstain or be faithful. Do people really believe it? Don't they see that sensible words are no match for the trump card of intimate, exquisite pleasures of the flesh? 'Use condoms until you've tested' might stand a chance, if test kits were as easy to get your hands on as condoms. But nobody's suggesting that. The vast testing endeavours now under way, with an army of counsellors and an army of non-governmental organisations (NGOs) and government posts, have become too vested in their own existence to consider allowing HIV-testing kits to be sold like pregnancy tests over the counter. Rather, we just carry on punting the failed line about condoms. Bafana and I make a small sample, but we are part of the world's largest-ever condom experiment. Millions upon millions upon millions of condoms are being distributed in South Africa every year but we can't dispute that even in their millions they have failed to stop the epidemic.

Bafana helped me see this once his true feelings about condoms came eventually into view. But what surprised me was the way in which his honesty disappeared from view again. I'd assumed that once we'd reached this level of understanding, the rock-bottom truth from which there was no further descent, then we'd stay there. Bafana and I would continue to share this understanding, even if he would keep up pretences when others were present. But it wasn't like that. On later occasions he'd happily give me the official line on condoms. Once he went into some detail as to how a couple should use condoms until they wanted to 'etsa (make) family planning' (i.e. to have a baby). That time would come, he confidently explained, when the couple knew that they were 'right' for a family. It was at these times that I was grateful for my notes and the tapes of our discussions to confirm that he had clearly outlined a more complex, and much more compelling, picture of condom use, even if only briefly.

Dancing in and out of view

Between interviews with Bafana, I was regularly driving between Johannesburg and Butleng in the Free State. It's a four-hour drive, but one that I enjoy. Coming out of Johannesburg, I pull into the Grasmere One Stop service station and buy the biggest black coffee they serve and sweeten it with white sugar. The coffee lifts my mood for the long, flat road ahead, giving me time to ponder problems that are otherwise crowded out from my schedule.

On this trip, with the caffeine kicking in, Jackson Browne's *Late for the Sky* on the car stereo, and the traffic of the city behind me, I was thinking through the complex truth of condom use. As the kilometres streamed past, I realised that this was not the only thing that was dancing in and out of view. I had to admit to myself that I didn't really know if Bafana was HIV positive. Not with a certainty that was unshakeable. I had started with that certainty, but it had loosened. Of course he was positive, I reassured myself with the macabre reasoning that there would be another health crisis. But, 'on the other side', to paraphrase Bafana himself, I had to accept there was room for doubt. There might even be dubiety over his status as we lowered him into the grave.

My attempt to have a penalty shoot-out and decide on a best out of three was as good a place as anywhere to start this meditation. I could see now that Bafana had absolutely no intention of testing again. As far as he was concerned, one HIV test was positive, but one test was negative. 'So,' he was suggesting to me and anybody else who was prying into his life, 'who can really say?' Perhaps it was not so surprising that we'd both started laughing, as he'd been telling me, very politely, to back off. What he didn't want was another test. What he needed was to throw up more obstacles to the veracity of his status, like earthworks around a fortress. He needed us and himself to be unable even to formulate the question that would challenge his citadel of doubt.

I was struck by the way he was telling me that TB and HIV were not really different. He never lost an opportunity to make this point: *Di batla di tshwana* (they're almost the same), *Ha di fapane haholo* (they're not very different). I was particularly struck by the way he had illustrated this once by holding his two index fingers together in front of him so that I could see them aligned. One was HIV, one was TB, '*Di haufiyane* (they're really close together),' he had said. The shared list of symptoms had grown from the original handful he had provided to encompass everything that had ailed him when hospitalised. Now, he was expounding how both TB and HIV attacked *masole a mmele* (the soldiers of the body or immune system). When I had asked him about TB, he had explained that there were different types. He'd once heard on the radio that there were three types, but a nurse at the hospital had said there were actually 17; he was not sure which kind he had.[32] What I realised he wanted me to conclude, because he never, not once, said it outright, was that the sum of his illness was TB. He couldn't say that he was negative, because he knew I'd baulk. But he could make me doubt myself. And, of course, this was not just about me; he had other audiences, the people he lived with day by day, to steer in the same direction.

I left off the question as to whether Bafana was positive or negative. I believed he was HIV positive, but I had to accept that he'd carefully constructed uncertainty around his status. Though this was slightly galling, I had to respect the choice that he'd made. But if this was the case, then how did I distinguish between the ambiguity he constructed around his own status and his beliefs about AIDS? The more doubts about AIDS, the more doubts there could be about himself. Witchcraft was a good example; he didn't believe he was bewitched, but if he kept open the possibility that, maybe, witches could send AIDS, or something that looked like AIDS, then there was another trench in the earthworks of doubt that I or anybody else who might be curious has to manoeuvre around.

As my journey came to an end, and Butleng township came into view, I made a decision. I was going to go along with what Bafana was doing. I was going to recognise what Bafana wanted me to see; that he had a unique form of TB that mimics HIV so closely that the two could not be distinguished, even with a test. Teasing myself, I named this new strain of TB *Bafanitus-FauxHIVarius*. I could see that there were ethical issues beyond anything remotely conceived in the project's ethics application, but I wanted to see if I'd got Bafana sussed. Although I hadn't gone looking for this, it lay at the very heart of my research. Was it really that under my nose, as we'd been talking, he'd been reconstructing his illness, using me to test out ideas and suggestions, to a point where it was no longer clear to anybody, including himself, what the problem was?

What is AIDS?
Back in Potlakong, and once again with Bafana, I made my move. I started by explaining that I wanted to talk again about his *boemo* (situation, though it also means status). I said that we didn't really know whether he'd got HIV or something similar to it. Could he

explain the situation to me?

Bafana smiled and then nodded to show that he was taking my question seriously. In this carefully waged campaign in which he'd been constructing meaning around his illness, I'd finally conceded ground to him. Yes, he confirmed, he had something that was similar to HIV, but it wasn't HIV, it was TB. He knew this because it hadn't returned. But, he continued, if he did have HIV, he thought that he was strong enough to keep at bay. That was why it was important that he look after himself. I waited, realising that he'd also given me ground, he didn't want to make too strong a case, he'd rather that his *boemo* lie in a middle ground of equivocation. He wasn't HIV positive, but neither was he categorically saying that he'd not got HIV. He continued, 'If it returns,' (he didn't say what 'it' was and I didn't ask), 'then I'll go back to the clinic.'

I thanked Bafana for this explanation and started to ask him about AIDS. It was an easy discussion. We were talking about AIDS, not about Bafana.

He wasn't sure, but his best hunch was that it was *bopilwe* (created) when different diseases were mixed together. Probably, he suggested, it would have been generated in a woman. It is harder for them to see that there is a problem than it is for men and they're less likely to get treatment. HIV was, most probably, some kind of a hybrid germ that had been incubated in a woman's womb. As to why there was so much HIV now, when there had been none before, well, he suggested, that was just the way things were with diseases. There were times when a disease was common, and then it decreased. Like the *drop*. When he was younger everybody talked about syphilis, it was common. Now you hardly heard about it.[33]

I wanted to test his account by running through some of the alternative explanations. I started with condoms: did he think there was anything in what people said about the virus being in condoms? 'No.' He dismissed the idea. People talked about the worms that you could see when you put hot water in a condom, but he explained that that was the oil (lubricant). He went on without being prompted, to outline why people *might* think that '*Makgowa a batla ho fokotsa batho ba rona*' (Whites want/need to reduce our numbers, i.e. Africans), but he didn't go along with these ideas; condoms could be used by any *setjhaba* (nation or people). If there was something put inside them, there wouldn't be a way of it killing only Africans.

'So why do people say these things about condoms?' I asked.

Bafana's response was straightforward. People made these stories up because they didn't want to wear condoms. And he topped this off by saying that not wearing condoms is the reason why people got diseases. I noted that we were almost back to the official condom message, but accepted that he really didn't think condoms had been contaminated by Whites. This might, he was saying, be a plausible argument, but it wasn't a practical scheme.

I probed his thinking about condoms as a prophylaxis and asked him whether they would prevent *mashwa*, a pollution-based illness resulting from sex with an uncleansed widow/widower.[34] He was clearly a little thrown and wanted to know exactly what I was talking about and checked by rephrasing my question, '*Ho etsa thobalano le mosadi ya aparereng thapo ya lefu?*' (Sex with a woman who's still wearing mourning clothes?). Yes, I confirmed. Rephrasing it, he'd put emphasis on the rituals and symbols of the mourning period in which the widow would be in black and cleansing her blood using *moriana* (traditional medicine). Thinking it would help, I suggested, by way of an example, that if he was visited by a woman still within the mourning period and sex was on the cards, would a condom ensure his safety. Bafana was shocked at my suggestion. It would, he outlined without hesitation, be dangerous, but more importantly, he wouldn't even think about sex with a woman who was mourning. He wouldn't have those kinds of feelings for her. She would be like a sister to him.

'Maybe she doesn't tell you that she's widowed.' I suggested, trying to rescue my line of questioning. But I was just digging the hole deeper. 'I would know,' Bafana replied, nodding towards the imaginary widow sitting on the chair where I'd placed her when I set up the scenario. 'She'd be in mourning clothes.'

My example had been revealing, but it wasn't the response I was seeking. I tried again. 'What about a woman who had an abortion and hadn't cleansed?' This is also widely seen as a dangerous state and one in which sex is perilous. Here Bafana conceded that a woman might not tell you that she'd recently aborted and you wouldn't be able to tell. Sex with her would be dangerous. But, again, I'd overlooked something. If you didn't know her well, you'd use a condom to begin with, and by the time you might want to *entsha*, you'd know more about her. She'd have to cleanse before the condom came off.

I still hadn't established if Bafana thought condoms could protect from traditional disease. 'What', I asked, 'if you were *tauwe* [drunk]?' He considered the scenario and accepted that it could happen. 'Yes, then you'd panic the next morning,' he admitted, indicating that you'd regret taking the condom off with a woman you knew nothing about. I was pleased to have regained some control over the discussion, even if I'd had to rob the characters in my example of their rationality to do so. Now, I pressed on, asking Bafana what he would do if he found out subsequently to the drunken sex that the woman had recently had an abortion. Bafana suggested *makgonatshole* (literally, that which is able to do everything, the Sesotho name for potassium permanganate). A few drops in a glass of water would take the *ditsila* (dirt) out, but he cautioned that one had to be careful, *makgonatshole* was strong and if you took too much it would *phunya mala a hao* (pierce your gut).

This conversation had not gone as I'd expected, but it did illustrate how Bafana held some traditional beliefs in current contexts. So I asked him about healers and AIDS. Did he think traditional healers could cure AIDS? The answer was 'yes' but only (he was citing Dr Tshabalala now) if they came early enough. I wanted to test this belief against his own status, but couldn't; we had agreed that we didn't know if he'd got HIV. So, I asked whether he'd recommended Dr Tshabalala to people who have HIV. He'd given Mosa Dr Tshabalala's number, but it had been too late. He now told me, what I hadn't heard before, that Mosa had died on the back seat of a car as his family, in a frantic last effort, tried to get him to Dr Tshabalala's surgery but got lost on the way.

'And *boloyi* (witchcraft)?' I was asking whether witchcraft could explain why there was an AIDS epidemic. This, like the idea of infected condoms, was dismissed, not on the fundamentals of the issues, but for pragmatic reasons. Witches could send something that mimicked AIDS, though it would not really be AIDS. That, he thought, might well happen. But to explain the epidemic in terms of *boloyi* simply wasn't credible, there was nothing to indicate such a massive increase in witchcraft.

I was now onto the last of the big three folk theories of AIDS. 'What about God?' Do you think there's anything in the belief that he can cure people with HIV?' Bafana blew this one off with a brief account of Kgopotso, a relative who had gone forward to an 'altar call'[35] and told the Lord he would stop smoking at the 'Universal ya Motsoeneng' (a Bafana Radebe conflation of the Universal Church of the Kingdom of God and the Miraculous Happening Church of Prophet Motsoeneng, both large Pentecostal-type churches operating in Gauteng). 'They', Bafana was referring to other family members who had gone along with Kgopotso, 'told me he'd given up cigarettes.' Though he wasn't going to say it in so many words, Bafana clearly knew better. He didn't need to go further: if God couldn't even stop Kgopotso smoking, there wasn't any substance to the more outlandish claims that people made about miracle cures.

It was hard not to smile at the way Bafana had snubbed Christianity by rolling two earnest churches together and simultaneously, with the lightest of touches, scorned claims of God's power. But before we finished for the day, I wanted to go back to his illness once more. We'd talked about AIDS and what it was, but what did he think was the cause of his own illness?

He paused, just for a moment, and then told me that the most likely thing was breathing in fumes at his workplace. The oil that lubricated the band saw would smoke as the machine, in use for hours on end, became too hot to touch. The ventilation in the building was not good and they, the management, didn't provide proper masks. He'd been forever coughing up thick dark phlegm stained from the smoke.

This had not come up before in our interviews. Then it rang a bell. He'd raised the issue of dust when Tokelo and I had visited him at his sister's home, now more than two years ago. Nobody had said anything at the time, but Tokelo had scornfully dismissed the idea as soon as we had left Bafana and were driving home. And there was the suggestion that the petrol fumes that Mosa had been exposed to while working as a pump assistant had 'somehow' contributed to his death. Bafana was back at work, busy throwing up the earthworks of doubt.

Wrapping up

In qualitative research, it's time to move on when themes start to be repeated. I thought that it was now time to shift my attention elsewhere. I accepted that there were things that Bafana had still not told me, but I had a clear picture of his account. There was, however, still the outstanding issue of Bafana's provident fund. Despite the promises and the follow-up with Ingrid, Bafana still had not been paid out. The matter had dragged on. Ingrid had phoned Bafana again. She had spoken in English to him and he reported that he'd struggled to understand exactly what she was saying, but he thought the money would be paid into his account the following week. But it wasn't. Nor the following week. I told Bafana he had to chase them up and ask when it would be paid. He said he would, but he didn't.

Weeks, then months, and nothing had happened. I was focused elsewhere and saw Bafana only occasionally. I stopped asking about the provident fund. Eventually, with time running out before the sabbatical leave when I would draft this book in Lesotho, I made a point of raising the issue. He said he'd thought maybe he should try and get an investigative TV programme to take up his case. Then he backtracked: people were going to make fun of him for causing that kind of fuss for the amount of money involved.

I rang Firstjob and got hold of Portia. She transferred me to a Mr Botha. He told me that Ingrid had left Firstjob. I rattled off the situation along with dates and promises we'd been given. He said he'd look into the matter. I asked for his direct number, but he said I could get him through the switchboard. I realised that it wasn't only Bafana whom they'd worn down. I didn't have the time or energy to keep this up. Mr Botha didn't ring me back and, when I tried again, I was told he wasn't in the office. Neither was Portia.

Being frustrated by bureaucratic inertia, incompetent administration and illogical procedures are things I'm familiar with; after all, I work at a university. But this, when I tried to frame what had happened, was different. They were not playing by the rules. Not the rules that operate in my life. If I can prove that I'm owed money, it will be paid to me. Probably with delays and probably after frustrating arguments, but if there's proof, it has to be paid. Not so with Firstjob. They didn't play by any rules other than those from which they could benefit. I should have let that chair go through the window.

The strength and weakness of informal cultures

Paul Willis in his book *Learning to Labour*[36] examines the informal culture of working-class schoolboys. Willis wanted to understand how a minority of boys, the 'lads', were able to build a counter-culture within an institution that was consciously attempting to mould them with the publicly proclaimed and dominant values of society. Such values can and do rival the values of the formal, dominant culture of the institution. Yet, at the same time, Willis saw how fragile these informal cultures were in any direct encounter with the dominant culture. When members of the group of lads that he was studying were prosecuted for theft, something which their counter-values condoned, their rebelliousness collapsed in the police station and magistrate's court. It was, Willis says, a 'decisive and irrevocable victory over the informal. The informal meanings do not survive a direct confrontation.'[37]

In talking to Bafana, I was forever aware that many of the arguments he was making were partial, spurious and very often bolstered by specious evidence. To suggest, for example, as Bafana did, that Mosa dying on the way to Dr Tshabalala's surgery supports the argument that traditional healers can cure AIDS, if the disease is caught early enough, isn't going to survive robust interrogation. I could have shot it down, as I could have shot down scores of similar suggestions that he made. Except that my logic and biological knowledge would have delivered only a pyrrhic victory. There would be no more confrontations to win. Bafana would have disengaged after the first encounter.

Informal cultures, such as the many and varied beliefs about HIV/AIDS in South African townships, are strong because people believe them, not because they can stand up to a direct confrontation with the power of allopathic medical knowledge. So, in line with my research objectives, I chose to listen and not to confront.

I hope that my commentary on the conversations I had with Bafana, and my attempts to agree with him without believing what he told me, do not come across as a belittlement of him. I can understand how it could be interpreted thus. But rather than condescension, I increasingly felt respect for what he was doing. Beyond the specifics of particular arguments or suggestions, since Bafana was every ready to retract if he sensed resistance, I started to admire the persistent creativity with which he worked his material, myself included. What emerged from this exercise was not what I had set out to find. When I elected to talk with HIV-positive individuals, my idea was that the salience of the virus would strip away superfluous arguments, idle chatter or bravado, that I would find alternative theories of AIDS that had been tempered hard.

Bafana had given me something different. It was certainly different from the biomedical model of HIV. But it was not a theory constructed in hardened steel. More like a tissue of suggestions, innuendo and hints. Of course, I could see that, when viewed as a whole, they served a purpose: to maintain doubt that bested biomedical power. Suggestions and allusions might, in fact, be more robust in any encounter with biomedical power than betting on a single, clearly laid-out alternative. There was nothing to be defeated, only opportunities to duck, dive and deflect.

7

The certainties of
Paseka Radebe

Paseka

Paseka Radebe, Bafana's sister, is a large, assertive woman who takes
no nonsense. The kind of person you'd want on your side if there
was a dispute getting out of hand. When Bafana was sick, she had
appeared on the scene and played a decisive role in Bafana's treatment.
Indeed, without Paseka it was clear that Bafana would not have made
it. She had saved his life. With resolve she had acted within a plethora
of explanations as to what ailed him. At the time of Bafana's illness,
she had appeared as a clear proponent of Western medicine; she had
got him to the hospital, she suspected HIV, though the hospital staff
had refused to reveal the results of Bafana's test, and she had nursed
him back to health at her home, making sure he took the prescribed
medications. As I started to talk to Bafana about his illness, Paseka's
championing of Western medicine became all the more significant.
Bafana told me that she had been a traditional healer for several years
but had now, he was quite adamant, *kwetse* (closed) that chapter of
her life.

One afternoon, I drove over with Bafana to Paseka's house in the
Matala Section of Potlakong to ask if she'd be willing to be interviewed.
After spending almost two months at his sister's house recuperating,
Bafana had only been back a handful of times. He put an empty plastic
Tupperware box in the car, hoping that his sister would have baked.

It turned out she hadn't. The box came back still empty and he was pointedly teased for only visiting her when he was hungry. Bafana was ready to leave as soon as we'd arrived. Almost immediately he complained of *bodutu* (boredom) and claimed to Paseka that I was *tatile* (in a hurry). But I wasn't, and said as much. So Bafana cadged a bottle of *Zamalek* and disappeared. I sat with Paseka in the front room of her house, which was now nearing completion. She listed what still needed to be done: a sink installed in the kitchen, a geyser (boiler) for hot water, and a ceiling so that we would not be looking up at wooden rafters and bare zinc sheeting.

The contrast with Bafana's shack was striking and it illustrated the difference between the two siblings: Paseka worked hard and had kept her marriage to Dumi together; the house was what she had to show for it. Getting the *setsha* (stand) had not been easy; it had taken almost a year of badgering at the municipal offices. Sometimes, she would be at the offices before it was light to make sure she got to see an official. When the stand had been allocated to them it was without electricity and water had come from a standpipe at the end of the dirt road. The road was still a nameless track, but they now had electricity and water. The original *ntlwana ya mokoti* (long-drop toilet) that they had dug had been replaced with an outside flush toilet that was kept spotlessly clean. They had put up a *mokhukhu* (shack) when they first moved onto the *setsha*. It had been their home for almost eight years. Now it was not much more than an outhouse. They could have rented it out, but Paseka preferred having only family on the property.

The house was within striking distance of being completed and she was happy to tell me how hard it had been to get to this point. For several years Dumi, her husband, had been unemployed. It was only her work as a domestic worker that had provided an income. Now Dumi was back at work, and their three children were grown up and working. Money was again less of a problem. She looked after several grandchildren, the oldest now 14, but their parents helped with expenses. She hoped to have enough money to fit a zinc sink into the kitchen next month, and, sure enough, when I arrived a month later to conduct the first interview, it was in place. The geyser, a much more expensive item, was now in her sights.

As we talked, it became clear that she'd been fortunate with her *lekgowa* (White person or employer, and of course, often both) of almost 10 years who had paid her well above the going rate, and was willing to help her here and there. When Bafana had been in the hospital, they had allowed her to finish halfway through the morning and had driven her to the taxi rank so that she could get to the hospital for midday visiting. Unfortunately, they had now emigrated and she was making do with a series of *dikoropo* (piece jobs). She complained that the taxi fares made it hardly worth her while on some days. One employee for whom she worked on Wednesdays insisted that she arrive by seven o'clock so that she could give instructions before leaving for work herself. That meant Paseka had to be out of her house by five o'clock. She shuddered at how cold it would be in winter. A five o'clock start also meant she had to *palama habedi* (take two taxis), something that wasn't necessary if she travelled an hour later when more taxi routes were operating. Yet, she told me that she intended to stick it out, at least until she could find something better. She knew that if she stayed at home it would be hard to find anything else.

In theory, the interviews I conducted with Paseka were in Sesotho. In practice she spoke to me in a Sesotho-heavy version of Sekasi (township hybrid language), laced with creative alliterations and grammatical innovations taken from English, isiZulu and Afrikaans. It could be very hard work. The transcriptions could be baffling, even to the township Sesotho-speakers whom I asked for help. Some of the language she used was unique to Paseka. Gradually I got used to her idiolect and the interviews became easier, but it remained hard to close the interviews on time. Paseka explained by examples, and examples became stories, and the stories had sub-plots that would turn on fine points of detail. On several occasions, well aware that we had not reached a natural conclusion to the point-turned-story-turned-saga that she was recounting, I simply had to plead exhaustion and say that we would pick up from where I had broken her off the next time. She took some pride in my submission to the 'Paseka Chronicles'.

Bafana

Paseka described herself as the *tjhobolo* of the family, the talkative and assertive one, and this description was confirmed as we talked in her front room over the next three months. Before she agreed to be interviewed, she wanted to know if we would be talking about Bafana or if I wanted to know about her life. I assured her that it was the latter. We would talk about Bafana, but not till I knew more about her. She had smiled broadly. Later, I realised it was because she wanted me to clearly understand her side of the story. At the time, I didn't realise how long it would take to hear her out.

Until we reached her account of Bafana's sickness, it was striking how absent he was from the account of her life. He was much younger. Too young to understand many of the things that Paseka went through as a teenager and young woman starting her own family. She had got pregnant when she was 15. Her father had been furious, but Dumi, her boyfriend, stood by her. However, when her father died, life had descended into chaos as his family descended to claim what they saw as theirs. Once the funeral was over, it was a free-for-all and the house had been stripped. It was not long before they were forced out of the property under threats that it would be set alight with them in it if they remained.[1] The family, now consisting of her mother, her older brother Maru, twin brother Naledi, Bafana and Paseka's newborn child, had lived in a succession of shacks and rented rooms. Before finding a permanent home Dumi had been working away most of the time.

Then her mother had been killed in an accident. Paseka took over looking after Bafana, but he was already gravitating to the street. He was out till late, even when he had school the next day. When he came back to the house, there were arguments, especially when he'd been drinking. It had culminated in a fight when Dumi, back on leave from work, had waded into the family dynamics, insisting that Bafana show respect to his older sister. With Bafana old enough to move out, the parting of ways had been a relief.

They had, however, kept in touch over the years. They were, Paseka pointed out, *bana ba motho* (children of one person). The phrase encompasses not only siblings, but also first, second, even third cousins.[2] While the term *bana ba motho* dilutes the privilege of a full sibling bond, it builds responsibility to a wider family or clan that in African tradition stresses both age status and the bonds within a generation that are kept vital by rituals of burial, unveilings (of tombstones) and *mesebetsi* (gatherings to thank ancestors).[3] Standing aside from these ritual events is a drastic step that few take, even if they feel uncomfortable about the prominence of the ancestors at these gatherings, with the shedding of an animal's blood and brewing of *jwala bo bosotho* (traditional sorghum beer). So, notwithstanding that it was a relief for the two of them to go their separate ways, they saw each other periodically and frequently heard of each other through the extended family.

Paseka heard the news that Bafana was sick from one of their aunts, the younger sister of their mother. When she had arrived at Bafana's *mokhukhu,* she recalled that people were gathering, concerned at the rapid deterioration in his health. There was a lot of sitting around and people were praying for Bafana, but nobody was in charge and not much was getting done. Bafana's blankets were filthy with excrement and the shack was dirty. She sent her niece to the shops and set other people to work, cleaning and cooking. She could see that Bafana was dehydrated and she started to try to get him to swallow liquids. She had stayed with him over the weekend. Bafana, she recalled, had been refusing to go to the hospital, saying that he would die there. On the Monday, with the help of a cousin who owned a car, they had gone to a local clinic, but there had been a long queue. So they went to the hospital, which is what she wanted all along; she knew that he needed to be put on a drip. Despite Bafana's condition, they spent all day in the hospital waiting room, with Bafana vomiting into a bucket whatever she managed to get him to swallow.

Once he had been admitted to hospital, she was able to go home. The following morning she was at work and, with the help of her *lekgowa,* back at the hospital by noon. Bafana had nappies on but they had not been changed, and diarrhoea was leaking out onto the sheets. There was an untouched meal at the side of the bed; the nurses couldn't be bothered to feed him. Paseka had asked for gloves and set about cleaning him up. She then tried to get him to swallow a couple of spoons of the cold *pap* (stiff maize porridge). That went on for two weeks. She washed and fed him every day, and, despite the indifference of the nurses, Bafana survived.

Batho ba motho

In describing how she had pulled Bafana through, Paseka outlined the importance of psycho-social support, not as a nice-to-have, but an integral and vital part of treatment and healing. Bafana was helpless by the time he was admitted to hospital. Not only was he doubly incontinent, but he was so weak that he had lost control of his limbs. Even if he had wanted to eat, he was incapable of lifting a spoon to his mouth. If Paseka couldn't get a few spoonfuls of food to stay in Bafana's stomach, his treatment wasn't going to stay down either. Yet even to swallow, he had to be encouraged and cajoled. He had to be loved enough for somebody to go to the effort of putting up with his soiled body and patient enough to feed him, when most of the time any success was soon vomited back. The nurses were responsible for getting him to swallow the pills after that – whether he kept them down, whether he managed to eat anything, or even whether he still had the will to live, was left to others. Paseka brought in different foods and found that he could keep down a few spoonfuls of *mageu* (a maize-based drink) and, later, mashed potato. Bafana was lucky that Paseka cared enough to nurse him away from the brink of death.

However, to see Paseka as stepping in to save Bafana as an act of unconditional love would be to simplify things. It was not as straightforward as that. When she had first got news that Bafana was ill, very ill, she had held back from going to see him. She still harboured anger from the past; Bafana was selfish and cared little for other people. Even the night that Paseka had spent frantically trying to find out what had happened to their mother, he had been out drinking with friends. Her mother had not come back from work, and by late evening Paseka had gone to the police station. They had told her to check the hospitals and the morgues. It wasn't till midnight that she had got home, having found out that her mother had been killed instantly under the wheels of a bus. Bafana was still out. He came back after one o'clock in the morning, drunk, even though he was supposed to be writing an exam the next day. Later in their lives, they had fought over erecting their mother's tombstone, over Refilwe, Bafana's wife, of whom Paseka disapproved, over his drinking, and over household expenses. She still had a burn mark on her arm when, drunk and angry at their remonstrations, Bafana had thrown the lit paraffin stove at her and Dumi.

Once they were no longer cooped together in the same small house, things improved, though the tension remained, as did the underlying differences between them. Paseka was determined to make something of her life, Bafana was determined to enjoy whatever he could whilst he could. I interviewed them concurrently and during that time served as a conduit for news that supplemented their otherwise occasional interactions. Once, when Bafana had got some work as a building labourer on a house extension, I had told Paseka and described the work he was doing as he had explained it: digging foundation trenches, mixing cement and ferrying bricks to the bricklayer. Paseka had laughed, '*Ke* [he is a] *daka boy!*' she had exclaimed, laying emphasis on the pejorative side of this argot designation for a builder's labourer.

When she had got the news that Bafana was sick, her feelings had been mixed:

> [I thought] now I would get revenge. It was time that, so to speak, he would be hurt, to feel pain ... He'd done things which hurt me a lot ... now I thought that I could make him feel that hurt [yet] at the same time I moved quickly to make sure that he was OK.[4]

In fact, she had not moved as swiftly as this quote suggests. Rather, she had wrestled with the competing emotions as the news of how sick Bafana was continued to come in from different members of the extended family. She was proud of having nursed Bafana through, but it was something that was laced with resentment at the unfairness it entailed. He was the one that had brought this upon himself. That it was HIV she was in no doubt; along with drinking and smoking, he changed girlfriends 'too much'. Yet she was the one having to rush from work to the hospital and beg for plastic gloves from the nurses so that she could change his fouled nappies.

But she had no choice, he was her *ngwanabo* (brother) and she had to take care of him. Their common parentage as *bana ba motho* also gave her the right to call the shots when she had arrived at Bafana's shack on the Saturday morning. Other family members had been dropping in for over a week, but despite her late arrival on the scene, they deferred to her. That position had, however, received no recognition at the hospital when it came to Bafana's HIV status. Paseka still felt resentful as to how the medical staff had stonewalled her, saying that the result was confidential. They were willing to let her change his nappies, but she wasn't good enough to be told what ailed him. That Bafana also chose not to tell her underscored just how tense their relationship was, even as she was nursing him back to health.

Paseka within a plural health care world

So far Paseka's role ran along conventional lines. Her interventions underlined the frequent indifference shown to patients within South Africa's public health care system. It revealed how, beyond the medical procedures of getting pills into a patient or keeping a drip in place, the burden of care often falls upon patients' families. Paseka's honest account also illustrated how such care, which could not happen without love,[5] was not without contradiction. She took on the burden of caring for Bafana even as she harboured resentment towards him, and saw his current problems as the result of behaviours that she disapproved of. HIV was for Paseka the result of drinking, smoking and casual sex.

It may seem that digging deeper into Paseka's beliefs was simply curiosity on my part; after all, she had stepped in to fill the permanent, ragged gap in the South African health care system. With enough Paseka Radebes in South Africa, 'we' (which really means 'they') would be able to cope with the epidemic. If Mosa and Ronnie had had a Paseka in their families, maybe they also would both be alive. It would be easy to conclude that we need more Pasekas. It could also be concluded that Paseka's deeds manifest faith in medical science. Such a conclusion would be mistaken. There is a difference between believing and using.

The first thing that struck me, from the opening small talk with Paseka, was how she was juggling plural responses to her own health. After being involved in an accident when she was travelling in a minibus taxi, her blood pressure had been taken and it was sky high. She emphasised how seriously this had been taken at the clinic – they had written down her blood pressure with a *red* ballpoint pen. She had been given medication and advice on diet. She was cutting down on salt, fish oil (cooking oil), sugar and spices.[6] Although her compliance with this advice weakened over the course of our interviews, as measured by how many spoons of sugar she put in her tea, it was something she had embraced with enthusiasm. Cooking without oil was imbued with cultural value as '*ho pheha ka tsela ya Sesotho*' (to cook the Sesotho way). Here Paseka found herself aligning what she did, under advice from the clinic sister, with what she understood to be her cultural legacy.

The medication was more problematic, and more varied. After being prescribed medication by the clinic, she had paid R200 to see Dr Sibonyani, a private doctor, with a surgery in Matala Section. Just to be sure. It was just as well that she double-checked, as it turned out that the clinic had been 'overdosing' her with the wrong prescription of hypertension-lowering drugs: Ridaq, Pharmapress and Aspirin. The doctor had halved her dosage and added a further drug, Simvotin, a cholesterol-lowering drug which may benefit people with hypertension. Paseka certainly felt better coming away from Dr Sibonyani with a fourth medication, but she didn't stop at four, and added a Chinese herbal tea picked up in a local shop to her treatment.

When I first interviewed her, she extolled the virtues of this tea and felt that it was the aspect of her treatment that was making her feel better. On the strength of this, she halved the dosages of the Western medicine set by Dr Sibonyani, now a quarter of that prescribed by the clinic. Initially, this seemed to work, her blood pressure had improved when she next went to the clinic. But by the following visit, it was back to levels almost as high as when the problem was first diagnosed. She went back to Dr Sibonyani's dosages, but more importantly, in her eyes, dropped the Chinese tea and started on Uzifozonke, a bitter, commercially produced cleansing preparation that can be bought for R20 a bottle off the shelf. The name, in isiZulu, means 'cure all ills' and is one of many that are used to clean the blood. [7] The recommended dosage of half a cup a day acts as a 'health tonic', though everybody knows that larger amounts will see a dramatic clearing of the bowels that will remove *nyoko*. [8] Paseka again put more store on Uzifozonke than the prescribed pills, and took it on a regular basis. In the days running up to her next clinic appointment, she kept the pills steady, but doubled the dosage of Uzifozonke. Her blood pressure, at 140/100, [9] was much better and she was praised by the clinic sister who saw her. Paseka did not tell her about the Uzifozonke.

Paseka's balancing of the clinic's prescriptions against the private doctors' opinion and her own supplements rested on two major considerations. The first was her distrust of Western medical establishments, particularly government-run hospitals and clinics, which were, in her eyes, unreliable. It was not simply that those running these establishments didn't care, but that they were incompetent. They were not professional. Hence her willingness to pay to see a private doctor to make sure that the prescribed treatment was not going to make her worse. Paseka saw what had happened over her hypertension as an example. [10] She was more than ready to believe that the clinic had got it wrong. In addition to her own experience of how people were treated in hospitals and clinics, she could draw on examples in the media of doctors accused of killing patients through mistakes or negligence. It was best to double-check.

The second consideration was that the Western medicine prescribed didn't address a key belief over health that Paseka held: the need for blood to be cleaned. Paseka took this seriously. Much more seriously than Bafana, although she had reduced the frequency of *ho kapa* (cleansing by induced vomiting) from the once a week of their childhood to once a month. Generally, she would use warm water with salt and vinegar added, though sometimes she would use a traditional herb, *ngwavoma,* which can be bought at the open-air street market in Potlakong. Occasionally she'd *sepeite* (administer colonic irrigation) if she felt that *nyoko* was building up, and for this she used Sunlight soap[11] dissolved in one or two litres of warm water. But unlike Bafana, she never used *dipidisi tsa ho sebeditsa mala* (laxative pills), as she worried that the tablets might do harm as well as good. Both the Chinese tea and the Uzifozonke fulfilled the role of adding this missing cleansing ingredient that she experimented with to deal with whatever problem in her blood underlay the hypertension. That the Uzifozonke had proved better than the Chinese tea was satisfying in that it showed the value of her African culture. She liked that this had come out trumps – as it had with the dietary advice, which had restated traditional Sesotho cooking used before people were distracted and corrupted by the *dintho tsa makgowa* (things of the White people), which it turned out are not always so good, bringing high blood, *tswekere* (diabetes) and heart attacks. Idealised exemplars of African culture were proving valuable in the here and now, in meeting the challenges she faced.

Paseka's calling

Paseka had *thwasitse* (trained and graduated as a traditional healer) shortly after the death of her twin brother, Naledi, although with hindsight, earlier dreams predicting events, including the murder of her father, pointed towards a strong connection with the ancestral world. She had been very close to Naledi. The next sibling, Bafana, came eight years later. She and Naledi had done everything together as children. She struggled to come to terms with his death. Every Friday evening the adults of the family that her mother now headed would pool their wages and the money would be carefully divided up for transport, for groceries, for the municipal rent, for paraffin and coal (there had been no electricity in their section of Potlakong till the late 1980s) and for the burial society policy. One Friday, two of Naledi's friends had come round for him and had stayed to chat to the family before the three of them had gone out in high spirits for a beer. Half an hour later came the news that they had been attacked and that Naledi was hurt. Paseka had rushed to the spot where the three young men had been accosted. It was only a few blocks from the house. Naledi lay with his arms outstretched. He was dead, shot through the heart. Nothing had been taken. The two *tsotsis* (criminals) had run away after the shot had been fired. Nobody was ever arrested. He left her life without reason.

Not long afterwards, a rash of symptoms started to plague her: she lost weight, she was unable to sleep at night, she heard people calling to her when there was nobody around. She had retreated into the bedroom and stopped doing the housework. She neglected looking after her young children. Her mother took her to dozens of healers and prophets in an attempt to resolve the problem. Nothing that they suggested helped, until one healer made the obvious diagnosis, following a disturbance in the house in which the kitchen pots and pans had mysteriously come crashing to the floor, that she was being called to become a healer. She had gone back to the house with her mother and, as instructed by the healer, sprinkled snuff on the floor and a mixture of ash from the stove mixed with *phofo ya poone* (maize meal) and water onto the walls while telling her ancestors that she had heard their call. That night, she had slept deeply for the first time in months. She was up the next morning, cleaning the house. Two weeks later, on a Saturday morning, she left the house and, following what she had seen in a dream, walked until she heard the sound of drumming. This was her *lethwasong* (place of training), where she spent six months under the direction of her *kobela* (instructor and mentor).

There had been obstacles along the way, but these had been overcome with the support of her family. Her possessing spirit was identified as a now long-dead family member. On occasions, her possessing spirit, a man, had been quite specific as to where she should turn for help. Once he told her to approach one of her uncles, a man who had been unemployed for years, and ask him to pay for the beads that she would wear as a healer. When she and her mother went to talk to him, he told them that he had put two rand on *dipere* (the horses) after a dream. His horse had been given odds of 50 to one. It came in first, just as it had in his dream. He handed the winnings over to Paseka without hesitation.

Once she had graduated, she started to pick up clients. She would *hlahloba* (examine) them either with *ditaola* (diving bones) or with a *spiel* (mirror). This latter tool became her speciality, and she would get referrals from her *kobela* as well as other traditional healers for this service. The *spiel* was especially popular when people had lost something. Lost was, in most cases, a euphemism for stolen. She would draw the curtains to dim the room and then give her client a drink of *moriana* (medicine). They would then sit together on the floor and she would ask what it was they could see in the mirror that she placed in front of them. They would be in a dreamlike state and would see into the mirror as though it was the *bioscope* (cinema). When the client had seen enough, Paseka closed the session. The client would then be induced to *kapa* (vomit) to take out the remaining *moriana* in their stomach and be given milk to drink. After sitting quietly for half an hour or so, Paseka would tell them what they had told her as their own recollections were often poor; they would frequently have recognised people that they had quarrelled with and see them enter the room where the missing article had been, open the wardrobe or look under the bed. Then the client would know what had happened.

Paseka also prescribed steaming as a way of cleansing and for a while she was running what came close to a township spa. Clients would be enrolled for a five-day course. They would come in the morning and *kapa* and return in the afternoon to *futha* (steam). For this the client would sit on a chair in the middle of the room, with the paraffin stove in front of them; on it rested a large pan of water to which *moriana*[12] had been added. A large *moseme* (traditional mat made of grass or reeds) was then placed tightly around the stove and the seated patient, who needed to keep his or her legs apart to avoid being burnt. A blanket was placed over the top of the mat and the steaming began. The person stayed there for up to an hour until, perhaps, half the water was boiled away.

Then it was straight into a cold bath, for which Paseka used a large zinc tub. Cold water was poured or splashed over the patient. There was more *moriana* in the water. When I suggested that what she was providing was similar to a sauna, Paseka pointed out that people didn't dry after the cold bath – other than wiping their faces – because the *moriana* needed to be absorbed and not wiped off. Rather they put their clothes back on. They would *ikutlwa bobebe* (feel light or good).

Paseka stopped her work as a traditional healer not long after her mother died. She had quarrelled with her *kobela* over new initiates, but more significantly she had joined a new church. It seamlessly accommodated the calling from her ancestors and provided a viable alternative to being a *sangoma* (traditional healer).

Drums, spirit and preaching

Paseka described herself as 'born again', but by that she meant she believed in God, rather than identifying herself with a particular form of Christianity. Lay taxonomies of Christian denominations vary widely, depending on what is perceived as important to whoever is doing the classification. What was important to Paseka, in describing the Jerusalem Church of Zion, was that they used *dikupu* (drums), that the *moya* (spirit) which enters church prophets was mediated via ancestors, and that they allowed women to *rera* (preach/prophesy).

She had joined this church after her mother had been given a low-key funeral, despite her active participation in the church and its *manyano* (women's group). Given her mother's standing, it should have been a funeral attended by the whole congregation. The women's group would be decked out in their uniforms and, during the service, come out to the front of the church and surround the coffin to see off one of their own. Instead, the minister had instructed that it be a 'private funeral' for which uniforms were not to be worn. Paseka put this slight down to conflicting political allegiances between the pastor and her mother. The year 1986, when her mother died, was one of tension between ANC- and IFP-aligned residents of Potlakong. Once the mourning period was over, she had looked for a new church. An uncle was a preacher in the Jerusalem Church of Zion, which at that time had a dozen branches in Gauteng, including one in Potlakong. She had joined and had not looked back.

The synthesis of Christian and traditional beliefs and rituals worked well for Paseka. Drumming and dance, which had been a central part of any gathering of traditional healers, were part of the Jerusalem Church's services. Even the ancestors were welcomed, though there was a distinction. As a traditional healer she had been in touch with two spirits: one from two generations back in her own family and the other a *sendau* spirit (a possessing spirit from outside the sangoma's family). The *sendau* spirit had attached itself to her because it had been killed away from home and the deceased family had never properly integrated him into the spirit world. Once possessed, she would talk in a man's voice and sometimes the possessing spirit would request *kwae* (tobacco) or, depending on which spirit was present, *matakwane* (cannabis). By contrast, at church the *moya* that entered her when the drums were beating came from the *badimo* (ancestors) collectively, rather than a specific possessing spirit. Now, there was no change in voice and no requests. Other things had also changed – the healers' herbal pharmacopoeia was replaced with ash – plain ash from a coal stove, sieved to remove clinker, mixed with water and blessed. The mirror and the bones had gone; that part of her life was *kwetse* (closed).

That the church allowed women to preach was important to Paseka. Not all churches, even those which had women prophets, allowed women to speak in services.[13] She spoke every Sunday. This was not giving a sermon to the congregation. If this was done it was the role of the male *moruti* (preacher) in the Jerusalem Church of Zion. Rather, it was that women could stand up during the service and say their piece Typically, this was a proclamation of God's word, the world's sin, and the need for salvation. When the climax was reached and, if it had been a good session, and the speaker was drained, the slack was taken up by another woman, who would begin a hymn which the rest of the congregation quickly joined. After such preaching, Paseka would feel much better. In fact, if for some reason she was unable to get to church and *rera* (preach) on Sunday, she would feel that something was wrong during the week, though occasionally if she used the Metro trains and there were enough women returning home in the afternoon, a service would be held in a carriage and she'd have a chance to *rera* mid-week.

The smooth transition for Paseka between healing and 'churching' points to the two institutions being able to meet Paseka's emotional and spiritual needs. Through drums, dancing and possession, she was able to give voice to her frustrations and relieve tensions. The death of her parents and brother, acrimonious family disputes and the constant grind of township life had caused Paseka to question why she had been given such a hard lot in life. Both traditional healing and church provided what Victor Turner[14] called 'cults of affliction' in which those struggling to cope within 'normal' social environments supported one another in breaking out of otherwise restrictive social norms of behaviour – such as collectives of middle-aged women releasing emotional energy by proclaiming to one another on crowded commuter trains the sinful nature of the world and the need for redemption.

Navigating the perils of the world

Explaining in psychological terms Paseka's career as a traditional healer and then membership of a Zionist church is not, however, to suggest that Paseka didn't believe in the ancestors or God. She believed in both. The good thing about the Jerusalem Church of Zion was that the two co-existed.[15] The result was a multiplication of beliefs, rather than one of conversion or change. Indeed, at home she continued to *phahla* (talk to ancestral spirits) when she needed help – if, for example, she needed something badly. Currently, she was asking them for help to find better work and the money to buy her hot water geyser. The appearance in dreams of deceased relatives, especially those she had communicated with as a healer, constituted warnings or requests from the spirit world. This contact was welcomed and needed to be nurtured, she kept pictures of relatives close to her bed, as this helped them to enter into her dreams, and during the time that we talked, she held a *mosebetsi* (event to thank the ancestors) after having been visited in a dream.

If, within Paseka's worldview, we were to reckon the forces that stood for and against her, on one side of the balance sheet would be *Modimo* (God) and the *badimo* (ancestors) and on the other side would be *Satane* (Satan), *botsostsi* (crime) and *boloi* (witchcraft). It was a dynamic balance. The more she was blessed, for example with the achievements of the house in which we were talking, the more this trinity of dangers would be looking for her vulnerabilities. The last danger, witchcraft, stemmed from those who knew you well and were jealous. This evil, Paseka feared least. It was the first two, Satan and criminals, that she really had to fear. Before, when she was a healer, witchcraft had been something she had taken more seriously; now she believed it was powerless against the combined *matla* (power) of

Modimo and the *badimo*. But the other two sources of danger were more difficult to counter, and emphasised the need for her to actively maintain credit on her side of the balance sheet.

Understanding illness

How did illness fit into Paseka's accounting sheet of danger and defence? We should be careful about hiving off illness from the other problems. Manifestations of *madimabi*, that is, bad luck as a condition rather than being in the wrong place at the wrong time, come in different forms: a car accident, unemployment, theft or illness. However, if we are to focus on illness, then we need a third column for our balance sheet: some illnesses are *disiki tsa thlaho* (natural illnesses), so although faith might be able to instantaneously relieve you of some ailments sent by malevolent forces, there are others that require medicine – either *sekgowa* (Western) or *setso* (traditional) or both. Paseka's high blood pressure would be an example. She did not put it down to *madimabi*; it was a problem disconnected from the protection that *Modimo* or *badimo* would provide and needed to be responded to with medications of both *sekgowa* and *setso*.

Drawing the boundaries between natural illnesses and those stemming from the forces arrayed against people is not easy. Individuals' balance sheets of danger and defence differ. Moreover, people's views change, sometimes over long periods, as their views of the world are remoulded, such as Paseka's transition in and out of traditional healing, or, more rapidly, around a particular case of illness, as new evidence emerges pointing more strongly towards one explanation than the other, such as occurred during Bafana's health crisis.

When I pressed Paseka on the nature of TB as an illness and whether there were different causes, her response largely omitted the complex balance of danger and defence that she otherwise invested so much time in. One way of explaining would be that she saw TB as a natural disease, in the third column of the balance sheet of life. However, as we'll see when she contextualised it within Bafana's story, that wasn't really what she was saying.

Paseka's explanation was not something that she gave me in

complete form when I enquired. We discussed TB and HIV on three occasions and her views developed as we went along. Not only did I deepen my understanding of her views on these diseases, but she, facilitated by my questions, enriched her own explanation. Despite repetition, there remained a degree of instability in her description. One way in which she explained TB was to work backwards from the prescribed treatment, whether the course of drugs was six or nine months. The six-month variety could be cured, as long as you didn't *jumpa* (skip) the medication. The nine-month variety could not be cured, though it could be stalled. This was because nine-month TB occurred when people had HIV.

Two forms of the six-month (curable) TB variety were identified by Paseka. To do this, she moved into a different taxonomical principle: the cause of the infection, rather than the treatment time. One six-month variety was TB *ya moya*, with *moya* being used here in its profane or secular meaning of breath or wind (rather than spirit). This form of TB was caught when somebody coughed in your presence. Different in origin, though equally treatable, was a six-month TB which was *lefusto* (hereditary). It ran in families. Not everybody in the family would have this TB, but if you were diagnosed, you'd find on inquiry that, say, your grandfather had also suffered from TB. This hereditary factor made this form of TB similar to *tswekere* (literally, sugar, i.e. diabetes) or cancer or *moya wa badimo* (a calling to be a traditional healer).

Her final example of a hereditary condition jolted me, but I should not have been surprised. Healing does tend to run in families since, with the exception of *sendau*, involving an outside spirit, possession is by a deceased relative, often a grandparent who was a healer. Paseka's long-dead grandfather had been a healer, and an open discussion within Paseka's family had taken place as to which of the younger generation would be called by his spirit. The collection of hereditary conditions that Paseka put forward illustrates well how different cosmologies can be woven together.

The key feature of nine-month TB was that it wasn't curable. Either a course of pills or the use of African herbs might suppress the symptoms, but it would not be cured. It could be *fodisa* (made better) but not *fodisisa* (really cured). That was because of the HIV inside the person. While Paseka saw that there must be different types of HIV, since she knew there were different types of antiretrovirals, HIV did two things: it attacked you from the inside, hence the presence of *diso* (sores or ulcers) and *mathopa* (boils or swellings); and it *iketsa* (masqueraded) as other diseases, TB included. Unlike six-month TB, which could be cured, the nine-month TB would be back. For Paseka the therapeutic parity that Western medicine and African herbs had over HIV was illustrated by a niece of hers who had been HIV positive for ten years. She took antiretroviral drugs and a range of traditional treatments, but was still constantly ill with one thing or another. Paseka thought that it was possible that a true cure might someday be found, especially, she stressed, among the herbs of Africa.

Grasping how Paseka understood TB had not been straightforward. Even during the interview period, her understanding was not entirely stable and it will, most probably, change further with new circumstances. Her construction of TB was as idiosyncratic as her linguistic idiom. Bafana had added his own *Bafanitus-FauxHIVarius*, which he proposed as a form of TB, to the possible 17 strains of the disease that a nurse had once told him existed. Now Paskea was adding another three varieties, using different taxonomies. I realised that, outside a willingness to defer to doctors and scientists, there was a potentially infinite number of TBs circulating in the township. And if this was true for TB, the same would be the case for HIV. Further, I could see that the materials used for these constructions were promiscuous, formed with shameless borrowing from different paradigms, including that of science. Yet this flexibility did not mean that there wasn't pride and competition over content, linked to individuals' priorities and beliefs.

Bafana's illness

Finally, I got around to asking Paseka about Bafana's illness. By now, I knew more about Paseka and how to weigh her words; to distinguish what were throwaway lines, and what was important. Around the third interview, she had told me she was enjoying our discussions, it was a chance to explain her side of things. Having an opportunity to speak your mind is therapeutic, especially in the contested everyday life of the township. These tensions increase when, like Paseka, you are making something of your life. At the bottom of the social pile, there is constant squabbling over the little there is; feuds can start with a bottle of beer or a few rands. As you start to accumulate wealth, even on a small scale, you pull away from this petty bickering of the streets and backyards. Increasingly, you inhabit the respectable privacy of a decently furnished living room in a house of bricks and mortar, and a geyser on the way. But the privacy comes only at the expense of greater scrutiny. You have to explain why it is that you are doing better than others. Although I was now asking Paseka about Bafana, what she told me was also justifying her own progress as well as his misfortune.

Paseka had already told me that Bafana's problem was obvious. It was AIDS. He had HIV inside him. Bafana had never told her so, neither had the hospital. It had, however, been confirmed in roundabout ways. There was the referral to the HIV clinic. Additionally, before Bafana started disappearing his status, he had shared the clinic test results with a niece whom he was close to and who was, within the family, open about her status. Word had got back to Paseka. In any case, she pointed out, his having AIDS was evident.

There were the girlfriends, the ones he changed 'too much'. And to be specific, she pointed to Thembi, a girlfriend Bafana had never mentioned to me, who had died of what was assumed to be AIDS a couple of years earlier. There was also the drinking and the smoking, which, along with unsanctioned sex, form a symbolic trinity of sins. Then there was the type of TB that Bafana had contracted; he'd been on treatment for nine months. It was the type of TB caused by HIV. Finally, there were the other symptoms that had presented: the *lethopa* (boil) on his anus was a clear sign of how the virus ate you from the inside, along, of course, with the diarrhoea.

Given this evidence, it was obvious to Paseka that Bafana had AIDS and, as far as she was concerned, when she had arrived at Bafana's shack on the Saturday morning, everybody knew what the problem was, though nobody said it in so many words. That did not mean they all saw it in the same way. Paseka knew that some saw it as witchcraft and others as a *moya o ditshila* (evil spirit or demon). She disagreed with both of these diagnoses, but the latter was particularly irritating to her as it had come from a cousin, Ben, who, along with his family, attended a Pentecostal church and to whom she was close. They saw eye to eye on many things: the value of working and saving, that they were born again, and the dangers of drinking, smoking and sex. But they differed over important details as to how the supernatural and natural worlds were linked. Ben, as a Pentecostal, rejected a role for *badimo* (ancestors) in the world of the living, but believed in *meya e ditshila* (evil spirits) sent by Satan; to his mind, this was clearly what had entered Bafana as a result of his desolate lifestyle. He and his family had spent considerable time praying over Bafana as he lay in his soiled blankets, trying to exorcise the evil spirit within him. Paseka had not approved. She believed in Satan, but didn't believe in *meya e disthila*. Paseka's understanding of AIDS might diverge sometimes from the medical explanation of HIV/AIDS, but it was, in contrast to Ben's diagnosis, much more practically aligned at that point to Bafana's health crisis. Ben's healing interventions only distracted from getting Bafana to hospital.

When, in our discussion, Paseka rejected witchcraft or *moya o ditshila* as the underlying causes of Bafana's illness, it appeared that we were returning to a simpler account of her actions, the one that I had initially seen when I watched her wrestle her brother from his death bed – a stalwart proponent of allopathic treatment. I had started to interview her on that basis. I had known that she had once been a healer, but also that she had closed that facet of her life. As our discussions progressed, a more complex picture of her beliefs had emerged. Now it seemed to be again simplified. Despite the plural but lucid worldview that she had described to me, when it came down to Bafana, it now appeared she was handing this over to Western medical science, and both diagnosis and treatment lay within its sphere of competence.

Running down my list of questions, with witchcraft and demons ticked off, I almost dropped the question of whether Bafana had been infected with HIV was the result of an ancestral *kotlo* (blow or punishment). I thought it would get the same response, but I asked it anyway for form's sake. What Paseka said was, 'Who knows?' But from the speed of her retort, the inflection of her voice, and the animated way in which the two-word response was delivered, she was clearly telling me that a *kotlo* was a distinct possibility. I had asked a pertinent question, one that deserved attention.

Bafana, Paseka pointed out, neglected their shared *badimo* (ancestors). The unveiling of their mother's tombstone was an example that she gave me – he had done nothing to help. She had had to pay for everything and organise the whole event. He had pitched up late on the day, drunk. Then there were the too many girlfriends coming in and out: that was disrespectful to the ancestors. Bafana, Paseka implied, was asking for it with his behaviour. She contrasted his behaviour with her own: she respected both *Modimo* (God) and the *badimo* (ancestors) and it showed. Her life was a success. Again, the leitmotif of her house demonstrated this; by contrast, Bafana was in a shack. And he was, when the chips were down, on his own. When he was sick, really sick, who did he have to turn to? He had nobody but his drinking buddies, his street friends. What good were they? In the end he had had to turn to her, playing on her goodwill and their shared blood. Now that he was better, did he keep in contact with her? No! Would he be back when he was sick again? Of course he would.

For Paseka, this lack of meaningful connection that Bafana had with his *badimo*, or with *Modimo*, was a reflection of his isolation in life and his transitory relationships with people. If he invested in respecting tradition, or church, this would not be the case. She illustrated the contrast in respect of herself. On the Sunday of Bafana's health crisis, a large group from her church, including the minister, had come to Bafana's shack. Her absence on a Sunday had been noticed and they had got to hear that she was looking after her brother. They came to support her. They had sung and prayed for Bafana. Clearly Bafana was close to a hopeless case for redemptive healing, whatever the exact nature of his illness; for that he would need to have faith, which Paseka dismissed with a laugh. Rather, the point she was making was that people were concerned about her enough to come over and give their support.

The contrast was clear. If you neglected others in this or the spirit world, you undermined yourself as part of a wider community. You, in effect, chose to forsake the support of others. Like Bafana, you would be alone and vulnerable. Nobody in such a situation could expect to succeed in life, Paseka explained. Bafana might make light of the suggestions that his problem was a *kotlo,* but Bafana's life spoke to his neglect of what was important.

And Bafana's treatment

In Paseka's account of Bafana's treatment, the pills he was prescribed by the clinic were important, though, given the type of TB, a full cure for Bafana could not be expected. Nor were they his only treatment once he had been discharged from the hospital. I had assumed that the *imbiza* (traditional medicine) given to Bafana by Dr Tshabalala had disappeared from the scene as his health rapidly deteriorated and he was admitted to hospital. This was not, however, the case. Paseka had rung Dr Tshabalala and spoke to her about the black powder prescribed for the *lethopa* (boil) on Bafana's anus. She had wanted to know how often it should be applied, as Bafana could not remember what he had been told. With this sorted out, the duty of applying the *imbiza* to this sensitive part of Bafana's anatomy fell to her husband. Paseka, however, made sure it was applied as directed and was emphatic that it was this preparation that had healed the *lethopa.*

Prayers also continued for Bafana. In particular, a neighbour who belonged to a different Zionist church came in every day. Additionally, there were prayers by visitors, even if Paseka didn't always agree with the requests these prayers made, such as those of their cousin Ben and his family. Such prayers were part of showing that you were concerned, but it was going through the motions, given Bafana's manifest lack of beliefs. Rather, Paseka was anxious to let me know that the thing that had really helped Bafana was the *motoho wa diherbs* (literally, herbal sorghum porridge) which she had bought for him. It took me a while to work out what it was she was referring to by *motoho wa diherbs.* *Motoho* is a slightly fermented sorghum gruel, but the term can be applied to any maize or sorghum porridge. The herbs, I twigged, were vitamin and mineral supplements. What she was referring to was the fortified *pap* that Bafana had once shown me in his shack. This was, indeed, the case.[16] Paseka credited the fortified porridge with giving Bafana an appetite. It also stopped the vomiting and diarrhoea. This provided the essential sustenance for his recovery.

That Paseka placed her own intervention at the centre of Bafana's successful treatment was consistent with her self-narrated role as the person who had, due to bonds of blood, stepped in as the primary caregiver – even if Bafana, the recipient of this care, had clearly brought about his own misfortune and showed little gratitude for what she had done. At least I was now listening to the true account of events.

But another point to note in this account is how the fortified *pap* was imbued with traditional properties with its herbal fortification – notwithstanding that these were actually vitamin supplements.[17] Paseka's desire to see synchronisation between different healing approaches extended from the case of her brother to the wider AIDS epidemic in South Africa. When I asked her what she thought would end the epidemic, she told me that it was a difficult question, but that she was encouraged by the recent emphasis on circumcision. She, however, used the term *bolla*, the verb to circumcise, but which also references traditional initiation processes in which young people graduate into adulthood.[18] Paseka had herself been to *lebollong* (literally, the place of circumcision, i.e. the initiation school), a female initiation school (which involved no circumcision). She pointedly noted that Bafana, unlike herself and her brother, had not gone to the *lebollong*. Her message here was not that physical circumcision might reduce the chances of HIV infection, but that the initiation school taught you about sex, its risks and how to protect yourself. Bafana's failure to attend *lebollong*, she was suggesting, had had obvious results.

Conclusion: Paseka's side of the story
In the opening negotiations over the interviews I conducted with Paseka, we had agreed that I would listen to her side of the story. That referred, in the first instance, to the differences between her and Bafana – their relationship as a whole, and not simply the role she had played in Bafana's illness. Looking back on this agreement, I realised that it

was exactly what I needed to know and that the story I had heard was also more than Paseka, Bafana and their relationship.

The death of Bafana's friends, as my interviews with him progressed, had brought home to me that the townships constituted a world saturated with death. At times, with yet another young adult's death implausibly explained, the sense could become overwhelming. I began to understand that there were limits to what one could shoulder. At a statistical level, it is easy to stand firm and to proclaim that these are AIDS deaths. It is not so easy when each death comes individually, embedded in suffering, tragedy and grief.

What Paseka's side of the story made me realise was that this has been going on for a long time. A continual liturgy of loss predates AIDS. AIDS has accelerated this process, but violence, accidents, suicides and illness have long been taking the lives of township residences while they are still young. Talking about 'the time of AIDS' or 'the era of AIDS' helps to highlight an unfolding tragedy, but it can suggest that the time before AIDS was without suffering. It wasn't. If we want to understand people's responses to AIDS, we need to account for how responses to suffering were developed long before AIDS added to the toll – those responses were never abandoned; rather, they were adapted in the time of AIDS. Or, perhaps more accurately, AIDS deaths were fitted into the existing ways in which suffering was understood, muffled and absorbed.

Seen in this context, we should recognise that the different perspectives over suffering are not going to resolve themselves anytime soon. There is going to be no decisive showdown – even should there ever be a medical breakthrough over AIDS. The baseline of misfortune will remain and has to be managed. Paseka was a proponent of Western medicine with Bafana's illness, but as a fellow traveller, not as a disciple. To the extent that Western medicine was useful, it was put to work, but it was trusted no more, and probably less, than several other explanations. In such circumstances, any sensible person will keep it jostling for relevance with Christian faith, traditional belief and whatever else can be mustered to assist.

8

The struggles of Grace Dlamini

Being positive

Bafana's status was always shrouded in some doubt and it became increasingly uncertain. Paseka's take on her brother's illness was clear. However, I now realised that she took a different perspective on his suffering from what those viewing sickness within a biomedical paradigm would assume if they had chanced, or bothered, to observe her saving Bafana. But with Grace Dlamini I was confident that she would not equivocate over her HIV status. She was openly positive – the only person in Potlakong who was.

Being 'open' or 'closed' about one's HIV status is usually neither exactly one thing nor the other. There are plenty of people who have disclosed their status, but disclosure takes place to different degrees: a single individual, perhaps a counsellor, peer educators, nursing sister, or close friend, then outwards to immediate family, good friends, antenatal class peers, colleagues, neighbours and so on. But at some point, for most people, it stops short of becoming something that *everybody* knows for a fact. Kept close to the individual, the boundaries can be maintained; beyond these borders their status is a matter of speculation. Lydia, a young HIV-positive woman whom I once interviewed, is a good example. She explained, after double-checking the confidentiality of our conversation, that she was HIV positive. She also told me the extent of her disclosure. She lived with her mother and two sisters. Her mother knew she was positive. Her older sister also knew. Both of them would remind Lydia to take her pills. The younger sister didn't know Lydia's status even though they all lived together. Those in the know collectively kept the news from the younger sister because she had a 'big mouth' and Lydia's status would end up being relayed beyond the household.

Grace Dlamini, by contrast, was broadcasting her positive status across the township, literally so – she had been on Potlakong FM Community Radio Station several times to talk about being HIV positive. I didn't imagine that she would give me an account of AIDS that corresponded 100 per cent with what a doctor would say, I expected to find some of the grit of township life mixed in, but, overall, I expected her account of her illness to be close to the AIDS gospel she proclaimed. When I first conceptualised a series of deeper conversations with township residents infected or affected by AIDS, I identified Grace as my 'control'. It would be against her account, the science of AIDS grounded in the realities of township life, that the alternative beliefs that others might raise could be measured.

Grace makes a splash

I first met Grace at a company workshop for peer educators in a slightly down-at-heel conference centre outside Johannesburg. Over a hundred peer educators had been brought in for the day from different company operations. The event was a mixture of training, motivation and feedback that the company HIV/AIDS manager had worked hard to organise. I was an invited speaker, and, keen to find out more about what peer educators could do, had offered to run an interactive session. I had sat with Grace and other presenters behind a cloth-covered trestle table at the front of the venue. We had microphones along with jugs of water, small glass bowls of mints, and wafer-thin notepads branded with the conference centre's logo. The peer educators sat in groups at round tables on which I had set them to work with flipchart paper and marker pens to map out the sexual networks that the HIV virus traversed. Hastily sketched diagrams in blue and red and green were now stuck to the walls with Prestik.[1] I had brought my session to a close, with some difficulty, more or less on time. Grace was scheduled to speak before we would go for lunch. This was not an easy slot to fill. It was clear we were all ready to eat; on the tables the bowls of mints had long been emptied.

Grace had arrived as I was on my feet hamming up the mock role of an interviewing journalist that I had assigned myself, questioning representatives from each group of peer educators on their multicoloured sexual network posters. Grace was a petite, spunky African woman in her mid-30s. Addressing the group, she was on her feet, hands gesticulating, engaging with her audience; she was a natural communicator. That day her hair was styled into short curly cones to give a studded effect. She could have just walked out of an avant-garde hair salon. We had been introduced and said a few words before she was called to the podium. The event's MC said nothing about her being HIV positive, but introduced her as a 'tireless worker in the community in the fight against AIDS'. Out-of-towners would not know her status and she played to this advantage by catching the men out when asking if they would like to date her. Nobody put their hand up or shouted out, but it was clear from the involuntary nodding that some of them would. 'Did you think I might be HIV positive?' she asked. 'Do I look positive?' She answered herself, 'No, you can't see that I'm positive and plenty of you would be happy to date me without asking that question.' The response was laughter. The women peer educators were teasing the men who had nodded to the first question. The men were laughing at themselves for being caught out so easily. I joined the laughter, relieved that, although she'd also caught me out, my nod had been imperceptible.

Now she had her audience's attention and lunch was, for the time being, out of mind. Grace built on her opening move to stress how antiretrovirals were keeping her healthy and attractive. They were effective in keeping the disease under control, contained, at bay. It was what the peer educators wanted to hear; on the front line they had to persuade people that knowing their HIV status didn't mean they were going to die. She continued, moving beyond her triumph over AIDS, to extolling others to empower themselves. She had a message specifically for women, she said, that she wanted the peer educators to pass on. Women needed to stop being 'parasites'. Rather than look to men for help when they were struggling, they needed to be financially independent. She explained that she wasn't lucky enough to have a job, but she didn't wait for a man to come and help her, there were many ways you could make money. You had to *zama* (try to help oneself), whether it was taking orders for clothes from neighbours, recycling bottles or selling fatcakes (deep-fried dough balls). You might start small, but it was better than doing nothing. She conceded that she liked men, but women could be their own worst enemies: instead of getting out there and making money for themselves and for their children, they sat waiting for a man and his pay packet. 'What do you get if you depend on a man for money?' she asked the peer educators and half a dozen responded loudly, 'AIDS!'

It was an impressive performance and, after she had brought it to a close, the MC asked if the peer educators had any questions. Several hands shot up even though we were well past lunchtime. One of the questions from a woman peer educator was about men not wanting to wear condoms. The problem, she explained, was that they said they couldn't get erections while wearing one. Another peer educator chipped in: other people complained that if they wore a condom they couldn't come (ejaculate). Grace was impatient to answer, and she gave the men behind such claims short shrift. 'You know where the problem is for those men?' she asked. There was a slightly uncomfortable silence. 'Here,' she shouted pointing at her head. We were all relieved and nodded our own heads in agreement. 'The problem is in the head. They tell themselves "I don't like these condoms." So they make these excuses.'

Grace knew she hadn't fully convinced the audience with this answer, so she continued. 'It's not about a condom or no condom. It's about what you do.' She selected a victim sitting at one of the front tables and asked her if she was married. She was. 'OK,' said Grace, 'You're negative, I'm positive. We share your husband for one month and we see whom he chooses.' Everybody is laughing again. We were not quite sure where Grace was taking us, it was clearly risqué, but we felt confident in her hands. 'You don't need to wear a condom 'cos you're negative and married to him.' We were nodding in agreement to this thought experiment. 'Me, I have to wear a condom with your husband because I'm positive. You know what? He's going to choose me at the end of the month. Why? Because when we do that thing, I'm working hard with that man. I'm spring cleaning. I say to him, "Papa, I want to do something special with you tonight." He says, "What, sweetie?" I say, "Let me show you, but we must use condoms." You know what? He doesn't even remember that he doesn't like condoms. Next day he's asking me, "Sweetie, how about we use the condom tonight?"'

Some of the peer educators were clearly on the edge of being offended by this explicit celebration of sexual power, but they had to go along with the majority who were whooping it up. The panellist and the MC were leading the way, clapping the finale to Grace's performance, laughing uproariously at the image of men being trained into a Pavlovian reaction to condoms via sexual excitement. Grace had got her point across well and the MC put a respectable spin on it, telling us all that the B in the ABC message is about being faithful, and that means we need to put effort into keeping relationships alive. It was now very much time for lunch; we all had a good appetite.

Grace had to leave shortly after the afternoon session started. It was a disruptive exit as she demanded a hug from all the panellists as she left, but she was making a point. She might be HIV positive, but that didn't mean we couldn't embrace her; you couldn't be infected by hugging. We hugged her in turn, in front of the cheering peer educators.

Journey to Potlakong

When I rang Grace to ask if she'd participate in my research, it was somewhat of a relief to find out that she was well. I was acutely aware that AIDS was killing people every day; it had crossed my mind that the phone wouldn't be answered. She was enthusiastic about the project and suggested that I interview her in her house in Masimong Section of Potlakong. It was, she explained, hard to find, so she offered to meet me at a major intersection to the south of Potlakong. We agreed that I'd be there at 10 o'clock the following Tuesday morning, a cold, overcast day.

The intersection was badly potholed and had wide dusty verges occupied by a handful of rickety stalls. On the Tuesday, most of them were empty. It was the middle of the month and there was little point in setting up shop. Two or three women sat hunched at one corner of the intersection with *dipaola* (braziers) in front of them; they had just been lit and heavy smoke was swirling across the road. When the coals were hot, they would start roasting *mielies* (maize cobs) to sell to those hurriedly changing taxis. I received a missed call on my cell phone from Grace and, when I rang her back, she assured me she was on her way. She arrived wrapped in a blanket, walking hurriedly. She'd been asked to counsel somebody at the clinic, which was why she was late, but it was fine. We could go to her home.

Masimong Section is a vast but orderly settlement that has sprung up in the last ten years and for the moment forms the south-western extremity of the township. Here it is hemmed in by one of Jo'burg's arterial freeways. Across the freeway there are open fields, but it is only a matter of time before people will be living there. The roads are laid out in a grid system, but they are not yet tarred and most are deeply rutted. We bounced along, past a mixture of shacks and occasional RDP houses that are being built in ones and twos among the existing structures. There are electricity poles along the streets, but no wires. The poles, Grace told me, had been there for two years. The electricity was coming, but there were problems with the contractor and work had stopped. We passed the contractors' depot on a corner with a large, faded sign and a high wire fence. Inside there are what remains of a burned-out truck and a prefab office. Local people had got tired of waiting and torched the place.[2] 'But what good does that do?' Grace asked me.

We turned several times and I was no longer sure if I would know my way out. Grace pointed to an RDP house, plastered and painted pink, one of two standing next to each other in the street. Otherwise, the street was lined by buildings of corrugated iron or raw breeze blocks. Most had some kind of front fence or wall. Most of these were symbolic markers of the owners' territory, less than a metre high. Once parked outside her house, Grace waved to a neighbour and shouted greetings. She was in no hurry to go inside, she wanted people to know that she was being interviewed by a professor from Wits. We chatted to her immediate neighbours in the other RDP house; they were introduced as Mazuma and her daughter Zanele.

There was little furniture inside Grace's house and the floors were bare. Grace apologised that she couldn't offer me anything to drink. Later, we walked to a nearby *spaza* shop and I bought a packet of tea bags and sugar. Grace heated water on a paraffin stove and made us both a mug of sweet black tea. After that, I always brought a few groceries with me as a gift, and so as to be sure there was something for a mid-way break, in what were typically two-hour interviews – Grace needed no prompting to talk.

Grace had grown up in what is now Limpopo Province.[3] Her parents had died when she was still young. Her mother was struck by lightning; witchcraft was suspected. She can remember her father telling her that his wife's brothers wanted to be rich and for this they needed to kill a member of their own family. They were Pedi,[4] he was a Zulu[5] and a stranger in the area. They had come to take back her mother's possessions after the funeral. A year later, he died in a hit-and-run accident, making his way home from a tavern. She and her brother went to live with their uncle – one of those her father had accused of witchcraft. They were clearly not welcome charges. She and her brother would go hungry. One afternoon, when she was nine or ten, her teenage cousin asked if she would like Sunday *kos* (a full plate of food). If she did, she must come to the bedroom with him. That went on for three years. What she remembered most painfully was the guilt of eating, while her brother was hungry.

When their uncle died, it was a chance to get away. After the funeral there was a family meeting. The two children were asked whom they wanted to live with. Her cousin had primed her to ask to stay, promising her even nicer things to eat. She had initially agreed, but in the meeting she spoke up and asked to live with the uncle that lived furthest away. Her brother chose a different house where he knew there was always food on the table. Things had improved. When she was sixteen, she met a boy she liked. He was three years older than her, and he said that he would love her and look after her. He said he didn't want to hurt her, but he wouldn't accept that she wasn't ready for sex.

When she got pregnant, he denied it was his child, but she hadn't slept with anybody else. The two families met and an agreement was reached. His family paid a fine and the boy, when he was born, took their surname. Four years later, despairing of finding a job, she left the child with the father's family and stayed with a school friend, Dineo, in a shack settlement near Rustenburg in the North West Province.[6] Dineo was living with Bomvu, a Xhosa man working on one of the platinum mines in the area. Bomvu and Dineo had been good to her, letting her stay rent-free and giving her meals as the weeks stretched into months and she still hadn't found work. But then Bomvu started to proposition her when Dineo was out. He became insistent, pointing out that she was eating from the money he earned. Grace moved on, this time to Potlakong where she had a friend she could stay with. This time there were no men. It had been three women sharing a house in Sizwe Section, far from where she now lived. They were just a couple of streets from a large hostel for migrant workers.

That's where we left off for the day, and as I wrote out the receipt for the research honorarium, Grace explained that she'd put the money towards a new 12-volt car battery to run her TV. There was a shop up the road with a generator that charged batteries for a few rands, but her battery was old and would be flat after a couple of days. She accompanied me to the intersection and I made a concerted effort to remember landmarks each time I turned the car under her instructions.

Clinic counsellor: truth and lies

Despite the memorised landmarks, I was grateful when Grace offered to meet me again at the intersection for our next interview. It was another blustery morning, but despite the cold, Grace was wearing a bright green dress and had only a black cotton shawl over her shoulders. She told me that after the interview, she was going to a church meeting. There was a freshly lit *paola* burning in her neighbour's yard. Other than for street-side hawking, these are normally only lit in the late afternoon. Once the coals are hot and the acrid smoke finished, the *paola* is brought in to warm the house. Grace explained that her neighbour, Mazuma, ran a *chaf posi* (drinking spot) from the house. A warm room would attract customers on a day like this. I waved to Mazuma, standing upwind of the smoking *paola*, but Grace hurried in without greeting.

We sat in Grace's cold house and I asked her about her work as an HIV-counsellor volunteer at the Bophelo Clinic on the edge of Masimong Section. When someone agreed to test for HIV, Grace was asked to counsel them; she explained what the test involved and asked them what they would do if the result was positive. Often, she told me, it wasn't hard to know that the result was going to be positive. She was familiar with the symptoms and many people came late to test. After the test, she explained what they must do to look after themselves. Particularly with the women who test positive, there were long discussions about what they should say to their partners. Usually they were scared about what would happen when they broke the news to their boyfriends or husbands, who usually did not know their own status. Grace had several tricks to share with these women; some she was taught by Sister Irene who ran the HIV/AIDS programme in Bophelo Clinic, some she had come up with herself. But if the woman was afraid to give these tricks a go, then there were strategies to introduce condoms into sex. An easy one, which sometimes worked, was to say that the clinic had taken them off contraceptive injections, a medical lie that the woman's partner wouldn't be able to counter.

I remembered her condom speech at the peer educator training and this seemed a good time to pick up on the issue. Away from an audience, she conceded some ground. 'OK,' she said, 'for some men that problem is there. They can't get an erection or maybe they can't finish in time. But maybe that's two out of 100. The other 48, they are putting that problem into their heads because they want flesh-to-flesh.'

'The other 50?' I wanted to know.

'They don't have a problem,' she said. 'But you know, Professor, men are stupid. They say they love you, yet at the same time, they're having that flesh-to-flesh with other women.'

'So it's a problem with men wanting flesh-to-flesh sex?' I sought to confirm, but Grace didn't answer directly; she was now on a roll, answering questions with explanations that begged new questions.

'Men, they think they're so clever, Professor, but they're stupid. It's not only them that are doing this thing of many partners. They tell you that they can tell if their wife has been sleeping with somebody else,' and she launched into a story to illustrate that they couldn't:

So before I get this house, I was in a room and you will hear what is happening in the next room. I remember there was a girl, Ntombi, who was busy too much. When Joe came out, James came in. One day immediately [after] she was doing it with someone, Sipho [one of Ntombi's boyfriends] comes and she never had a chance to wash [before he arrived]. I was scared thinking, 'This one's going to get angry.' But when they get out they were happy. We sit around chatting. Sipho says, 'I see other stupid men, their wives are busy doing it, but I can tell if my wife is doing it with another man. I can feel it when we are doing it [having sex]. I can tell it's different. You know what [referring to Ntombi]? You are not the same, sleeping around. I can feel it.' I agree saying, 'Yah, yah, Ntombi is not like those other women.'

'You see, Professor,' Grace appealed to me after telling the story, 'people put all sorts of things into their heads. Like with this Bactrim [antibiotic tablets, used as a prophylactic with HIV-positive patients to prevent opportunistic infections], they were complaining about it in the clinic the other day. They were saying it makes them dizzy, it makes them sweat, it makes them what-what. Now they're putting this idea into each other's heads.'

Grace explained that she had taken on the ringleader. Asking what pills she took, she had put one of each in her hand and demanded of the woman how she took them. The woman had to confess, she took her four medications together, morning and evening. If so, Grace pointed out, how did she know it was the Bactrim that was causing the problem? That, Grace indicated, ended the minor waiting-room rebellion.

I was getting the picture now. Grace was engaged in a constant battle with people who were trying to get away from what had to be done. It was often an encounter in the shadows, as motives were hidden and excuses put forward as reasons. But Grace could read it for what it was and wasn't scared to take people on. Still, it could wear her down.

'You know what, Professor? One of the big problems I have is people not believing I'm HIV [positive]. They say I've been paid by the government to tell them that.' She was referring to those in the clinic waiting room when she was holding impromptu education classes on HIV/AIDS.

'They say that, because you look healthy?' I asked.

'No, Professor,' she answered, 'because they don't want to listen to what I'm telling them.' Then she looked wistful, 'Especially before when I still had my figure. Before I was having those hips, back seat, but now I'm shapeless. Now look, I'm having stomach, no figure, no hips, no back seat. My legs [are thin], I can't wear even a [knee-length] skirt.'

I had been struck at how her shape had changed since I had first seen her two years previously.

She went on, in a disappointed tone, talking about her problem, not the problems in other people's heads. 'It's the antiretroviral drugs; it's the only thing which they're doing which I don't like. They told me that this shape I've got, it's a side-effect. The first time I see my body changing like this, I *amper* [nearly] kill myself, it's not easy. First thing you have to change is your wardrobe because those clothes you were wearing before can't fit you now. Then, [secondly] you were having that nice body and you feel shame and you say, "OK, that means I'm not going to find a partner now." You see it's not easy to accept the body, knowing very well what you were like before, but what I told myself is to accept it. Now I've accepted my body as it is, the only thing I have to do is to know what kind of clothes fit my body.'

As she explained to me the process of coming to terms with the way her body's shape had changed, she also got back to her role as the public face of AIDS in Potlakong. 'Some people when they see me and my shape, they're afraid to take the treatment, but I lie to them, Professor, I say, "The problem is that me, I made a mistake, I forced them to give me the treatment without checking if it's okay for me or not."'

I was to find out that Grace had indeed forced her way onto a HIV-treatment programme, bypassing the start-up protocols. But it was clear she was making up this explanation about rushing into treatment to hide the drug's side-effects from people she was persuading to follow her. I said as much and she agreed. 'I'm lying. Yah, I'm lying, you know what, Professor? You know why I lie? Sometimes you have to lie to fix things, to help others. You have to lie to help other people, you see.'

After the interview I took pictures of the training certificates she had proudly pulled out when explaining her work as a clinic counsellor. The sun had emerged and I took the documents outside for better light. By the time I'd finished, she was ready to go and I took her picture. Smiling for the camera, she posed in front of her house, clutching a large black Bible and wearing the long green dress that hid her skinny legs and no back seat. Then we bounced along the rutted dirt roads to her church appointment.

Earning a living

As my interviews with Grace continued, I worked out that the time she had spent living in Sizwe Section was longer than she initially implied. The timeline that I drew for her life in my notebook didn't account for her 36 years. Even if I added on a margin to compensate for misremembered dates, the time in Sizwe, before she had become the only openly HIV-positive person in Potlakong, must have been between six and eight years. She had never had a job and, although she talked about selling children's clothes, which she would buy at the *maindia* (Indian, i.e. wholesale, shops) in Johannesburg, or hawking sweets and s*imba* (crisps),[7] she never portrayed these as fulltime occupations. Rather, they had been sidelines, as they still were, to the monthly volunteer's stipend that she received for her counselling work at the clinic.

She never fully clarified the dates, but as the interviews progressed, she opened up about how she had made a living in the taverns around the hostel in Sizwe. Initially, it was that men were happy to buy her drinks. She was hot stuff then with a big back seat and hips. When the night warmed up, she would take to the floor and men would offer to buy her what she wanted. She drank Redds cider.[8]

But you can't live on Redds alone. In later interviews, she was much more candid about the way the business worked. Like any trade, there is an initial investment that needs to be made and she would head out with money to start the evening off.

'I will buy two Redds from the tavern. You know when I first come, no one's saying, "Hey, I love you," I must get two, and then I started dancing, then they will come. You see, when I started dancing, I'm showing my stuff. I'm showing my nice stuff.'

Grace clicked her fingers rapidly to imitate the beat of the music in the tavern as she continued her account.

'Then I know they will come and say, "Hello *sisi* [sister], how are you doing?" Then if they want to talk with me [they] go and buy something for me or he puts money in my hand. Maybe he pops out R50. "Grace, please go and buy what you want." I buy maybe one or two, I go to the toilet, I'm always wearing *takkies* and socks, because I dance too much. I put the paper [notes] in the socks, even when I'm going to sleep I'm only taking off the *takkies*, not socks, it's [the money] still there [in the morning]. Only the loose [change] I put in my pocket. And before I'll go [back to my room] with him, although I was drunk, I'm asking him one question, "Are you going to give me money? Remember where we are going, I'm renting, I'm eating, I have to work, I have a child to look after." If he asks me to go to his place I say, "Remember, I'm not going to stay with you permanent, I'm having my place, a room to rent."'

Getting drunk made asking for money easier. So, too, was thinking about her son or, as she referred to him, her baby. 'Immediately you put money in my hands, I just started thinking about my baby. When I put money in my socks, I say [to myself], maybe this one is for my baby, I'm going to buy something for my baby. I used to buy expensive

205

clothes for my baby. My baby started wearing a leather jacket when he was six years old.' With pride, Grace explained that she used to buy clothes for her son at an expensive men's outfitters in town. 'They will tell you about that shop, it's men's clothes only and from younger [ages] too. Only expensive clothes there, Professor, too expensive! I didn't want my child to suffer the way I was suffering, I wanted him to wear what he wanted to wear, to be nice, not like me. I was suffering, although I was staying with my uncle who was rich, but I never get, sometimes I was even crying, asking my uncle to buy what I want, but he won't get it. So [when men wanted to sleep with me I would ask], "What are you going to give me?" Sometimes I wake up with R300, sometimes R200, sometimes, if maybe he told me that "I'm broke," maybe R100. If it's R100, I'm going to spend R50 for my baby, I keep the other R50.'

Grace's son was now a teenager. He had come to live with her when she moved into the RDP house, but things had not worked out. He still harboured resentment over having been left with relatives. He had moved on to live with friends. She continued to demonstrate love for him by giving him what she could spare. She had only contempt for his father, who failed to support him. 'I don't care that he dumped me or whatsoever, [but] I hate one thing, my son keeps on begging. I hate that thing, he keeps on complaining to me, "My Papa doesn't want to give me even R100." He [the father] says he don't have money, but he's working. He's driving a taxi.'

Once when she heard that he was taking credit for how well turned out his son was, she had gone to the taxi rank and publicly humiliated him in front of the other drivers.

'I find him in the taxi rank where he was working. He resigned that day.'

'Because of the scene you made?'

'Yes.' Grace was proud to take responsibility for his downfall. 'I asked the other drivers, "Why is he proud of my boy, but he can't tell you his (clothes) size? Why is he talking lies?" Me, I'm always telling the truth.'

'But you know, Professor?' Her voice dropped dramatically. I was now used to Grace's sudden change in mood. One moment she had been on her high horse, berating the useless father of her baby. Suddenly, she was reflecting on the past and concerned about the future.

'I was a prostitute ... now I'm HIV positive, sometimes I used to sleep without the condom because of money. I don't want a cure [for HIV]. The only thing I want is to get a permanent job and for my son to get a good future ... for [him to go to] university.'

A treatment odyssey

Yet Grace had wanted to be cured. It had taken a long time to accept that she had to live with the virus. Things had not got off to a good start. She found out she was HIV positive when she was referred to hospital because of bleeding from her vagina. The doctor had talked about fibroids, a nurse took blood and she was given a date to return for an operation. When she came back, it was a different doctor, an Indian. He said they couldn't help her; there would be no operation. He told her she had AIDS and left the consulting room.[9] That was in 1992. She'd walked out of the hospital crying and was nearly hit by a lorry as she crossed the road. As far as she was concerned, she was going to die. That was all she really knew about HIV and AIDS, which to her, at the time, was one thing. Drinking became more than just Dutch courage for the dance floor; it meant she could get to sleep. If she was sober she'd lie awake the whole night. Sometimes she'd get morose and start weeping. Then she'd have to cover up when people asked her what was wrong. She'd tell them she was an orphan. She knew she should be using condoms, but men didn't always want to wear them. She conceded if they insisted, she didn't want them to suspect that she might be infected. That was something she needed to keep hidden from everybody, especially those whom she was making a living from.

Over the next few years, Grace was cured of HIV, several times. She'd consulted several traditional healers. Her orphan status led several of them to diagnose that the necessary cleansing rituals had not been followed after her parents' death. Her mother being a Pedi and her father a Zulu complicated matters, but clearly things had not been done properly at the time. Several times she followed the detailed, but differing, instructions given by the healers. These involved buying two white chickens. Their blood was then mixed with medicines and the mixture was smeared over her head and shoulders. With the first healers, the chickens were to be left in the *veld* (open country) where the pollution (dirt or bad luck) causing the problem would remain. He told her to go back for an HIV test, she would be negative. The second healer said the first healer hadn't used the right medicines. The third healer said that the chickens should not be left in the *veld*, rather he would take them. She didn't test again, but she kept getting ill after each cure. The fourth healer disagreed with the previous three and diagnosed that she was being called to be a healer herself. She got through three months of training, before she was sick again.

This time it was TB. She was admitted to a sanatorium where she stayed for six months. There had been classes about TB and about HIV/AIDS. TB and HIV, she was told, went together; they were friends of each other. Years after being told she was HIV positive she was still struggling against her status. 'Every time I was fighting with my teacher, telling my teacher that "Okay, you are telling us that we are HIV positive." He said, "No, I'm advising you to go and test." I said, "Not me, I can't do such a thing."'

After six months she was TB-free, but she still wanted to get rid of what she knew was inside. In Rustenburg, Dineo had been a ZCC member and Grace had gone to church with her. She started to go to ZCC services in Potlakong. A church prophet diagnosed her as having too much anger inside. She would go to his house where he would brew a bitter tea for her to drink. She would drink several litres. After that, her urine ran clear and didn't smell as it often did. She liked that, she felt it was a sign that it was cleaning her blood. Usually, several people would attend the prophet's sessions, but one day the others had gone to a nearby *spruit* (stream) to pray. There had been a strong smell of *spirit* (i.e. methylated spirits) when the prophet was brewing the tea, but she told herself that he must have spilt some. That day he added copious spoons of Klim[10] (milk powder) to the tea. Her head started spinning. She had gone outside to the toilet but, hearing music thumping in the township night, had made her way towards the sound. The prophet had caught up with her as she opened the *shebeen* (tavern) door and had laughingly explained to those around that she was drunk. He'd led her back to the house where he raped her.

Her life was falling apart. On the Monday morning, she'd gone to the nearby government Bophelo Clinic in Masimong Section, where she now lived. A friend had spoken highly of it; the nurses didn't shout at you. Sometimes they would serve tea and bread to the women who arrived early. Sitting in the large waiting room, Grace had heard a nurse talking in the Sepedi dialect of Pulane that her family spoke. Her name was Sister Irene. She'd got up and gone over to the nurse. '*Sisi* (sister),' she said, 'I've got a big problem.' Sister Irene had seen the tears welling up in her eyes and taken her into one of the consulting rooms. Without Sister Irene, Grace doesn't think she'd be alive today.

Toyi-toying for treatment

Sister Irene had organised counselling for Grace. Then she'd given her R300, with instructions to find somewhere else to live. It was a break with the past. If Sister Irene saved Grace's life, Grace was now saving others. Sometimes it was hard. People could be stubborn, just like she had been. Sometimes she would get them onto treatment, only to lose them as they abandoned the pills and threw their lot in with traditional healers, church prophets or charismatic preachers in the township. It was a battle without end. During our interviews, there was a national public sector strike that closed down the clinics in the area. The strike was about pay. At Bophelo Clinic, strikers had forced their way into the building and let off the fire extinguishers. Everything was covered in white powder, which remained until the strike ended. Patients who were unlucky to have their appointment that week were running out of antiretrovirals. Grace has a stash of the drugs and she rationed these out to people who were short as the strike dragged on, pointing out to me that the drug's expiry dates had not yet passed. She was being careful to show me that there was nothing wrong in what she was doing.

After the strike, Grace moved our interviews to the Bophelo Clinic.

By now she was confident that I was not going to embarrass her and she was keen to parade me elsewhere. The clinic is a large, one-storeyed, red-brick building standing alone in the middle of a field, surrounded by a heavy concrete palisade fence. A dirt track leads across the field to the gated entrance. Sometimes the guards were friendly and waved me through with a smile, sometimes they made a point of keeping me waiting while they finished their conversation. When they were finished they would thrust a visitors' log and a pen though the car window. The first time I met Grace at the clinic it had been raining overnight. I had carefully weaved the car past the worst sheets of soft mud and pools of water into which the dirt roads of Masimong had turned. The waiting room was full of people, mostly women, sitting on wooden benches and plastic chairs. Grace, engulfed in a large red-and-white tracksuit festooned with AIDS badges, had been watching out and greeted me loudly in Sesotho so that everybody's head turned. Then she addressed her waiting-room audience and told them that I was her boyfriend and that we were getting married. There was a disbelieving but curious pause, which I broke by telling them, '*Yena o bua maka*' (She's fibbing). This became our stand-up routine each time I came to the clinic.

With my credentials presented in the waiting room, I was taken around and introduced to everybody working in the clinic. It was clear that I was being shown off, just as I'd been shown off to her neighbours. Finally, I was able to say hello to Sister Irene in her dark blue skirt and nurse's jacket with maroon epaulettes. I explained the research project to her and she said it would help their work. We agreed that Grace was doing a wonderful job. Then she asked me if I was going to buy her something from the small stock of snacks that Grace peddled in the waiting room: sweets, biscuits and nuts. The small packets of peanuts were *ponto* (R2) a piece and I bought three, one for each of us.

Once we were alone, Grace's mood had subsided and she started to cough. She told me she was ill. She was worried it might be TB again, she had not been sleeping well and she was tired. One of the nurses had taken a sputum test and they would get the results in a few days. 'It's hard, Professor,' she told me. She was talking about her constant health scares; over the nine months that I interviewed Grace there was rarely a month when she wasn't ill. Sometimes it was just flu, but she would always be worried that it might be something more. As each of these infections cleared up, I realised that she was only in remission before the next problem would come along. Once she was hospitalised for a week with pneumonia. Alongside this catalogue of infections, there were her three-monthly CD4 counts, which she knew off by heart: 198, 302, 221, 245. When it went up she was pleased, when it dropped she was disappointed. That it fluctuated worried her; she could always think of reasons afterwards, but she fretted that she didn't really know if it was going to be up or down before she tested.

But she always bounced back and put her doubts aside to convince others. 'Even in the chat rooms, I'm a peer educator, Professor!' she enthusiastically told me. I had to ask her what she was talking about. She showed me the chat room application on her cell phone. Mostly she entered the chat room for Potlakong. There are chat rooms for most large settlements: it allows people to text, and perhaps meet with, people nearby. It's something she'd just got into, using the nickname 'Orphan'. Now she had over fifty 'contacts' – people who asked to text directly with her privately. Some were curious to know if she really was positive, as she told them. But it was in the 'HIV support' chat room she also visited that the rough-and-tumble happened. As Grace explained:

> It's for the people who are HIV positive. It's like a group to support each other, those who are affected by the HIV. Like, maybe you ask me, 'When did you take ARVs?' I told that person, 'OK. My CD4 count was maybe this, now it's this.' Others will ask and say, 'Please help me, I don't know how to disclose to my boyfriend.' But, there are those people who will say, 'Ah, leave him and come to me, baby.' If I find a shit talking about HIV and saying [for example], 'All women in this room, I hate you, you've got HIV, because you were sleeping around,' whatsoever, I kick them out of the room.

Kicking somebody out of the room meant reporting them to a

moderator. The offender would be suspended for a few days but would be back to take 'Orphan' on. Now, Grace had a string of user names and played a cat-and-mouse game in the HIV chat room with these 'shits'.

After watching her thumb a short, highly condensed text conversation in the Potlakong chat room, I decided to move us on and asked her how she got onto treatment. She had started in 2005, the national antiretroviral drug programme was finally under way,[11] but it would still be years before they got to Bophelo Clinic, given the rate at which this huge intervention was progressing. Sister Irene had given her the taxi fare to go to one of the initial roll-out sites.[12] At that point her CD4 count was only 27. Sister Irene had told her to go and *toyi-toyi*[13] (i.e. cause a scene) if she wanted to get treatment. She had got up at four the next morning to be first in line. At the ARV clinic, they had made a file for her, then she had asked where the antiretrovirals were. They explained she first needed to be seen by a social worker. So she started crying. The doctor came out, an African woman who knew Grace from previous admissions to the hospital. She explained that they needed to know her CD4 count. Grace already knew her CD4 count. They needed to start her on prophylaxis treatment before the antiretrovirals. Grace had no problem with taking the prophylaxes but she told them, 'You can give me both [prophylaxes and antiretroviral drugs], but not one. Both now. If there are two, give me both.' They said they needed to know if her liver was healthy enough to deal with the antiretrovirals. Grace told them that they wanted her to die. They got the blood tests done that day.

She left the hospital with both: the prophylactics and the antiretrovirals.

Her CD4 count rose tenfold. She continued to be ill, and she continued to worry about her health, but she was no longer dying. She had hope – initially, too much hope. One of the reasons that she'd determinedly *toyi-toyied* to get antiretrovirals that day was because she thought the drugs might do more than suppress the virus. 'I thought maybe it's a treatment to *finish* it in my body,' she had whispered to me after concluding the story.

Faith and secrets

I wanted to backtrack to the time before Grace had started treatment. She had told me about the repeated attempts of healers to finish this thing in her body, but I wanted to know if, notwithstanding her disillusionment with them, she might still hold to some of the cosmologies their folk theories were based upon. It seemed not. She dismissed the ability of ancestors[14] to help people, out of hand. Using her own life as an example, she demonstrated why: she'd been orphaned, she'd been infected with HIV, she was suffering. What were her ancestors doing to help her? It was a rhetorical question. She went on with a wider criticism of cultural practices that she saw as nothing more than superstition. She gave the example of how Africans washed their hands on returning from a funeral to remove contamination picked up at the graveyard. A bowl of water with cut pieces of aloe leaves would be waiting when the mourners returned to dip their hands in it before joining the queue for food. She ridiculed the practice as unhygienic; with 200 people sharing the same water, it was simply a way of spreading germs.

Traditional healers, she now concluded, were just people. They said they could cure illness, but they themselves died. They said they spoke with the ancestors, but they had their own problems. If, as some claimed, they could help you win the Lotto, why didn't they simply play it themselves? They were just people. Church prophets were the same: they claimed to cure people but only God could do that. God was not a person.

It was impossible for me not to ask, 'Do you think God can cure HIV?' We ended up discussing God and AIDS several times. It was a difficult question for Grace to answer unequivocally. She understood that it was the antiretroviral drugs that were keeping her alive, but she wanted very much to believe that God could do anything.

Some aspects of this question could be dispatched easily. There were people who chose to believe in God so as to deny that they had AIDS. This included relatives. A cousin had come to her asking what she should do if she was positive. Grace had been generous (the same cousin had shunned her when she had told her family that she had

HIV). Grace told her that the very first thing was to accept that you had the virus.

Not everybody could do that. Grace's cousin never got past first base. Instead, she'd joined a charismatic church. The change in her life had been dramatic; she was never out of church and never missed an opportunity to pray. Her health also improved. So much so that she'd discontinued the TB treatment and declared that she was cured of HIV and that the TB had merely been a chest infection. On that belief she stood; God had cured her. And on that belief she had died, asking visitors at her bedside to read Scripture when she was too weak to read herself.

Grace had a grudging respect for the way her cousin had died, but thought that what she'd done when alive was akin to the Gospel account of Satan tempting Jesus in the wilderness. God wasn't asking you to throw yourself off a cliff, in the expectation that he catch you. It was easy to say that you would be cured by faith, but in doing so you not only condemned yourself, you also undermined the efforts of others, like Grace, to get people onto treatment.

Rather than testing God, Grace explained to me that you needed to ask for God's help. That's what she liked about her church – *Moruti* (Preacher) Puleng told her to pray and to take her tablets. What *Moruti* Puleng didn't want was for Grace, or anybody else, to 'mix systems'. If you were praying to God for help, you shouldn't also be seeing a traditional healer. If you were doing both things, how would you know that it was God that had helped you when your request was granted?

'But,' I quibbled, 'isn't taking tablets and praying to God mixing systems?'

'Professor,' Grace explained to me, 'God gave us minds. We have to use those minds. We have to use everything that God gives us. If you drop treatment, you're being lazy. But you must have faith that God will help you. It is God who helped those scientists discover the ARVs. He will help the ARVs in your body also.'

This was more complex than I'd expected. To me it was mixing systems, but Grace was explaining it differently. I'd already met *Moruti* Puleng when dropping Grace off at her church. Now I asked Grace if she'd mind if I talked to her. Grace was pleased by the suggestion and said she would set up a meeting.

'The thing I like about *Moruti* Puleng', Grace stressed, 'is that whenever I'm angry she says I must use my knees [i.e. pray]. It helps a lot. Sometimes the stress is so much. But if I shout, the situation gets more stressed.'

This was easy to categorise. It was sound advice in a situation where resources are tight and squabbles can easily break out. 'What else do you like about the church?' I asked.

'She's', Grace was talking about *Moruti* Puleng, 'not too much hard on us that aren't married. She accepts that we need somebody. She says it's OK to have a boyfriend, but she says we should stick to just the one. That men play around too much, so we should bring him to the church so that they can be shown the way.'

There was a pause. In between her long and fluid monologues, Grace could be hesitant. I'd learned to wait these gaps out.

'You know what, Professor? Sometimes I'm ashamed. I took my boyfriend with me when I started churching with *Moruti* Puleng two years ago, but I'm no longer seeing him. I just say, "No, he is fine," when they ask after him. But, really I'm no longer seeing him. They've only seen the one boyfriend.'

That there had been other boyfriends was not the only thing she couldn't tell *Moruti* Puleng.

'You know, Professor, I changed, but not exactly. What I can tell you is that's my secret, I'm having everything, everything that you want from a Christian, but ...' There was a long pause, nine seconds on the transcript. 'I can stay six [months] or a year or sometimes two years, but the day comes and I'm going to tell myself that now *I'm going to drink*, [whispering] I'm going to drink like a man ...' A six-second pause. 'I'm telling you the truth and the other thing ...' (four seconds) 'I'm doing, but is not supposed to be done by a Christian, is that I'm having sex before marriage ...' Eleven seconds. 'You see, I'm doing that thing of chatting, [to] find a boyfriend, when I'm going to meet one, if I like him, I will end up doing it with him.'

I waited.

'OK, although I'm using condoms, but that thing is eating me. It's a sin to me. Sometimes, I think *Moruti* Puleng can see right through me, like when I used to think that people could see the HIV inside me. Once, when we were praying next to each other [with each person praying individually out loud] I hear her asking God to help her control her body, her flesh. You know, Professor, her husband died and she's on her own. So she's praying to God to help her. But, I think maybe she's really talking to me. I become so scared, thinking, "Oh, maybe she's seeing me through the spirit; she sees that my flesh is busy controlling me."'

Grace had even peeked. *Moruti* Puleng's eyes were tightly closed, but Grace was still not entirely convinced that her sins were not visible in some way.

Moruti Puleng

Moruti Puleng was waiting for us in her living room when we arrived. We had gone around the back of the large, slightly dilapidated house in one of the older sections of Potlakong. Grace had knocked and we had gone in. *Moruti* Puleng's voice had called us into the living room. It was spacious and carpeted. She sat in her blue-and-white Apostolic Church uniform in the centre of a large black vinyl sofa. It had seen better days and the covering was brittle and cracking. A large handbag was by her feet and she was clearly ready to leave the house. She told us that she'd been asked to pray with a member of the church who was very ill; she would go as soon as we had finished talking.

I had intended to ask *Moruti* Puleng some questions about her church, the Holy Apostolic Church of Christ's Forgiveness, or Church of Forgiveness as it was referred to in short, to ease us into the discussion. From Grace I knew that between two and three hundred attended her Sunday services, and that the majority were women. I also knew that the Potlakong church was one of 20 branches across the country which fell under the authority of an archbishop based in Pretoria. I started off double-checking that I'd got the church's full name correct. I had a list of other introductory questions, but *Moruti* Puleng leaped immediately into an explanation of the church's mission. We were off, straight to the question of forgiveness, healing and God's power.

The church was about helping people; it was a church for people who had problems, for whom things were not going well. They came to the church for help and the church directed them onto the path of God's forgiveness. Problems were a *pontsho* (sign) from God that you were sinning, that you were moving away from God and the way He wanted you to live; if you repented of your sins, asked for forgiveness and mended your ways, your problems would be solved.

It was, I came to see, a cycle. Sinning came from not having God in your heart. Sin leads to suffering. Through repentance, suffering brings you closer to God. This cycle would be repeated, since when things were going well you would forget that it was God who had given you these blessings; even as your health and life prospered by his grace, you would forget that this came from Him, you would be moving from Him and He would again send a sign.

When you pray to God, *Moruti* Puleng explained, 'You will feel better, you will sleep deeply, other people will cease hating you and will start to love you. If you do not have work, you will find employment.' That was a wide-ranging and important set of problems that could be turned around, but I wanted to be sure that she really meant all problems were a sign from God. Did this include sickness? '*Jehovah ha a hlolwe ke letho*' (Jehovah is beaten by nothing) was her response; all diseases are signs from God. And in an oblique reference to Grace, who was sitting with us in the room, she explained that was why in the church there was no problem in sharing a glass or a plate with other members.

What *Moruti* Puleng was putting forward was a profound democratisation of affliction that was being reduced to a single common denominator – one we all shared. I could see why it was attractive to Grace.

Moruti Puleng wasn't saying that the different forms of suffering were randomly allocated to those who drifted from God – the signs were specific. She made this point very clear by asking me to read from her Bible the letter to the church in Thyatira that is found in the second chapter of Revelation. The last book of the Bible is better known for its indecipherable prophecies, but the letter to the church in Thyatira is a direct chastisement of church members, from the Apostle John. Members of the church were tolerating 'that woman Jezebel' who has led them into 'sexual immorality'. Since there has been no repentance, Jezebel is to be 'cast on a bed of suffering and I [the Lord] will make those who commit adultery with her suffer intensely ... I am He who searches hearts and minds and I will repay each of you according to your deeds.'[15]

As I began to read the passage I had no idea that the words *Moruti* Puleng had asked me to speak aloud would be so harsh and so direct. But once I had started, I had no option but to carry on till the reading was finished. I was surprised to see that Grace seemed quite happy, nodding in approval as I concluded. Direct as the message might be, her HIV status was a sign from God that served as a rebuke for her sins, but it was a sign like any other *pontsho*. All suffering was a corrective calling from God. God sent these signs because He wanted to forgive. Anything could be forgiven.

If the Church of Forgiveness's theology was so tightly constructed, I wanted to check if there was any room for witches, ancestors, Satan or demons – all of which are incorporated into the explanations of suffering and healing put forward in other township churches. The answer was precise: No. No. No. And No. None of them existed. *Moruti* Puleng was clear. In comparison with other cosmologies of suffering, that of the Church of Forgiveness was a stripped-down affair with a single reference point. It's a significant point to note. Not simply because of its attractiveness to Grace, but because it warns us not to generalise and then essentialise the beliefs of others working with different paradigms of belief.

To illustrate the foolishness of ancestor belief, *Moruti* Puleng employed the metaphor of a can of fish – when the fish is eaten the can remains, there is nothing left inside and it is thrown away. When we die, the body is like the tin, it is lifeless. The spirit has gone. How can the empty tin now do anything? The body that is left on earth can neither harm you nor protect you. What she was saying, indirectly, was that the church was staking a claim on what happened to a person's spirit after death. This was an important claim that she was able to use not only to strip the ancestors of agency, but also to sidestep conflict with Western medicine.

When I asked her how medicines fitted into what she'd told me as to the cause of illness, she explained it as a division of labour. They, the doctors and nurses, were attending to your body; the church was attending to your spirit. It might be that God sent illness as a *pontsho* and that repenting would heal you, but the objective was to get you back to God, not to heal disease. She had no problem with *dipilisi ya sekgowa* (literally, White people's pills). On the one hand, she was conceding ground and it struck me how different on this point was the Church of Forgiveness from the Apostolic churches studied by Bengt Sundkler in the 1940s, which rejected Western medicine as, '*not a cure of disease, but the cause of demonical possession*'.[16] On the other hand, *Moruti* Puleng was claiming far more than Western medicine. God was, she said, more powerful than pills; she had been trained in the *Univesithi ya Modimo* (University of God) to work with the spirit. 'Which [Western] doctor', she asked as she brought her explanation to an end, 'can cure somebody of not being loved?'

On that note, I drove *Moruti* Puleng to pray with her sick parishioner.

Director SA

It struck me that that while Grace received support from the Church of Forgiveness, what she couldn't give to the church was honesty. The next time I drove over to the clinic to meet with her, I'd been unable to get through to confirm our appointment. I went anyway and found she was expecting me. Her phone was 'on charge' (i.e. left at an outlet that charges phones, for a fee, for those without electricity). Once we had settled down, I asked her how the chat rooms were going. She said she had stopped. In fact she now saw it as an addiction. She had left the phone on charge deliberately. She was telling those contacts whom she might meet outside the world of text messaging that she had lost her phone and had done a SIM swap, but that the new phone wasn't able to download the chat application. She promised them that she'd start again as soon as she got another phone, but her intention was to stop completely.

This had been precipitated by one of her chat room contacts,

'Director SA', whom she'd met the previous week. She'd been chatting with him for almost two months and they had exchanged pictures. Director SA knew her HIV status. He had been supportive and kind. But, when she met him she realised that he'd sent her old pictures of himself. What she saw now was Stavudine. The 'camel's hump' at the back of the neck and pot belly were telltale signs that he was taking this antiretroviral drug. But she had decided to say nothing. They had gone back to his house. It was taken for granted that they would have sex. After they had settled down, he'd put on a pornographic movie. She'd asked him if he had condoms. He hadn't. He told her he didn't need to use them since his only problem was that he had an ulcer and that he wasn't worried about getting HIV from her since it was not possible to get AIDS having sex once with a person. They went ahead, without a condom.

Afterwards, he had showed her his antiretroviral treatment and mocked her for thinking that he'd have slept with her if he was negative. Back in the chat room all hell had broken out; she'd posted her version of events and people had started accusing him of spreading HIV – Grace, it emerged, was not the only person he had hidden his HIV status from. He'd started sending her messages, calling her a bitch and a cunt. She switched her phone off and left it on charge.

In telling me this, Grace presented herself as a victim of Director SA. He was, she was saying, a public menace. He knew that he was HIV positive but lied about it and didn't keep condoms in the house. Grace was clearly genuinely upset by what had happened, but to me she'd gone along with the deception from the moment she saw his Stavudine-shaped body. As for the story about not being able to get AIDS if you only slept with somebody once, in a public forum she'd have ripped the assertion to shreds. Since she knew, really, that they were both positive, her advice to others would have been to use a condom to prevent mutual reinfection with their different viral strains.[17] Finally, if before she had seen Director SA, she thought he was negative, but she knew herself to be positive, why had she not taken condoms with her? It was hardly as though sex was not in the offing. When I asked her, she could only tell me that she had forgotten them.

Grace's confessional syndicate

As much as Grace was guiding others, she was herself struggling, but she kept this hidden from all but a few to whom she selectively confessed. I was now incorporated into the segmented confessional syndicate that she had put together.

Never mind what *Moruti* Puleng might think about Grace yielding to her sexual desires for a man she'd just met, Sister Irene would, I was quite certain, be a very unsympathetic ear for confessions of flesh-on-flesh sex. But Grace clearly needed to tell somebody beyond the condensed, fast-paced angry texting of the chat rooms that she now, in any case, eschewed.

What she got from *Moruti* Puleng was unending love and support. It was always the same message, 'Use your knees, and ask for forgiveness.' At times that helped: Grace needed her spirals of frustration to be checked. But there were things that she could not bring to *Moruti* Puleng. Things that were too deep and too dirty to be open about. Confessions that would reveal her to be unworthy as a Christian and erase the hope that God would, in some way, free her of HIV.

Neither could Grace talk to *Moruti* Puleng about her medical treatment, which belonged to another realm, that of Sister Irene. Though Grace thought the world of Sister Irene, she too had her limits. Grace complained to me several times that for all the support Sister Irene gave, she would dismiss Grace when she tried to tell her how hard it was to manage without drinking or sex. She told Grace she must be patient, hardly words that would quench Grace's cravings as they bloated inside her. But at least Sister Irene was a woman of the world and Grace could talk to her in a way that she would never be able to do with *Moruti* Puleng. As Grace explained to me, with Sister Irene, when there was a boyfriend on the scene one could bitch about him. You could say, 'You know what that shit of mine did yesterday?' and you would be listened to with sympathy.

I heard the secrets that Grace was unable to raise with Sister Irene or *Moruti* Puleng. Research is not supposed to be about confessions, but confidentiality and researchers' curiosity can make us a repository of last resort for confidences. Such talk is likely to be important components of understanding an individual, so I listened carefully to Grace's account of how there had been no condoms when she met and slept with Director SA. It was not the first time she'd told me about sex without condoms.

Before she had come to terms with her status, there were the men who had paid extra for flesh-on-flesh sex. She regretted that she must have infected some of them, but she could put this down to the way she'd been first informed that she was positive. Told that she could not be helped, and cut adrift to stumble out from the hospital crying, was hardly the way to ensure that she took responsibility for her status. But even when things had come right, there had been others. She told me how the boyfriend she had taken to the Church of Forgiveness had told her he wanted to show how much he loved her. She had thought that maybe he was going to present her with a ring, but rather he was pleading with her that they stop using condoms.

He knew her status well enough, she had told him many times – though quite what this meant to him she could not be sure. He had gone to a traditional healer and given her a two-litre (bottle) of *moriana* (traditional medicine); she was to drink half a cup a day. When she'd finished the two litres, he'd asked her to test. She did and she was still positive, but she didn't like to upset him and told him that the clinic had run out of testing kits. Short of this proof of the *muti's* effectiveness, he had asked her if she felt better. She said she did. 'You know, when you love someone. I didn't want to … to disappoint him.'

She had asked him to test. He told her that he had and that there was nothing to worry about; he hadn't told her the result. She thought that maybe he was positive and unconcerned about being infected by her – people didn't just jump into fires because they were in love. She pointed out that she might get pregnant if they didn't use condoms. He had no problem with that. He told her again that he loved her.

Aware of our previous discussion on condoms and her own public stance on them, Grace had struggled to conclude what had happened. Only after she'd double-checked that our interview was confidential did she confirm that the condoms had been left in the bedside drawer. 'You know, he convinced me because he said he wanted a baby and because I loved him and I trusted him ... I don't know how to explain love. Have you ever loved someone in your life in the way that you can trust that person? Ya really, really, it happened to me, I'm a human being.'

And with that frank confession, which applies to all of us, she had moved swiftly to a second. When the boyfriend had left her she'd been distraught, she'd prayed to God, but she'd also sought the help of a traditional healer, who'd promised to bring him back. For R500. Grace didn't return with the money. She'd felt ashamed for going and was convinced as she left the healer's house that she would be seen by somebody.

Too much context?

The next time I interviewed Grace, I had to abandon my planned questions. Writing up the interview that evening, I started by noting that it had been a case of 'too much context'. A deteriorating relationship with her neighbour had erupted into a violent dispute the previous weekend, and Grace had an ugly gash across her forehead as testimony to the climactic fight that had taken place late on the Saturday night. It was Tuesday when I arrived at the clinic and the conflict was still as raw as the wound. I had listened to her account of events before trying to move on to my prepared questions. She would begin to answer them, but would quickly return to the still unfinished business of the dispute. Her mind was gripped by events and I realised there was little point in trying to talk about anything else.

Although the fight itself had been triggered by accusations of slander, what underlay the tensions between them was economic competition. As a way of supplementing her volunteer stipend, Grace had started grilling chicken feet at weekends and selling them to her neighbours as a snack for a rand a piece. Mazuma had copied suit, serving similarly cooked chicken feet to her *chaf pozi* (informal drinking venue) customers and anybody else hankering for a tasty snack and with a rand in their pocket. A neighbour, who reported back to Grace, had pointed out that Mazuma was selling exactly the same thing as Grace. Mazuma's response had been to point to the Potlakong Mall where shops competed to sell customers the same thing – she was free to do the same.

Grace took her up on this, and on the Friday afternoon invested in ten crates of beer and enough ice to fill a *waskom* (plastic washing bowl). The two neighbours were now going head to head. On the Saturday night, Grace had won hands down. It had been a party with people parking cars in the street outside and pumping music into the night. She'd sold almost all the beer by the time Saturday night turned into Sunday morning. There was a novelty factor at play, but that would do little to cushion the signal that it sent as to which of the two neighbours was most popular. Something snapped in the empty Mazuma house and her daughter, Zanele, came around accusing Grace of badmouthing her mother. How else had she stolen their customers? Having made the allegation, she had left but returned to smash two of Grace's windows. Grace had run outside with a frying pan in her hand. She was too late to catch Zanele, so instead sent the pan through Mazuma's window. That brought both Mazuma and Zanele out. Eventually, neighbours separated them, though not before Grace and Zanele had been blooded. Grace's wound had been inflicted by Mazuma with a bottle while Grace was pummelling Zanele, whom she'd managed to wrestle to the ground. The police arrived, but were reluctant to get involved. In the end, they threatened both Mazuma and Grace with prosecution for selling liquor without a licence if they didn't go back inside. Then they drove off into the township night, hoping to find something better to do than referee a neighbourhood squabble.

The next morning it was cold war. Grace could hear Mazuma shouting across the street to neighbours about 'that thing which is having AIDS' and who was infecting young boys. But there were 'things which is having AIDS' on both sides of the fight. Zanele was also HIV positive. Grace knew because she had counselled her at the clinic. 'Only now', Grace explained to me, 'she's in denial.' What's more, Grace was sure that Zanele had not told her new boyfriend anything. As we talked, Grace outlined to me how she was going to get her revenge. Zanele's boyfriend was working out of town and Grace had already sent him an SMS that she needed to talk to him. When he rang, she told him that she had to see him at the clinic with Zanele once he got back to Potlakong. Zanele rang her a few minutes later. She was worried and wanted to know what Grace was going to tell her boyfriend. Grace had hung up; she wanted Zanele to suffer. 'Professor,' Grace told me, 'I'm not Jesus.'

In the end, Grace didn't follow through on the final steps of her planned revenge. *Moruti* Puleng helped, telling her to pray and forgive. She should put things into God's hands. Grace took the advice, and she pointed out to me the next time we met that this was a good example of how *Moruti* Puleng helped to break the cycles of anger that would otherwise escalate into tit-for-tat conflict. Grace held her tongue. The relationship with her neighbours was now one of mutual contempt, neither talking to the other. The cycle of conflict was for the moment stilled. That was something, but it was hardly as though Grace had found it within herself to forgive; she liked to think that her silence had thrown her adversaries. She was doing the right thing *and* making them worry about what she was up to. Grace heard later from another neighbour that Mazuma thought she'd gone to a traditional healer, and, in response, Mazuma had shelled out money for her own protection against the witchcraft she suspected Grace had initiated. Grace laughed when she heard that; she'd forgotten her lapse of faith over the lost boyfriend and was again confident that God was more powerful than any traditional healer. Mazuma was wasting her money and Grace was not going to tell her otherwise.

Was this falling out between Grace and her neighbours a case of too much context? It certainly derailed my research agenda, but it also helped me to see how people's HIV status becomes embedded within the often unhappy relationships of community life. Vinh-Kim Nguyen has outlined how, within contexts of economic hardship, the 'confessional technology' of HIV-status disclosure can become an asset for survival.[18] This was true for Grace, because she was willing to talk openly about being positive, and therefore as a PWA (Person With AIDS[19]) she was in demand on World AIDS Day and other events that needed to have a face of AIDS. Such appearances were flattering for Grace, in part because they did not catalyse what those of us working on AIDS stigma had hoped PWAs would achieve – disclosure would become the norm, and the silent, strangling grip of AIDS would be loosened. Yet, rather than leading a deluge of disclosure, Grace remained one of a few brave individuals willing to talk publicly about being positive.

Paradoxically, however, her status also restricted the economic value of her disclosure; brave individuals aren't supposed to be in it for the money. Once she complained to me how she'd been palmed off with R250 in supermarket vouchers after a speech at a local government AIDS awareness event. She knew it wasn't much and, since she asked, I confirmed that a motivational speaker, who might be a bit more polished around the edges but would essentially be doing the same thing, could well receive ten or even twenty times that amount. She was also insulted that she had to go and buy groceries; at least with the R250 in cash she could have used it to buy stock and increase the value of her appearance fee or, depending on how you saw it, token of appreciation.

Yet, notwithstanding the complexities of 'AIDS entrepreneurship' through public disclosure performances, the violent neighbourhood spat revealed a more closely woven relationship between AIDS status, economic survival and the moral economy of the township. Selling beer from a township house is as much about popularity as it is about prices – popularity with men in particular. This was not the first time Grace has been singled out in township gossip, a syndrome that culminates in accusations of sleeping with other women's partners and, integral to the process, taking their money. That was perhaps not surprising; Grace was a vivacious single woman, with a history. Her defence, when accused, was that she was openly positive, but that only worked to a degree. Whether a man would balk at sex with her would depend on what he believed about AIDS in the first place, the central issue that we are engaging.

The problem with context is that it defies the simple, clear solutions for which we yearn. Arguing that you can abstract from particular contexts answers that will serve everyone is a fallacy that serves only to blunt our response to AIDS just as it dulls our understanding of the world.

Sweets and styling

Grace's attempts to *zama* (try to help oneself) suffered another blow when she was barred from hawking in the clinic waiting room. The clinic manager had introduced this as a 'policy', explaining that it wasn't directed at Grace, but nothing was to be sold on the clinic premises. Grace had been the only person selling and the waiting room queues had been a captive market. It had made a significant addition to her income. She'd buy R200 worth of stock – mainly sweets, biscuits and peanuts – from one of the Indian shops located in the scruffy end of town that sold in bulk to hawkers. She would sell this on to waiting patients over a week for around R500. That multiplied to a monthly profit over R1 000, a sum that almost matched her volunteer stipend.

The slack had been taken up by two women with a stall just outside the clinic entrance. Grace knew the two women, as they went to the same church as Sister Irene. It was, as far as she was concerned, a conspiracy. She was being punished for not joining Sister Irene's church as several other clinic staff had done. Sometimes, she told me, she'd go to see Sister Irene for advice, only to find her talking about church matters and with no time for her. Grace became increasingly direct as our interviews progressed over how she felt abandoned by Sister Irene. 'She's forgotten about me now,' Grace told me. 'She's never got time for me now, even though she's the only person I really trust.'

Given how Sister Irene was so central to Grace's survival, I asked if she had ever been to her church. She had, two or three times. 'And?' I asked. She didn't like it. 'Why not?' Two reasons emerged. The first was their theology of AIDS, the second was style.

Perhaps, Grace suggested, Sister Irene didn't fully understand her church, the Pentecostal Tabernacle of God's People. Grace was softening the blow she was about to deliver. But, she told me, she didn't like the way they interpreted the Bible. To Grace, what the preacher said was pointing fingers. He didn't mention names, but he told them about other people who were doing bad things. Members of the congregation had filled in the gaps, warning one another, 'Beware of Mrs So and So.' This, Grace thought, was not healing, it was adding to whatever problem you had. Grace contrasted this finger-pointing with her own church where affliction was a sign from God and the response was to pray, not to point fingers. Grace had no intention of abandoning the democratic interpretation of suffering that *Moruti* Puleng preached, to enter a congregation where fingers could be pointed, just as they were in her neighbourhood.

In any case, she couldn't keep up with the women in Sister Irene's church. They wore seriously nice clothes, different clothes each week that she could not afford. Again, she compared this with the levelling spirit of the Church of Forgiveness. The blue-and-white Apostolic uniforms that church members wore helped disguise who was getting by and who was struggling to make ends meet. Not so in Sister Irene's church. 'Yoh!' Grace exclaimed, 'different hair styles. Today she [an exemplar congregant of the Tabernacle of God's People] comes styling it like this, next day she's styling it differently.' I was surprised. I'd always been impressed by Grace's hairdos. But I had been looking with an untrained eye. When I told Grace that her hair was differently styled each time I saw her, she paused for a moment, then lifted up her wig. Underneath her hair was short and greying. To the trained eyes in Sister Irene's church, it would all be quite apparent.

But what about, I asked, the women selling sweets at the clinic gate, the ones who had taken over her income-generation opportunity? Surely, they could not afford styling either? Grace had to concede the point, but it only made her feel worse. Sister Irene had abandoned her and transferred her patronage to others. She felt she was out in the cold.

The Bible tells me so

I'd arranged with Sister Irene that I'd interview her at twelve on a Tuesday morning. But when Grace and I knocked on her office door, the corridor was crowded with patients hoping to see her. She was so busy she wasn't even going to have time for lunch, but she would find time for me once her work was done. In the meantime she told me she liked KFC. This was not a hard hint to pick up and I took her order for a Streetwise Two Piece meal and a Coke. Grace and

I drove to Potlakong Mall and returned with a bulging plastic bag that we brazenly took through the waiting room. We were following Sister Irene's instructions and could not be faulted. We ate our chicken and chips in the consulting room that we used for interviews. I was hungry and finished quickly, but Grace was careful to leave one piece of chicken untouched. She wanted the neighbours to see the takeaway box and know she'd been treated. We left Sister Irene's Streetwise on the desk. It got cold as we waited for her to finish with her patients.

Sister Irene had worked in various Potlakong clinics for almost 15 years, working her way up the nursing hierarchy from Enrolled Nurse to Sister. Her current focus was the antiretroviral drug programme that the clinic had recently started as part of the unfolding national treatment programme. She started to give me the month-by-month statistical breakdown for those newly enrolled on the programme, their gender, those under 15 and those co-infected with TB. When she realised that she no longer knew all these figures off by heart, she paused. 'Let me bring my statistics,' she suggested and returned with a large file. We settled into the interview by filling two pages of my notebook with six months of carefully recorded enrolment statistics. So far defaulters were few, but then Sister Irene had done her best to pre-empt defection. Once somebody was on the programme, she personally told them that her community volunteers would come knocking on their door if they didn't collect their monthly supply of drugs.

The clinic ARV programme was only the latest in a series of HIV initiatives that Sister Irene had led. Back in the late nineties, she had been trained to run an HIV/AIDS peer education programme. She'd replicated the model she'd been shown and recruited sex workers as community peer educators. Not, she pointed out, that she went around actually recruiting sex workers. She knew well enough how the business operated in Potlakong and that nobody called it sex work, let alone prostitution. There was a level of dignity that was being maintained via a carefully constructed collective fiction. If she wanted her peer education programme to be successful, she had to respect that fiction. So she recruited women without ever asking if they supported themselves through sex work. Instead she went around looking for houses in which the curtains in the windows didn't match.

When she saw one she'd knock on the door and enquire where the owner was. If the owner lived elsewhere and there were only women, each renting a room in the house, but with none of them working, she knew she was talking to her target audience. She'd then explain the peer educator project and ask if they'd like to join.

That's how Sister Irene met Grace. It didn't tally with how Grace met Sister Irene. But then there were several things that didn't correspond between Grace's and Sister Irene's accounts of each other. In the end, I resigned myself to not being able to work out where the truth lay. As close as the two of them were, there was room to hide things that didn't fit into how each saw the world.

Despite these differences, it was clear that Sister Irene and Grace formed a genuine partnership. Both were smart. Sister Irene was close to the ground and Grace was even closer. They had riffed together over how women could introduce condoms into sex or persuade partners to test. Then they had tried to get these ideas activated. Although Sister Irene had saved Grace, Grace was something of a gift for Sister Irene. Sister Irene pointed out that Grace had opened her eyes as to how women had to break their cycle of dependence on men by generating income independently. Without this, women competing with one another for men and men demonstrating love and commitment through flesh-to-flesh sex, would always undermine condoms.

Sister Irene was a wonderful example of someone engaged in thoughtful grassroots AIDS education within the public health system. If you were a donor-funded AIDS NGO seeking to publicise best practice response to the epidemic, you might well nominate Sister Irene for an award.

Unless you asked her what the Bible said. Which I did.

I started this line of questioning by asking her about her church. She was keen to tell me she was 'born again'. She now regarded her previous membership of a mainline church, the church she had been brought up in, as not really engaging with God. She had been going through the motions on a Sunday. Now she was part of a dynamic

Pentecostal church and, to show the extent of commitment, she now tithed, whereas before tithing had just been something talked about by the minister. The Tabernacle of God's People had just put up a new building that could hold 500 worshippers. It was already crowded on Sunday mornings; soon they would have to find larger premises. 'Why?' she asked me rhetorically 'Because our pastor doesn't keep quiet and tell people nice things. He preaches what the Bible tells us.'

So, I asked her what the Bible tells us about illness and she told me:

> The Bible tell us that we are a conqueror of sickness because Jesus Christ died for us. The Bible gives us hope that you can live with diseases and conquer diseases. Jesus Christ died for us ... so the Bible tells ... that if you can give people hope, [if you] can really give us hope, like my pastor does, people can live with diseases and they won't even feel them.

For Sister Irene the real battle over sickness and health was in the mind. If you had faith, illness would be conquered – not, she was careful to say, cured. The point is that you wouldn't even know it was there. You could be a diabetic, but with faith it would not affect you. High blood pressure was the same. I didn't even have to prompt her on HIV/AIDS. The compromise she was constructing, implicitly, between her professional role and her faith was easily juggled. She outlined how somebody's viral load would be undetectable and their CD4 count would rise. It would stay that way: if you trusted in the Lord Jesus Christ.

Faith, Sister Irene explained to me, can achieve anything. 'The Bible tell us to have faith, the faith that makes us live.' She gave me an easy example that I would understand. 'Like for instance I might leave home without food and I will tell myself that tonight I'm going to eat. And through Him [God] I'm really going to eat because David comes by in that dilemma, and says, "You haven't eaten." And then you'll tell him, "There's nothing [at home to cook]." Then he'll give me something, because God provides.'

We both looked at her Streetwise box at the end of the desk. I supposed that she must have left home that morning worried that there was nothing in the fridge. I didn't recall that our earlier conversation about KFC had gone quite the way she now recounted, but narrative differences can be over-emphasised. The point is that she had nothing in the fridge when she left home, and now she had something to put in the microwave when she got back. The chicken and chips I had bought from Potlakong Mall had, I reflected later, gone almost as far as the five loaves and two fishes that fed the multitude in the New Testament miracle. The KFC fast food had assuaged my hunger, provided a status symbol for Grace and vindicated Sister Irene's faith in God.

But I was not yet satisfied. How, I wanted to know, does the Bible help us understand where AIDS comes from? Just as Sister Irene had gone for her file when the specific details of her antiretroviral programme had escaped her, so now she went for her Bible. She wanted to make sure she gave me the correct verse references. After thumbing through the well-used book, she gave me Hebrews, Chapter 13, Verse 4, 'Marriage should be honoured by all, and the marriage bed kept pure, for God will judge the adulterer and all the sexually immoral.' And Corinthians I, Chapter 6, Verses 16–20, which warns church members of the dangers of sexual sin, which, unlike other transgressions, is committed inside the body as two people become one.

'So,' I asked hesitantly, 'HIV is a punishment for sin?' I was probing, not wanting to lead too much, wanting to know how, away from her training as a nurse, she understood AIDS. If I asked too sharply, I was afraid I'd jolt her back into a medical account.

I need not have worried. I was touching on a matter that Sister Irene had thought deeply about and was keen to explain. Initially, she told me, she had liked HIV and assumed it was something that God had sent to bring people closer to Him. But then she had seen its effects and concluded that it came from 'the enemy' – that is, Satan. What had been particularly convincing in bringing her to this perspective was counselling discordant couples. However hard you worked, it usually ended in divorce and she knew God hated divorce. She had concluded similarly on mother-to-child transmission: it could not be God who allowed the child to be infected for something he or she had not done. On this basis she had to conclude that HIV must come from the Devil, at least in these cases. 'Sometimes I hate HIV, sometimes I like it,' she elaborated. She liked it when it brought people to God and the life He wanted for them. HIV could in this way serve God's purpose, though she made it clear that it did not come directly from God; rather, the Devil was slipped into a theology of HIV that, excluding discordant couples and mother-to-child transmission, went along these lines:

God does not send HIV,

But He may allow Satan to

Tempt me do the things

That will put me at risk of

Becoming infected.

It was this message that her pastor preached at the Tabernacle of God's People and the weight of his words rested on the need to avoid temptation. Perhaps *Moruti* Puleng did not see the sins that Grace kept hidden, but Sister Irene did. She told me so directly when I asked why it was that Grace had not joined her church despite being invited. 'She didn't join the Tabernacle because my pastor is always killing sin, talking about the sins that she's still practising. She's still practising sex, yet she's not married, she's having sex with boyfriends. The Bible says this is a sin.'

On this point Grace and Sister Irene gave me the same story, though they did not share it with each other. It's a narrative that illustrates their differences. Both reasoned towards an understanding of HIV that enabled them, subject to caveats, exceptions and doubts, to hold together their own experiences, medical knowledge and beliefs. Their experiences were of course very different; a prostitute turned PWA and a nursing sister. It is the Christian faith, not medical science, that provides the malleable component which allows them to produce their respective models of HIV that they are able to believe and act upon.

Stories without end

As I started to wrap up my discussions with Grace, I drew up a list of outstanding issues that I hoped to finalise. For what I'd billed as the last interview we met as usual at the clinic, but she suggested that we talk at her house. As we made our way slowly though the narrow dirt roads, the electricity poles remained without cables, but they were festooned with election posters for the ANC. Grace announced she would, after all, be voting for the ANC in the upcoming municipal elections.[20] Up till then she had told me she would be staying at home. The council was run by the ANC and what was there to show for the promises of delivery? Dirt roads and darkness. Once, when driving through Masimong, she had pointed to a new VW Golf. It was the councillor's car. He was, Grace said, inside the tavern drinking and playing cards. He spent every afternoon there, he didn't care that she was suffering.

But, it seemed that the ANC were finally making good on their promise of electricity; a meter had been installed on the outside wall of her house and a cable run through to the kitchen. She would have electricity before the elections. In return, she was going to vote the card-player back in. She was excited about having electricity, but the meter was not what she'd brought me to see. The house was now well on its way to being furnished. She had bought a large TV and a DVD player that occupied the centre of a veneered bank of display shelves and cupboards bejewelled with monstrously large wrought-iron handles divided the main area of the house into a living room and kitchen. I sat behind this divide at a kitchen table with matching chairs, made of white vinyl-covered surfaces and grey enamelled steel tube, that were still wrapped in plastic delivery sleeves. Grace lit the paraffin stove to make tea and told me that when she had electricity and was no longer dependent on her 12-volt battery holding its charge, the first thing she wanted to buy was a fridge. Then she would be able to keep milk and food fresh.

The money for the furniture had come from the two *mekgodisano* or revolving credit schemes paying out to her on the same month along with help from a new boyfriend. She paid R1 000 into both schemes each month; one had four members, one had five. When they both paid out to her on the same month, she was the recipient of R7 000 with which she had gone to the Fair Price furniture shop in town. When everything had been delivered, Mazuma from next door, who had stood with the crowd of watching neighbours, had asked how long it would be before the goods were repossessed. She was assuming that Grace had bought the goods on credit. Grace was avoiding a 30 per cent mark-up by not buying on credit from Fair Price, but she now had three months ahead of paying R2 000 before her turn came around again with the saving circles. This was, she said, a worry, but her boyfriend had given her R700 and she had gone to Johannesburg and bought children's clothes that she could sell at a 50 per cent mark-up. Meeting her *mekgodisano* obligations would depend on her turning the stock around fast enough.

As this account continued, I realised that this probably wasn't really going to be the last interview with Grace. As much as I wanted to wrap this up, Grace's story was never finished. She was now back in the chat rooms; that's how she had met her latest boyfriend. 'Seriously, Professor,' she told me, 'he loves me.' Then she giggled, 'He's Mr Right!' That was his chat room name, but she was bubbling about their relationship. He'd told her that he loved her while they were still texting and she'd challenged him by asking how he could say that if he'd never met her. He told her to text her bank account number and he'd prove he loved her. Three days later there had been R700 deposited into her account. She was impressed, enough to visit him. Another woman had rung Mr Right while she'd been with him. He'd explained to Grace that he'd gone out with her for three months but had ended the relationship. He also explained that he'd taken the phone outside to speak to her because he didn't want to speak harshly in front of Grace. He had, he told her, been telling his 'ex' to never, ever, call him again. Grace wanted to believe him. She had told him her status from the beginning and, since he said he didn't want to use a condom, she assumed he must be positive also – though, when I pressed, she was unsure. She had seen no medication, not even the prophylactics and vitamins handed out to those who are HIV positive but not yet needing to start antiretrovirals. But she was sure he loved her.

A treatment holiday

One thing I did re-visit, in what turned out to be the penultimate interview with Grace, was the time she had come off treatment for four months. They had been out of stock of her medication. At first she had been told not to worry, they would ring her when the drugs arrived. It would be any day. Then she had been told they would receive it only in a month. In the end it had been four months. When the drugs were in, she'd been sent to the hospital pharmacy with a script which also had an antifungal cream written on it. The cream was prescribed on a repeat basis, but the pharmacist was careless and also entered the antiretrovirals to be repeated. When Grace went in for a repeat of the cream a week later, she was asked if she was collecting both medications. She thought quickly and said 'yes'. That way she cycled three extra months' supply of her antiretrovirals. When the error was spotted, the pharmacy rang her and demanded that she bring back the drugs. She gave them an earful – they had not been concerned when there had been no drugs available and her CD4 count had dropped from 325 to 174. She kept hold of her buffer stock in case she was left in the lurch again.

During the stock-out she had started to feel weak and suffered a string of complaints: a running stomach, rashes, itching, coughing. Once she was back on the drugs, her CD4 count had risen and the complaints subsided, though they had never left her completely or for long.

So, on the surface, it was a clear-cut case of inefficiencies in managing the supply chain of drugs that had proved, again, to Grace that it was antiretrovirals that were keeping her alive. But still, I was curious and asked tentatively whether, at the time the drugs stopped, she might not have also welcomed the opportunity not to have to take the pills. She had once told me how she got fed up with having to take them every day and that even the sight of pills made her feel fatigued. If she had a headache she chose to use the common Grandpa Headache Powder, rather than a Panado; it was one less pill to swallow in her daily treatment choir.

My hunch was wrong, but not completely so. My question opened up a longer account of this treatment holiday. She had seen it as an opportunity to really and finally get this thing out of her body. *Moruti* Puleng had told her that maybe this was part of God's plan and that

He intended to show her His power. They prayed that she could live without the treatment. It had been an optimistic first month in which she had prayed daily; the second month she managed to shrug off her complaints as normal problems that everybody had; but by the third month she could no longer convince herself. Her prayers and her hopes trickled away. When the drugs were back in stock, she didn't hesitate to return to them, though she wished it hadn't been necessary.

A reputation to maintain

The day of our final interview Mr Right was still on the scene, though I got the sense the initial shine was dulling. I was anxious that it really was the last interview as I had to wrap up the research and start writing. I didn't inquire much about Mr Right but rather tackled her on some of the ways she *zamile* (enterprisingly made money). As well as selling beer, briefly and with dire consequences, she also had been selling *loose draw* (single cigarettes) from her house. Buying *loose draw* is by far the most common way to purchase cigarettes in the township, and there is a good mark-up for the *morekisi* (seller).

The point I raised with Grace was that she was advising people to live healthily when she counselled them at the clinic, but she was selling tobacco to them from her house. It was something of an unfair question, but I was probing how an individual makes decisions within contexts that consistently drive them in other directions. It was particularly unfair because Grace is poor and has limited options to establish economic independence. She told me as much, throwing the choices back at me; what she was doing was better than stealing or selling her body, wasn't it? I conceded, though remembered that she had justified selling sex in order to provide for her son. Then she tried some other arguments, such as people knowing the risks of smoking well enough but choosing to ignore the warnings and that she didn't force them to buy from her.

But she still felt uncomfortable, because after her response she told me she'd stopped selling *loose draw*, so the matter was no longer relevant. I was curious to know why she had stopped since I now understood that she was in a never-ending struggle to juggle the ways in which she could make ends meet. She had stopped selling them, not because it wasn't profitable, or because she couldn't fit it in with her other income-generating activities. She was afraid of being caught. The cigarettes she had been selling were *moqwenati* (counterfeit) and smuggled into the country without tax being paid. She had simply been one of many outlets of a network across Potlakong. She only knew the person whom she bought them from, but she knew well enough that they were counterfeits – they had been splashed across the television several times in crime-watch programmes.

Her decision had been tempered by pragmatism: if it had been a major source of income, she would have had to carry on with it despite the risks. But she had weighed up the amount it brought in and the risk of people, Mazuma for example, who would be happy to see her in trouble. If someone did *mo pimpa* (informed on her) and the police came, she doubted that a bribe would get her out of the situation. Right now the profile of counterfeit cigarettes was too high. There was a brief moral panic generated over this smuggling at the time I was talking to Grace. This was fuelled by the tobacco industry and the South African Revenue Service, which were both losing out. Public concern was whipped up by suggesting, somewhat ironically, that these counterfeits posed health risks since they 'did not comply with the strict government regulations to which legal manufacturers and traders adhere'.[21] In this environment there would likely be charges and she was a public figure. 'I'm working with the community,' she said. 'This thing is going to give me a bad name.' This thing was not selling cigarettes, it was being caught selling fake cigarettes, which had been turned into an infringement of public morality. It was of course a malleable morality; the cigarettes continued to be sold throughout Potlakong via a supply chain that worked better than that of getting antiretroviral drugs into public hospitals, but Grace was pointing out that as the face of AIDS in Potlakong, she had to abide by the morality of the establishment to which she was aligned. In the era of AIDS, that morality includes proclaiming the use of condoms.

Grace told me again, that it was easier to counsel people than to take your own advice. She went back to cigarettes to illustrate her point. When she was asked, in the clinic, how to quit, she would tell them that it was all in the mind and when they felt the cravings they should rather eat fruit or a sweet – she knew that quitting smoking wasn't easy. However, she assures me, with condoms it was different. She maintained that she was proof. She used to let men have flesh-on-flesh if they paid extra, but that was before. Now she assured me, and herself, it was different. Mr Right, she was telling me, was the man she loved, it was OK for them not to use condoms. Mr Right was the latest in a string of boyfriends that she had convinced herself over. Each one was the last.

Reputation always has to be fudged by the poor. Getting money from Mr Right demonstrated love and commitment and got rid of the condom in a more respectable way than making choices over R100 or R200, the differential for commercial-as-it-gets sex. It's not enough respectability to be displayed honestly, but enough to shore up appearances that will do ... that will have to do.

Conclusion: doubts and deceit

The more Grace stood for something, the harder it became to stand by those beliefs. Once she stripped away alternatives by rejecting traditional healing and rubbishing the concerns of others over condoms or treatment, she was left with little room for manoeuvre. There remained limited scope for shuttling between the various environments that Grace was embedded within: her church, the clinic, her neighbours and, as a PWA, the wider community of Potlakong. All of these allegiances make demands in different ways; some could be mitigated through selection, such as her choice of church; some, such as her neighbours, were something that she had little choice over. To the extent that Grace was unable to fulfil the expectations of membership, whether codified or understood, meant that she had held secrets and that she needed excuses when confessing them. These excuses included her botched diagnosis, responsibility for her son, falling in love, the necessity of money, and, when all other excuses ran out, that she was a human being and not Jesus.

Aligning herself publicly with antiretroviral drug treatment meant

Grace was incorporated as an auxiliary of allopathic medicine, even if she was denied the benefits of a professional salary. Yet, as much as she was an auxiliary of the health system, she also had to battle it, whether attempting to fill in for its supply chain shortcomings or lying about side-effects. She was always fighting on two fronts: attempting, on one side, to convince sceptics that they must use condoms, that they should test for HIV and that treatment was their best bet to beat AIDS, while, on the other side, being not infrequently in conflict with the system that promoted and delivered this response to the epidemic. But of course the biggest threat came from her own vulnerabilities: her 'sins', her public profile, her material needs and her doubts. Grace's struggles were without end.

9

The salvation of
Neo Pakwe

Secrets and news

The Pakwes' kitchen was warm and inviting. Outside the sun had long set and a cool night was gripping Butleng Township. The room was brightly lit by an unshielded globe and the large enamelled stove had been alight for hours and was now belting out heat. A big kettle quietly bubbled on the edge of the hob with steam ascending from the curved spout. Mathabiso, the family matriarch, was sitting on a chair to one side of the stove. She had a small tub of *seneifi* (snuff) in her hand and was tapping out a measure onto the lid of the box, preparing to *tsuba* (inhale or snort). Her oldest daughter, Mpheng, was sitting next to her. Mpheng doesn't like snuff and teased Neo and Holekane, her two younger sisters, when they disappeared into the bedroom to *tsuba seneifi* in private. Their departure from the kitchen was to maintain the fiction that they, as young women, don't *tsuba*, but when they rejoined those in the kitchen, their shiny eyes gave the game away. Mathabiso's older status means she doesn't have to bother about such appearances, at least not in her own kitchen.

The evening meal of *pap* (stiff maize porridge) and cabbage had been eaten and the plates washed. Now Neo was demonstrating a card trick. Her audience comprised Refilwe, her eight-year-old daughter, 15-year-old Simon, and myself. The deck of cards was worn with use and everybody knew the Eight of Hearts – it had a blue ink stain across

241

the back which lent laughter to family card games. Neo shuffled the cards noisily, slapping them down as she broke and recombined the pack with a circular motion of her hands. In Sesotho, to shuffle cards is to *tjhova*, a verb that is also used for pedalling a bicycle. Once the cards were thoroughly shuffled, Neo opened the pack and, turning away so she couldn't see, invited Refilwe, Simon and me to lift the top card of the split deck that she was holding out to us in her left hand. We lifted the card to peek at it, being careful that Neo couldn't see. It was the Three of Spades. Neo put the deck back together and ostentatiously *tjhovile* (shuffled) the cards. Then she started lifting the cards from the top of the shuffled pack. Each one was checked, then placed, face up, on the table for us to see – Hearts, Dice, Spades, Fly.[1] We got through some 15 cards when, instead of putting the card on the table, she held it out for us to see. The Three of Spades! We gasped. '*Jwang*? (How?)' Neo laughed and told us it was her *sephiri* (secret). The trick was repeated with the three of us paying close attention. Our astonishment brought others in and the game competed for a while with the soap opera on the small TV at the end of the kitchen. Again Neo baffled us by revealing the card that we had seen but she had not. And again. She refused to tell us how it was done. It was her *sephiri* and she was keeping it … right under our noses.

This card trick was not Neo's only secret. The secret about her being HIV positive is, however, akin to her using snuff out of sight. People can draw conclusions, but it still remains a secret despite close observation; neighbours, friends and extended family members know, or think they know, or assume they must know, but they are not certain, they do not know for a fact.

There is a difference between knowing something for a fact and something being obvious but never being confirmed and always vulnerable to doubt. I first realised that Neo was, probably, positive when Simon, her nephew, sought my advice late one afternoon in November 2009. Meeting me by chance, he had accompanied me for a while as I made my way across the township. As we were about to part, he had asked if it was possible for somebody to get TB twice. Neo had told Simon she had *sefuba feela* (only flu[2]), but other people said she had TB. What he was really asking me was whether Neo had HIV. He was using me to verify what he had been told by friends, that having TB more than once meant you were HIV positive.

Simon had reason to ask. His mother Violet had died five years earlier after returning ill from Gauteng. She had been dismissed by her *makgowa* (Whites/employers) from her work *kitjhining* (in the kitchen, i.e. domestic work) when she was too ill to work. Violet had conceived Simon while living in Potlakong and working in a nearby White suburb. Like other Butleng women, Violet brought back children, but not their fathers, from Gauteng. And like others, Violet had returned from Gauteng with HIV to die of AIDS. Since then Simon had grown up in his grandmother's house. His three aunts, Mpheng, Neo and Holekane, had taken the place of his mother in rotation as they also spent long periods working *kitjhining* in Gauteng.

News of Neo's illness had travelled fast. Just before I met Simon I had been told, 'Neo *wa kula haholo. Wa kgohela*' (Neo is very ill. She's coughing). This really was news. I'd bumped into Neo only half an hour earlier. We had chatted for five minutes. She looked tired, but she had not coughed once. The news that was racing *ka pele* (with speed) from the clinic and along the township's streets was not that Neo was sick, but that she'd been diagnosed with TB, again. Details, about how sick she was and that she was coughing were filled in from past episodes.

I was not sure what I should say to Simon, who was still a teenager, but figured that since he was asking a question, I should answer as honestly as I could. So, I confirmed that you could get TB twice. Then I went further, saying that, although I did not know what was wrong with Neo, if infections kept reoccurring it might mean she was HIV positive. I continued, unsure if I was going beyond what Simon wanted to know or what I should speculate about, telling him that if Neo was HIV positive, it was not a *molato* (a sin or something wrong) and that HIV could be treated with *moriana wa sekgowa* (literally, medicine of the Whites, i.e. Western medicine).

That evening, reflecting on the conversation with Simon, I realised that I was joining another AIDS waltz – a slow choreographed dance in which we would circle our way towards an understanding that it was, once more, 'this disease'. At that point, I did not yet know that HIV underlay Neo's TB infections, but that is was I suspected. I reflected that, despite saying we had to speak openly, I had chosen carefully what to say; I had cautiously speculated, maybe guessed, but had not been truly direct, and said what I suspected but could not verify. I noted how frustrating these slow and clumsy waltzes were and I wondered how many more I would have to join.

At least the AIDS waltz around Neo's status came to an end in July 2010 when she agreed to take part in my research. She told me that she'd been on antiretroviral treatment for more than three years. I also found out that she disagreed with me about HIV not being a *molato* (fault or sin). She believed that her HIV and her sin were one and the same thing.

Sharing secrets

I worked out Neo's card trick when I watched what she was doing, rather than watching that she wasn't peeking to see the card we were checking. Then I saw her clocking the card at the bottom of the pile that she'd taken from the pack. It was easy for her to do as she arched her right hand back while deliberately turning away so as to show she wasn't looking. The card in her right hand was the one that would be placed back onto the scrutinised card when she reunited the pack. Then she had to *tjhova* the reunited pack ostentatiously, but not thoroughly. If the shuffling is not comprehensive, the chances are that the two cards will remain together. The upper card is now your cue to amaze the audience by flourishing the following card.

Once I was sure, I asked for the pack of cards and pulled the trick off to acclaim. Twice, just to be sure and because it's nice to be on the inside of a trick and not puzzling on the outside. After that the card trick was *sephiri sa rona* (our secret) which Neo and I maintained as fellow members of the Pakwe Guild of Card Trickery for the rest of the evening. The secret was shared, not revealed. As was the secret of her status. Asking directly if she was HIV positive was a lot more difficult than taking over the pack of cards. In both cases I was confident that

I knew, but the consequences of being wrong were very different – laughter if I failed to crack the card trick; an awkward, and probably angry or hurt, response if I was wrong about her status. It was a relief when she'd confirmed that she was HIV positive. My research had already started even if it had not formally begun and might not yet proceed any further, as Neo still had to agree to the interviews. She said she'd think about my research and let me know when I next came to Butleng. We ran through the information sheet that explained the purpose of the research and the conditions. She didn't put it in so many words, but she laid down conditions of her own. Among those was that, if I wanted to know what she thought about AIDS, I would have to come to church with her.

This stipulation was not so much to help me understand her, or because she wanted a lift to church, but because Neo had her own projects to advance, and evangelising was one of the most important. She was striking a bargain and not simply accepting the terms that I was offering, which were approved by my university research committee. I told her that I was happy to go to church with her, but that our visits would also be a part of my research. That was OK, and the next time I was in Butleng we went to church together.

The Living Waters Church

The tin roof of the Living Waters of Jesus Church, usually simply known as the 'Living Waters Church', was still throbbing with the afternoon's heat when Neo and I entered and took seats in the second row. The first row, as I was to find out, was always filled with *bontate* (the senior men). The *bontate* arrived with large Bibles to read scripture and *waslaps* (facecloths) to wipe away sweat. Worship in the Spirit Church was a full-on affair and soon we were on our feet. *Moruti* (Preacher) Mofokeng, the church's founder, was a tall man who towered over me with a warm smile when he made a point of welcoming me during the service. He was dressed *trekile* (smartly) with a blue-striped shirt, dazzlingly white tie and sharply cut, black, three-quarter-length frock coat. He was wearing white *kick'n bhoboza* shoes (literally, kick and puncture, i.e. sharply pointed footwear). The *bontate* sitting at the front were also smartly dressed, though their attire didn't match the élan of *Moruti* Mofokeng. Smart clothing was a sign of success and success comes from God. Wealth was embraced by the Living Waters Church.

Wealth, however, was still an aspiration for most members of the church. Sitting behind us in the eclectic mixture of second-hand office chairs and plastic garden furniture were the women who made up the bulk of the congregation. There were well over 100 people on the first evening I attended. Most of them, *Moruti* Mofokeng told me later, came from the new sections of Butleng; many used to live and work on surrounding farms. Now they were no longer needed on the land, except for seasonal fieldwork for which they would be picked up at dawn as day labourers. Some were clearly very poor, shoddily dressed, even in this church in which prosperity was seen as a blessing from God.

Around the township, the church was also referred to as *Polosong* (Place of Salvation), the generic term used for Pentecostal or Charismatic churches, of which there were several in Butleng competing with numerous Apostolic congregations and the mainline *dikereke tsa* (churches of) *Roma* (Catholic), *Fora* (Lutheran), *Tjhatjhe* (Anglican) and *Wesele* (Methodist). Some of the Pentecostal churches, like the Living Waters Church, were home-grown around local pastors. Others formed part of larger Pentecostal brands – the Universal Church had a branch, though the initial popularity that it started with had faded. Distinguishing Living Waters from other Pentecostal churches, if necessary, was done by reference to *Polosong ya Moruti Mofokeng*. That this was the church of *Moruti* Mofokeng was not an exaggeration; he had built it.

Living Waters Church emphasised the importance of personal communication with God. In this, *moya* (spirit) was stressed over *kellelo* (intelligence). The point was that you can forget things studied, but you would never forget *Moya o Halelelang* (the Holy Spirit). Despite the big Bibles and the constant scramble to find verses that *Moruti* Mofokeng would pepper his sermons with, this was a church firmly within the spiritual tradition of Pentecostalism, not an erudite analysis of the Scriptures. That spirit could be uncompromising. I was

struck by how the services of Living Waters ran largely independently
of the Christian calendar that was followed by mainstream churches.
Christmas was an opportunity for more back-to-back services, but
there were no decorations in the church, no Bethlehem crib, and
hardy a mention of the Nativity. Rather than celebrating the story of
Jesus' birth, the congregation stuck enthusiastically to the radical and
repeated narrative: Jesus is my Saviour, hallelujah! Amen!

The low stage at the front of the Living Waters Church hall was
covered with a red carpet draped over the two steps that led to the
pulpit, which could be moved aside when more space was needed.
At the back of this low stage, the breezeblock wall of the building
had been covered with net curtains, and tacked onto these, in purple
cloth, were the words '*Jesu ke Modimo*' (Jesus is Lord). Even before
the service has started, the church was filled with the low, hard hum of
electronic amplification equipment on standby. When the women who
led the singing took the microphones, backed by two keyboard players,
they were amplified to the limit ... it was a wall of sound.

We warmed up by singing, followed by a chaotic period of individual
prayer in which everyone called to God in their own way. Some stood
with heads bowed, others paced the aisle, other were on their knees.
Some talked in whispers, others cried out. The room was filled with
a cacophony of sound. Then the babble subsided and there was more
singing. Then there was dancing, lots of dancing. Like most of the
audience, Neo and I were constrained within the rows of chairs, but
the *bontate* stepped forward and, showing that the spirit was with
us, synchronised their moves to the catchy song '*Holy Fire, Come
Down on Me*'. Soon we were all at it, our arms high in the air, then we
brought them down, hands waving to imitate flames, as the holy fire
descended upon us. Everybody was happy. The sweat was flowing and
the *bontate* were wiping their brows.

Finally, after more than an hour, we got to the sermon. *Moruti*
Mofokeng read from the Gospel of John: *Bonang, Konyana ya
Modimo e tlosang dibe tsa lefatse* (Behold the Lamb of God who
takes away the sin of the world).[3] That we were sinners was taken
for granted that night. The message was that Jesus, and only Jesus,

could show us the way to heaven. This was illustrated with a long story about the misadventures of a Butleng resident who, not knowing the route to his planned destination, ended up travelling in a circle. The story mapped the journey to Gauteng that the audience knew well. Even if they had never been to Gauteng, they would have received in-transit updates from family members on the road. *Moruti* Mofokeng listed the familiar names of Free State towns that travellers pass before reaching the bustling taxi rank in Vereeniging, where you must *palama hape* (board again) for Jo'burg or Potlakong Township or other destinations. But, because of a mix-up, our traveller ended up returning on the same route that he had come, thinking all the while that he was still Jo'burg-bound. The audience loved the story, especially the local detail as our *Moruti* took us on a final meander past familiar shops in Butleng's town of Plaasville. The traveller's puzzlement, played deadpan by *Moruti* Mofokeng, brought the house down. He underlined the message: our hapless wanderer lacked direction and never reached his destination. Did Jesus guide our lives? Or were we simply going in circles?

During my next attendance at Living Waters, the visiting preacher's message was to 'position yourself'. The phrase, in English, was repeated many times during the evening: 'Position yourself! Position yourself! Position yourself!' Positioning yourself for what? For riches! How? By accepting Jesus as Lord! The riches for those who accepted Jesus were illustrated as arriving at a Shoprite supermarket in the latest model car to buy whatever you wanted. *Moruti* Mofokeng was particularly approving of this image and repeated it in his word of thanks to the visiting preacher. In fact, Shoprite caters for lower-income consumers and not the rich. But the image was made all the more powerful by trading accuracy for experience – there was a Shoprite supermarket in the regional town of Wittenburg. As the nearest large store, most of the audience have shopped there. What was being offered was a transformation of that experience in very tangible terms. You were to arrive at Shoprite, but, unlike your neighbour, who deliciously was going to be there on this occasional to witness your success, you would not be balancing what you needed to buy against the money in your hand. Rather, you would choose whatever you wanted to buy. Nor would you have to wrestle heavy bags into a crowded taxi for the journey home.

That weekend I also attended a service in a Butleng mainstream church and cars again featured in the sermon. Only this time they were the latest model cars that people had acquired through their corrupt activities. It was a condemnation of ill-gotten wealth, a principled message from the pulpit that critiqued secular order in South Africa. It was a message that everybody knew to be true, but it fell for the most part on stony ground. People would rather position themselves for that car and arrive at Shoprite to buy anything that took their fancy.

While *Moruti* Mofokeng knew his audience and how to rev them up, he also made it clear that God's blessings were not something that could be taken for granted. Once you'd accepted the Living Waters Church's message of hope, there was more that you needed to understand. *Moruti* Mofokeng often got this over with humour, especially in the church's Bible study classes. Somebody who prayed earnestly for a BMW when he wasn't even working was gently mocked, *Modimo ha a sebeste jwalo* (God doesn't work that way). Rather, you needed to ask for help *ho rekisa dikota* (to sell township fast food) or some other, realistic way of earning money. The BMW would come, it was implied, but not *hang hang* (all at once). Alongside practical messages, the raw power of prayer was emphasised. *Ha o sebeletsa Modimo full time, o patala full time.* (If you serve God full time, He pays full time.) You had to be consistent with God if you were to *winahela* (be successful); it was no good praying at church but then forgetting God at home. To make us laugh *Moruti* Mofokeng reinforced the point by acting out a home visit in which he hears a furious argument inside as he approaches. He waits for a lull in the shouting before he knocks. When the door is opened, domestic harmony is feigned and he is warmly welcomed in. That was not, he explained, how we should live. We laughed because from the way *Moruti* Mofokeng told the story we knew it had happened, more than once, to him as similar situations had happened to us, here in Butleng.

Moruti Mofokeng was critical of rote prayer, which was a thinly disguised criticism of mainstream church practice that failed to get people to forge a personal relationship with God. Prayer needs to be directed to *Modimo wa ka* (my God), and not, it was stressed, *Modimo wa rona* (our God, or perhaps better translated as 'our Father'). Prayers should be directed to *Modimo* (God) in the name of Jesus – not any other agency such as saints, *badimo* (ancestors) or indeed *baruti* (preachers).

Neo, on the way back from the first service we attended together, explained that for her the communication with God that *Moruti* Mofokeng preached meant first being able to forgive people and then thanking God for what you had. Only then could you ask God for His help. When I dropped her off she told me that I had to pray before I went to sleep.

The messages of the Living Waters Church cannot be dismissed as Marx's opiate of the masses. The singing and the dancing and the praying are not just about fleeting happiness or dreams. It's also a way of making things better for those who otherwise have little social power. David Martin[4] has made the point that Pentecostal churches allow members to rally against destructive behaviours prevalent within communities. As such, Pentecostalism is a struggle against the enemy within. That enemy is identified as sin. The Bible talks of many sins, but the particular sins that are focused on again and again, by those in the townships seeking to improve their lives around the standard of Pentecostal churches, are drinking and adultery.

Neo

The first thing I found out about Neo when I started to interview her was that she had two surnames. I noticed this when she completed the ethics consent form as Neo Pakiswa, not Neo Pakwe, the name by which I knew her. Her details had been incorrectly captured when she applied for an ID book. For official purposes she was Neo Pakiswa. Neo had categorised the consent form into this official category. Her real surname, Pakwe, was retained for day-to-day matters. This was put up with as an inconvenience more easily managed than rectified. Given the capacity of South Africa's Department of Home Affairs, Neo might well have been justified in letting her official life as Pakiswa continue. Neo shrugged it off; the spelling of her surname was not important.

Likewise, she shrugged off other things. Her father had been largely absent from her childhood. He had been working in Gauteng and only returned irregularly. When I asked about his work, she didn't know. Similarly, Sera, the father of Refilwe, her daughter, had worked on a platinum mine in Limpopo province, but she had no idea what his job there had been. She didn't think he worked underground, but she couldn't be certain about what he did. This was not the only time I came across women in the township who knew little, and cared less, about the work that their men did away from Butleng. There are a number of factors at play here. Work is not a source of pride. As Africans growing up in a rural township in Apartheid South Africa, few got beyond secondary education and the jobs they would be inducted into far away from home would most likely be manual, menial and without promotion prospects. The value of work was instrumental – it was for *tjhelete* (money). As has been documented elsewhere,[5] for many migrant men in South Africa the focus of their lives is on *mahae* (their true homes), not the urban centres or mining areas where they work. The frequent oblivion of Butleng women such as Neo as to what exactly their menfolk did away illustrates the highly gendered nature of African society. Work, other than women's work (*kitjhining* as domestics), was the domain of men. Home was the domain of women. The connection between couples lay not in knowing about each other's sphere, but in honouring a gendered pact: the man provides the money and the woman runs the home.

Refilwe's father, Sera, had failed to keep his side of this bargain. Neo had met him when she was 19, when he was already working in Limpopo. They would see each other when he came back to Butleng at the end of the month. Refilwe was born two years later. Sera had never given her money for the child. Whether Sera had another woman in Limpopo, Neo didn't know. Refilwe was not even six months old when Sera died. The taxi he was travelling in was in a head-on collision just outside Vereeniging. The driver and all 14 passengers had been killed after the taxi crossed a double white line to overtake a truck as a long-distance coach crested the low rise ahead of them. But she had already given up on Sera as husband and father; Refilwe's name, translating as 'We were given', had not been realised. Five months after Sera's death, she started a relationship with Kenny, a local man with a decent income as a tractor driver on a nearby farm. The short period between Sera's death and taking up with Kenny was to hang over Neo's life ever after. She knew that it was interpreted by some as breaching traditional periods of mourning. She also knew that people branded her as promiscuous.

She had joined Kenny's church as part of her commitment to him, but he had not been committed to her. He had other women. Living in Butleng and bringing in a regular salary made that easy. He had a child by one of them. Neo had no children with him, but he did infect her with HIV. She was sure of this because she had tested negative when Refilwe was born. She found out she was positive when she first contracted TB. She'd been referred by the clinic to an AIDS counsellor. They both expected the result to be positive and it was. She took the TB treatment for three months and then started antiretrovirals. Kenny refused to test. It irked her that she was continually ill, she had had TB four times, but Kenny was still fine. She was the one that people would *jaja* (judge), not him. Every time she walked out of the house, she felt that people knew she was positive and made their assumptions. Butleng is a small place and her path crossed Kenny's from time to time. Then she would feel a flash of anger.

Few people knew first-hand about her status, but she told her mother and sisters and she confided in a friend, Dorothy, who was also positive. They bumped into each other in the ARV clinic in Wittenburg. It was a lucky accident, as Dorothy was the only person she really felt comfortable with talking about being positive and the problems it brings. She thought some people in her church must know as two women in the congregation worked in the clinic, but nobody had said anything. Otherwise, it was only I whom she had told, and that was because I had asked her directly. She has not told her daughter Refilwe, who she thought was too young to understand properly. 'She'll interpret the news by the standards of "street knowledge"', by which Neo meant that Refilwe would think she was about to die. When I asked about Simon, her nephew, she told me that she would tell him when he was 18, three years away. I did not tell her that he had already come to confide in me his concerns, but I suggested that he might already be hearing things from friends. She shrugged, she would tell him when he was older. I thought she was avoiding the obvious. Or maybe, I later wondered, she was hoping that in three years' time she'd no longer be positive.

O se ke wa feba (Thou shall not commit adultery)

Neo's understanding of the cause of HIV was not complicated, though the cure that she hoped for was far from straightforward. For Neo, HIV/AIDS was not really different from other incurable illnesses such as *kankere* (cancer) and *tswekere* (diabetes), but could be managed. She thought that HIV had come to South Africa around 1995 from a foreign country. She hazarded a guess at Nigeria, but was not sure. Where it had come from was not important. How one got HIV was. You got it from breaking *Molao wa Modimo* (God's law), it was the *mophutso* (reward or wages) for adultery.

God's law is to be found in the book of Exodus, Chapter 20: the Ten Commandments, which we discussed several times. She insisted that all ten were equally important. There were, she said, ten, not nine, not eleven. Ten had been given and they should all be kept. But despite her assertion as to their equality, it was always *O se ke wa feba* (Thou shall not commit adultery) which she listed first (though it's seventh in the Exodus list). Stealing usually also got listed (coming in on the Exodus list at number eight). Generally, when referring to God's law, her list of commandments didn't go beyond adultery and stealing. But she talked a lot about *jwala* (traditional beer or, generically, alcohol) being a sin. In fact, it usually got slipped in after adultery and before stealing. So I asked her why drinking was wrong if it wasn't one of the Ten Commandments. Since she'd tied the commandments down to *ten feela* (only), I wanted to see how she'd get out of this one. She wriggled free by explaining that there were different ways in which a commandment could be broken. Stealing provided an easy example.

253

She illustrated this with my cell phone, which was on the table in front of us – she could steal the phone or she could use the phone and steal my airtime should I leave the room. Both would be stealing, both would be wrong.

That still didn't explain why *jwala* was wrong. *Jwala*, she explained, led to the commandments being broken. It was a thing of *nama* (flesh) and not of *moya* (the spirit); this already placed it in a category of things that one should be wary of. But *jwala* caused people to seek things of *nama*, not of *moya*. Most significantly, those who drank did not *hlompisa batho* (respect other people). Without respect, God's laws were not going to be kept. As we will see, Neo used the importance of *jwala* within funerals and *mesebetsi* (ceremonies) as a platform to attack *setso* (African/Sesotho tradition). But her positioning of *jwala* as the supercharger for sin also pointed to a vision of how life should be lived. The first requirement was sobriety, because everything else rested on this.

Neo was able to categorise the things that would lead people astray. Only sniffing glue, which she had little direct contact with, was placed in the red-hot danger category alongside *jwala*. Other drugs that I listed – *kwae* (tobacco), *seneifi* (snuff) and even *matekwane* (cannabis) – all went into different and minor classes of *dibe* (sins). In Neo's experience, though these drugs were things of the flesh, they were *dibe* of a lesser order. By going out of the room to *tsuba seneifi* in private, Neo explained, she was respecting people by being discreet. That was not the case with *jwala*. She didn't have to labour the point. Only a few nights earlier, I had been in the Pakwe kitchen when Tshepo Nhlapo, a neighbour and relative, had burst in drunk. Probably he had cadged the drinks, because he had no money of his own. He had staggered around the kitchen repeating questions, even though they had been answered and even though we knew he would remember nothing of what was being said. He must have fallen earlier in the evening as his hands were grazed and his clothes dirty. An attempt to urinate had been only partially successful, and one trouser leg was soaked from his crotch downwards. He stumbled around the kitchen and it was a relief when he finally sat down on a chair that Mpheng and Holekane manoeuvred him onto. He still kept trying to make his way across the kitchen, disrupting whatever conversation restarted. Eventually he ended up unconscious on the floor, half under the table. In the warmth of the room the smell of urine was unmistakable.

This division of drugs into two categories by Neo is a lay taxonomy that we might quibble with, but it is one that is based on her experience of the most critical of categories: their impact on people's relationships. The cost of *jwala*, in particular its prioritisation over other, more important needs, was frequently wheeled out by Neo as a criticism, but that was a buttressing argument to the real objection to *jwala* ... it was the pathway to other sins.

Respect was, for Neo, critical in a relationship. She wanted a boyfriend, but only one who would value what they shared. She explained this by remarking how two people in a relationship needed to be honest with each other. For example, you would say that you were going to see a friend and you would tell your partner when you would be back. That way your partner would not end up spying to see if you were being unfaithful. You would trust each other. Of course, if you drank, then such a relationship was not possible; you would end up sleeping with other women and hiding what you were doing. That was how it had been with Kenny. In this she portrayed herself as wronged, but in the moral code that she constructed using the Bible she could do no other than recognise her own sin. She had slept with both Sera and Kenny without being married to either of them. This was prohibited by the Bible. Sex was, she said, like the forbidden fruit in *Tshimong* (the Garden of Eden). She might hate *jwala* for driving sinful behaviour, but the sin that obsessed her was the one for which she was being punished with HIV.

For Neo, that HIV was the wages of her sexual sin was foundational. It was on this foundation that she built her hope of salvation.

Ho winahela (To succeed)

I wanted to grasp the scaffolding of sin and salvation that Neo had outlined, an edifice as real to Neo as the breezeblock building of the Living Waters Church. Since *Moruti* Mofokeng was the architect of this structure, I asked if we could talk. We met in his small office in the accounts department of the municipality building, where we were interrupted every now and again by knocks on the door. Half of those coming to see him had queries about bills and payments, the rest came to pick up the religious CDs that he distributed.

The first time we met, *Moruti* Mofokeng outlined the history of the Living Waters Church, which was interwoven with his own spiritual journey. He had been brought up in a mainline denomination and had been an active member of the church, but two concerns plagued him. He didn't understand why the *badimo* (ancestors) were accepted in the church, which at that point was acculturating its liturgy with traditional African beliefs and symbols.[6] The priest had explained that the church had found the *badimo* when they came to Africa and that to work with the people they had to work with their beliefs. *Moruti* Mofokeng had also struggled with the church's saints and martyrs being White when every member of the church congregation was African. The two concerns may appear different: the church was too African, and the church was not African enough. But this racial analysis misses what the young Mofokeng was driving towards, that the relationship with God should not be mediated.

It was, however, only when he was 25 and his life was engulfed in a crisis that he actively started looking for answers to his concerns beyond the church he had grown up in. His marriage was falling apart, he and his wife hardly spoke, he had an affair, he was dreaming of sex with people he hardly knew, and he suffered constant stomach pains. With the benefit of hindsight, *Moruti* Mofokeng was now quite clear that all these problems came from one thing: he did not have God in his life and the Devil had entered.

One day, desperate and on his knees praying in his bedroom, he had a vision of a Christ-like figure bathed in light, his hand pointing to a distant point. *Moruti* Mofokeng took this as a sign that he had to find a new spiritual home. He started exploring the churches in the area, settling for the Damascus Pentecostal Church in the regional town of Wittenburg. After only a few weeks he was healed of pain, the dreams stopped, as did his affair, and his relationship with his wife turned around. He was insistent that what he had found in the Damascus Pentecostal Church was the source of his restoration. He pointed out that the various pills he had been prescribed by doctors and the clinic didn't work. He had had to keep going back for more. It was, in summary, necessary to *phahamisa matsoho* (raise one's hands or surrender) to Jesus if you were to *winahela* (win).

The Damascus Pentecostal Church was growing rapidly and within a year he'd been asked to start a branch in Butleng. But a couple of years later, the church's founder, Bishop Mokoena, had started moving the church towards the Apostolic emphasis on uniforms, symbols and rituals such as baptism and anointing. At a meeting he had told his pastors, including *Moruti* Mofokeng, that *batho ba batso ba rata dintho tse tshwarehang* (African/Black people like things that can be grasped or held). For *Moruti* Mofokeng this was a troubling return to the problems of his past in which the relationship with God was mediated. 'Christ', he emphasised, 'is all.' There had been another vision. This time God held out His right hand to him, but the hand was closed and what was held within it could not be seen. *Moruti* Mofokeng took this as a sign that he should act on his convictions. He left the Damascus Pentecostal Church and established the Living Waters Church.

When I interviewed *Moruti* Mofokeng, the Living Waters Church had been established for five years. Of the membership of some 250, he estimated that 200 were women and 50 men. In services, the gender ratio was closer to 10:1. *Moruti* Mofokeng explained this imbalance as the result of women who had lost their husbands joining the church, that women were more open to the message *ya efankgedi* (the evangelical message), and that men believed more in *meetlo* (traditions). These reasons point to the church being a rallying point for those marginalised within poor communities.[7] They were welcomed without reserve, and visitors were always requested to stand and God would be asked to help them.

It was, however, the youth that were *Moruti* Mofokeng's hope. There was a vibrant group of some 50 teenagers that met two nights a week at the church and attended services, where they would often put on a performance of choreographed songs. The group was roughly equally boys and girls and *Moruti* Mofokeng placed emphasis on teaching them what he called the *seriti sa kereke* (dignity of the church). He believed they could be moulded differently from their parents, particularly their fathers. His key advice was for them to respect themselves by paying attention to their behaviour and appearance. While God looks at the heart, *Moruti* Mofokeng explained, such an attitude shows to the world that the person is making an effort and truly does want something better for him- or herself. People would seek them out, even among the sea of unemployed youth in South Africa.

As I wound up my first interview with *Moruti* Mofokeng, the working day was coming to an end. He packed up his things and, since I'd arrived on foot, he gave me a lift in his shiny black Volkswagen Jetta sedan. We stopped at his house, as he wanted to introduce me to his wife. She was in the small neat living room of the brick-built house. He greeted her with a light kiss on her lips while his hand rested briefly on her shoulder. It was a small gesture that I would think nothing of outside the township, but it was something you rarely saw between a married couple in Butleng or Potlakong. It was a symbol of what Neo wanted: a partnership between a man and women who constantly reassured each other of their intimacy and fidelity, and a relationship in which they were answerable to each other and to God's expectations.

A system of sin and sickness

Moruti Mofokeng's Living Waters Church gave guidance on succeeding in business[8] or in getting a job.[9] It made little, if any, social critique of mass unemployment, poor services in the township or inequality in the country. What it encouraged was for church members to join the ranks of those who were successful, by emulating success. By contrast, when it came to sickness there was a rich and particular explanation of its cause. What *Moruti* Mofokeng put forward was a distinct version that constituted his and his church's worldview, which I distilled into six clauses.

1. Sickness comes from sin. That is from not obeying God's laws. Sickness is a *thohako* (curse) that came into the world as a result of the original sin of Adam and Eve.

2. Sickness, as well as other misfortunes, tests the righteous and unrighteous alike. The example of Job illustrates how sickness could be a test when it strikes those who are not obviously in breach of God's laws. As such, it might warn that you are separating from God. Thus, it can be seen as a blessing in that it can strengthen your faith.

3. Doing things in secret, things that you are ashamed of, will increase your vulnerability to sickness. You are moving away from keeping God's commandments.

4. We live in a world of *matimona* (demons) or *meya e ditshila* (evil spirits) that cannot be seen but afflict us. *Matimona* are the cause of sickness, but they do not represent specific sicknesses. They can manifest themselves in different ways and can shift within the body. Thus, while a doctor might try to help somebody with a heart problem, if the underlying cause was a demon, they could operate 20 times, but unless the demon was removed it will be to no avail; the problem will either return or will take another manifestation. Ill health is a sign of affliction and the specific diagnosis provided by the doctor or clinic is not sufficient to enable successful treatment.

5. We live in a world of *boloyi* (witchcraft). Witches are people used by *matimona* to help enter a person. This can happen through your dreams. A dream of eating, or waking up with the sense that you have eaten something, is a sign that a *matimona* has entered you via the medium of witchcraft. Even going to consult a traditional healer makes you vulnerable to *matimona* since healers are not separate from witches – the entire spectrum of *sangoma–baloyi* (traditional healers–witches) is used by *matimona*. The Living Waters Church, while denying the value of traditional beliefs, takes witchcraft seriously.

6. We live in the *Mehleng ya Qetello* (the Last Days) as described in the biblical book of Revelation. This is a time when there are *mafu a sa foleng* (incurable diseases). *Moruti* Mofokeng pointed to Timothy 2, Chapter 3, which describes how, in the Last Days, people will turn from God and act without love and without self-control, but will disguise what they are doing. Thus, the Last Days

are not just about the world being brought to an end, but also about people's behaviour in the earth's final epoch.

These six clauses of the Living Waters Church's worldview make for an open system of explanation,[10] which, because of its multiple and malleable explanations, is impossible to definitively falsify. Of course, if you don't believe the six clauses to begin with, then the whole perspective is patently mistaken. The opposite is equally true: with faith this system, or one of the multitude of variants on offer, is obviously correct.

Moruti Mofokeng's schema was a bio-moral explanation in which sickness was a punishment for sin, but also a sign of faith being tested. Such diagnoses point to alternative routes to restoring health. But the linking of sin with sickness also allows the rejection of whatever is classified as sin – this is usually an aspect of township life that congregants despise, even if they are not free of them. It validates certain social structures, such as patriarchal power, while denying other aspects of tradition, such as polygamy, through a fundamental reading of selected biblical texts. Such selection and rejection allows the construction of precise moral claims; it might, for example, be right for a man to head the household, but not right for a man to drink or to have girlfriends. The particular choice of values also allows church members to deny African traditional practices, such as the use of traditional healers or the holding of *mekete* (celebrations) for the *badimo* (ancestors), while continuing to believe in witchcraft.[11]

Healing through faith

Moruti Mofokeng outlined the system of sin and sickness after I asked him whether God could heal sickness. I knew full well that his answer would be 'yes', but he went immediately and unprompted to the hardest test of all: not only could God cure people, he could even cure AIDS. He knew somebody whose HIV-positive status had been reversed as a result of prayer. That *Moruti* Mofokeng should respond to my questions with the example of AIDS should not, with hindsight, have been surprising. If nothing is impossible for God, then getting straight to AIDS is simply putting your cards on the table.

What was needed for healing AIDS or anything else was, *Moruti* Mofokeng outlined, repentance for one's sins and faith in God's power to make happen what you were asking of him. This was not, however, a process that could be followed formulaically. You had to be sincere. This meant that a person would not only be healed of sickness but also spiritually saved. Indeed, for *Moruti* Mofokeng, for all his confidence about what illnesses God could cure, spiritual health was the important thing. Physical healing followed salvation. Only if the possessing *matimona* (demons) were driven out, could you be truly healed.

The Bible has many verses testifying to the power of prayer to heal. *Moruti* Mofokeng referred me in particular to James 5, Verses 14–15; 'Is any one of you sick? He should call the elders of the church to pray over him and anoint him with oil in the name of the Lord. And the prayers offered in faith will make the sick person well; the Lord will raise him up. If he has sinned, he will be forgiven.' As these verses indicate, the role of *baruiti* (preachers) or church elders was prominent in the healing processes of the Living Waters Church. Despite emphasis on a personal relationship with God, the *bontate* ([senior] men)[12] were regarded as conduits for God's power when they 'laid hands' on those who sought help.[13]

Altar call

During the services I attended at the Living Waters Church, several 'altar calls' took place. Towards the end of some services, congregants were urged to come forward to the altar, where they would be ushered into line below the wooden pulpit on the low carpeted stage by marshals who stood behind them with outstretched arms. There was little room at the front of the church, and Neo and I would end up helping to pull back front row chairs which the *bontate* had vacated. Up front, *Moruti* Mofokeng, supported by the *bontate*, worked as the congregation sang. He would talk briefly to each individual and grasp one hand, which he would raise up while placing his other hand on the person's head.

Then he would pray, really pray. The privacy provided by the congregation's singing meant little could be heard, but *Moruti* Mofokeng would be rocking back and forward with the intensity of his efforts. Sometimes one of the *bontate* would lean forward with a *waslap* (facecloth) to wipe away the sweat dripping from his forehead. As the process intensified, the *bontate* would stand behind their *moruti*, place their hands on his shoulders and themselves start to pray, creating a relay for the power of the Holy Spirit. Sometimes *Moruti* Mofokeng's intense prayer would last several minutes before, in a final dramatic gesture, he would push hard against the head of the supplicant to transmit a last thrust of holy power.[14] Sometimes it didn't get that far, the intensity of the emotions would be overpowering and the *mokopi* would collapse before *Moruti* Mofokeng was finished. When this happened, the marshals were ready to catch them before they had a chance to hit the ground. They would be gently laid out in the little space that could be found at the front; occasionally they would writhe and have to be restrained.

My own religious upbringing had not equipped me to immediately understand these altar calls. Initially, I overlaid my own experiences, dredged from 30 years previously, onto events. I assumed that the calls were for congregants to convert, to turn from sin and to take up the Christian faith. Indeed, some altar calls were primarily aimed at people who were asked to *inehela ho Jesu* (give oneself to Jesus). The first altar call I watched was led by a visiting evangelist,[15] whose energetically delivered sermon had included the deliberate repeating of each of the sins listed in Galatians, Chapter 5, Verses 19–21. These three verses constitute a comprehensive inventory of transgression. The New International Version of the Bible lists: sexual immorality, impurity, debauchery, idolatry, witchcraft, hatred, discord, jealousy, fits of rage, selfish ambition, dissension, factions, envy, drunkenness and orgies. Finally, just in case anything has been omitted, this list is concluded with 'and the like'. The Sesotho translation used by the church[16] differs slightly, most noticeably with more variations of sexual immorality.[17] The evangelist made a meal of the list, repeating each sin several times and asking the audience if they knew what it was. They did and noisily, sometimes raucously, assented to its being present in Butleng. Once he had concluded with an invitation for people to *phahamisetsa matsoho ho Jesu* (surrender to Jesus), there was an altar call and half a dozen people had come forward.

But not all altar calls were the same. Not long after this event, a second altar call, held after *Moruti* Mofokeng had preached, attracted well over 20 people and I realised that this could not be entirely a process of conversion. The church wasn't growing so rapidly and though nobody expected everybody who *inehela ho Jesu* to stay the course, I didn't think that *Moruti* Mofokeng would be willing to see the altar call conversions treated so lightly. I met with *Moruti* Mofokeng and two of the *bontate*, the core of the church leadership, one Saturday morning to clarify these calls. Squalls of rain were hitting the building as I ran in from my car to the shelter inside. The men took a break from re-wiring the building's lighting – a series of naked bulbs connected to flimsy wires that looped between the wooden rafters that supported the zinc roof.

They quickly clarified that while somebody might use an altar call to *inehela ho Jesu*, others would approach to ask for God's help with a problem. *Moruti* Mofokeng reminded me that his sermon, before the altar call, had been on the *tsietse ya batho* (suffering of people). His text had been the parable of the lost sheep in Luke's Gospel, how the shepherd searches for the lost sheep and brings it back on his shoulders, rejoicing. The message was that Jesus would help you with your problems – if you asked him.

It was these problems that *bakopi* (supplicants) had brought forward. *Moruti* Mofokeng would listen to the request for help and then pray for God's help. The altar call allows each *mokopi* to show his or her faith while standing at the front of the church. Asking for help only 'in your heart' indicated that you were unable to *bontsha* (show) faith. Raising their hands indicated that they were surrendering to God and that they believed he could do what they were asking of him. It was then up to those in authority in the church to channel the Holy Spirit. The Holy Spirit's presence was evidenced by those who collapsed. This was not simply fainting, but rather one of two things.

It could be the manifestation of an evil spirit. When people writhed on the ground, it indicated a demon was being subjected to the power of God. More sedate collapses indicated the power of the Holy Spirit which the person's body, with its *dikodi* (small sins), buckled under.

What did people ask God to help them with? The church leadership came up with a list that reflected common problems confronting members of the congregation, particularly women and young people who formed the bulk of the *bakopi*.

- Family problems, such as fighting;
- Trouble sleeping at night;
- Not finding a job;
- Needing help with school studies;
- Trouble finding a marriage partner;
- Problems conceiving children;
- The confession of sins, such as drinking and adultery;
- Depression/tiredness; and
- Physical illness ranging from headaches to cancer, strokes, diabetes and HIV.

Most of these problems had little to do with physical health. Some might appear banal. The instantaneous lifting of headaches was stressed as something that regularly occurred during the laying on of hands. Such releases might be explained by the intense emotional process that the *mokopi* (supplicant) immerses themselves in when responding to an altar call; but shedding a blinding headache is a welcome relief not lightly dismissed. But beyond such benefit, the routine blemishes of everyday life were, within the cosmology of the Living Waters Church, imbued with importance. At one of the church's Bible classes on demons, *Moruti* Mofokeng summarised how you could tell if somebody was possessed. It was striking, at least to me, how everyday the symptoms of possession were. Possession accounted for people who were angry, people who refused to listen, and people who refused to *kopa tswarelo* (apologise). People who could not sleep at night because of angry thoughts about others, or had angry dreams while they slept, also had a demon within them. There were, we were told, more dramatic manifestations of possession, such as being able to lift a table by simply looking, but what predominated was the tension of daily life: being snapped at, snapping at others, fuming over daily slights and conflicts.

AIDS was something of a special case, even among the class of more serious afflictions that God could heal. God could, of course, cure AIDS just as he could cure anything. He could even raise the dead, but AIDS was not straightforward given its link to sexual sin and its status as a disease of the Last Days. The *bontate* agreed that with AIDS it would be important that the preacher was 'live' with God and acting as a direct and unresisting conductor of God's power. With such high-performance ministry, AIDS could be cured, as God, I was reminded again, can do anything.

A critical point in understanding alternative explanations of AIDS, which can be drawn from this exploration of altar calls, is that curing AIDS is no more than the logical extension of a healing system that works with a broader, often mundane but still pressing set of concerns. If we engage only with one part of a larger system, if we interrogate the healing of AIDS out of context, then we fail to see the value of this system to its adherents. It is the engagement with daily concerns that brings and holds people to the healing promise of the Living Waters Church. This is the foundation of the church, not the claim to cure AIDS.

Though your sins are like scarlet, they shall be as white as snow

One reason for my research with Neo and others was to provide a counter-balance to the ease with which beliefs about AIDS could be bandied about if the disease is publicly salient, but privately distant – discourses of bravado. At this point, I imagine many readers regard the Living Waters Church's views on AIDS as exotic. But given how the church's system of belief is rooted in the conditions and challenges of life in Butleng, we should recognise that these beliefs are exotic from the outside, not the inside. Or, put another way, what has been constructed, with a great deal of care and effort, is a system of belief that makes sense, once you accept that there are *madimone* (demons) and that God can do anything. Indeed, with these beliefs in place, the Living Waters Church's doctrine makes more sense than the biomedical response to disease which only, and with many imperfections, scratches at the surface of township conditions and challenges. To decisively demolish this system of belief and truly turn its adherents, you would need to prove that demons do not exist and that God is not omnipotent. Good luck should you try.

But it could be that the Living Waters Church's views are not wildly shared and that I had stumbled across an extraordinarily febrile cult in Butleng that cannot be regarded as reflective of AIDS beliefs in the township. Given the diversity of township residents, it would be wrong to suggest that the creed of the Living Waters Church was typical. A key theme running though this book is the diversity of systems of thought that underlie the more visible plural health care system in South Africa. Yet, the views put forward by *Moruti* Mofokeng were not isolated. We have seen the perspectives of other churches in earlier chapters. There are enormous variations in the details of these systems of belief, but these alternatives systems, in this case Christian perspectives on sin and salvation, have a significant presence within townships.

I realised this was true in Butleng when I attended a World AIDS Day event organised by the township's church women's association. Women drifted in slowly to the cool relief of the large stone building that shielded us from the hot afternoon sun. We started half an hour late, by which time there were some 50 mostly middle-aged or older women, with more slowly trickling in. I was the only man who, billed as a speaker, had a seat at the front. Those from the mainline and Apostolic churches came in their uniforms which marked out the denominations: red and white for *Kereke ya Wesele* (Methodist Church), purple for *Kereke ya Roma* (Catholic Church), black and white for *Kereke ya Fora* (Lutheran), various blue, white and yellow combinations for the Apostolic churches, and so on. Those from Pentecostal churches were dressed in their usual attire of best dresses and hats.

The women represented a critical group that helps hold the township together. It was these women who wove the strands of social fabric with their practical emphasis on family, responsibility and service. It was these women who cared for sick neighbours or helped organise funerals when a *mofutsana* (poor person) died. Simultaneously, they frequently judged township residents who did not hold to their values. Notwithstanding that this was a remembrance service for those who had died of AIDS, judgement pervaded many of the afternoon's speeches and contributions – never as condemnation of those with AIDS, but as condemnation of the behaviour that led to AIDS.

Speeches were interspersed with singing and the lighting of coloured candles representing different aspects of the epidemic. Once all the coloured candles had been lit, we each lit the candle we had brought with us. The singing subsided and we bowed our heads for a minute of silence. When it was over there were tears running down the cheeks of several women – AIDS had staked its claim among their families and friends. The seven speakers sitting at the front of the church represented the largest churches. In addition, almost double that number of women spoke from the floor, not only making sure that every church was heard, but also giving women a chance to *rera* (preach) and speak their piece. The text used for the service, to which many of the speakers from the platform and floor referred, was Isaiah, Chapter 1, Verses 17–20:

> Learn to do good; seek justice, correct oppression; defend the fatherless, plead for the widow. 'Come now, let us reason together,' says the Lord: 'though your sins are like scarlet, they shall be as white as snow; though they are red like crimson, they shall become like wool. If you are willing and obedient, you shall eat the good of the land; But if you refuse and rebel, you shall be devoured by the sword; for the mouth of the Lord has spoken.'

Drawing directly from the text, it was outlined how AIDS had come because God's laws were not being observed. For many of those who spoke, it was, as Fraser McNeill and Isak Niehaus[18] suggest, an opportunity to rail against social ills; the scarlet stain of AIDS stood in for many sins. A second theme, also drawing on the text, was that God can heal. Indeed one speaker, standing with crutches following a fall, opened by thanking God for help in the rapid healing process she was experiencing. Thirdly, and emerging later in proceedings, was AIDS being a disease of the 'Last Days'.

The key speaker, Sister Maurine, who worked in a nearby clinic, re-read the text from Isaiah and also added Chronicles 2, Chapter 7, Verse 14:

> If my people who are called by my name humble themselves, and pray and seek my face, and turn from their wicked ways, then I will hear from heaven, and will forgive their sin and heal their land.

This shorter text, like that of Isaiah, pointed to the need for humility and obedience to God's laws. It also puts forward a wider social pact: individual repentance will cure social ills, the country will be healed. Sister Maurine outlined a list of ills that ailed South Africa, the Free State and Butleng. She started by explaining that failing to keep the commandment that 'o se ke wa feba' (thou shall not commit adultery) was why lefatse le a kula (the world is sick). The list of situations that contributed to AIDS went on to include domestic violence, men sleeping with young girls, girls selling themselves to men, the provocative way girls dressed, men not respecting women, and women not being humble as they were commanded by the Bible. She then moved from issues of gender relations and roles to some of the socio-economic contributors to the epidemic, particularly the lack of work, low wages and migrant labour, the product, she pointed out, of Apartheid. Lastly, and bringing the list full circle, there was jwala (alcohol) and the resulting thobalano (sex).

If you were to read a translated transcript of Sister Maurine's speech, it might well come over as a comprehensive, if conservative, outline of the co-factors that drive the epidemic. If a few of the more difficult lines were massaged away, it might be lauded as an example of how the epidemic should be explained in a way that linked the biomedical transmission of the virus via sex to key underlying social determinants, particularly around gender and socio-economic conditions. A local nurse, in touch with the community, she could paint the bigger picture of how developmental challenges in the township contributed to the

AIDS epidemic. An enthusiastic monitoring and evaluation report might even highlight Sister Maurine's address as a good example of how the South African National AIDS Plan was being communicated to communities. Yet, it was absolutely clear that this was not what was happening. Gender and socio-economic challenges were being articulated in ways that the audience understood. But the dialogue fitted socio-economic conditions into a religious and moralistic understanding of the epidemic, not the other way around. What was being explained was a sick world that needed to turn to God, not the social determinants of health.

The difference, between a morally sick world and a structurally determined epidemic, can turn on relatively small shifts of emphasis, by framing, for example, the problem as adultery and fornication, rather than multiple concurrent partners, or with an emphasis not on gender equality, but on traditional, Bible-justified gender roles.

Many of Sister Maurine's concerns were brought together in her warning as to what we were about to face – Christmas. Christmas means the long holiday stretching over three or four weeks of hot sunny weather. It is for many people what the year has been leading to: a time to see family and friends, a time to relax, a time to shop, a time to eat, to drink and to be merry, a time for gifts, a time to *enjoya*. People, however, enjoy themselves differently – some drink, some go to church, some do both, openly or in secret. But what Christmas highlights more visibly than at any time of the year in South African townships is the internal divisions of the township. Crudely, the church looks down on the tavern and says as much from its citadels, and the tavern accuses, generally *sotto voce*, the church of being hypocritical and defies criticism by drinking till dawn.

Sister Maurine, by raising the problem of migration, with its roots in Apartheid's racist labour laws, could well have been pointing to the sexual networks that extend between, for example, Potlakong and Butleng, through which the virus is transmitted. But what she actually highlighted for her audience was that men from Gauteng would be returning for Christmas and departing again in January. It was now December and Christmas was fast approaching. She was pointing to the cocktail of moral hazards that would present in Butleng: the materialism of Christmas, men returning flush with money from Gauteng, the girls who *batla kaofela* (want everything) and will dress to get it, and the catalyst of *jwala* (alcohol). Nurse she might be, but Sister Maurine was speaking as a prophet. The land was sick and it was only through repentance that healing would come. Her address went down well.

Toyi-toying for Christ

That Christmas the youth *toyi-toyied* for Christ. I went with Neo to the evening service at Living Waters Church on Christmas Day. The congregation was already high with the elation of enthusiastic singing, dancing and prayer, when a visiting evangelist's sermon set everyone on fire. The visitor's star turn had been to ask two young men to assist him at the pulpit: one was asked to crush an empty Coke can, the other an unopened can. We were told in anticipation that the liquid inside the can was like the Holy Spirit; if we were full of the Spirit we would be strong. True enough, the empty can buckled. The other young man was left red-faced and unable to make any impression despite his best, two-handed, efforts. The point was made amid laughter, cheering, applause and the regular punctuations of 'Amen!' and 'Hallelujah!'

When we finished it was late and outside it was dark. As we milled around organising who could be given lifts in the half-dozen cars parked outside the church, I could hear music pumping from the California Tavern a couple of blocks away. By now the place would be heaving and men would be spilling out of the building and taking over the street with their drinking, talking, laughing, joking and jostling. Quite probably there would be arguments and, in the small hours, a fight. While the taverns are magnets for those who drink and have money, plenty of people make detours so as to avoid passing the handful of large Butleng establishments when they are in full swing. Since nearly everybody's route took them past California, the lifts were not only a welcome ride, but also offered an easy way past the milling crowd, sections of which might well entertain themselves with returning churchgoers. Since I had come with Neo, I had only the back seat to offer. It was eagerly filled with *Ntate* Matjinini and his wife, who held one of their grandchildren on her knee, and Florence, a friend of Neo, all of whom lived on the other side of the township.

By the time this had been organised, the *batjha* (youth) had set off accompanying one another. On the *skontiri* (tarred road) they had coalesced into a dancing troupe of around 30, roughly equal numbers of young men and women, many with Bibles in their hands. I put the car into first gear and drove slowly behind them. The car's headlights shone through their dancing figures and illuminated the road ahead for them. They were in no hurry and neither were we. *Mme* Matjinini pointed out that her daughter was among the group. Their dancing was spontaneous, but drawing on their chorographic repertoire they had soon established a complex *toyi-toyi*. They would step forward a few steps, stop, stamp their feet in rhythm to their singing, step back and then take a step to the side before moving forward again in unison. They took their time, especially with the emphatic sideways steps which they executed in slow motion, and then paused for a moment before proceeding. As we came alongside the tavern I could see that it was overflowing with drinkers, many of whom were standing outside with quart bottles of beer. As the youth came level with the tavern, their steps become slower, their stamping beat more emphatic and their singing louder; they were challenging the tavern. The drinkers stood their ground and did their best to ignore the defiance of the church youth posed only a few metres from them.

Beliefs in context

Two very different segments of the township had, albeit fleetingly, faced off, but it was the Living Waters Church *batjha* that had made the better showing. Such open displays between church and tavern are not common; African culture stresses public harmony, with tensions within communities often dissipated into more private spheres and more opaque conflict such as gossip, reputational assaults and innuendo. The youth's defiance of the tavern tells us something about what values are in circulation. They are far from homogeneous, but what should give those concerned with health education food for thought is that the behavioural options available in townships rarely correspond with the choices that health promotion campaigns offer.

The split between church and tavern is not the only major social fracture in African townships, even if it is one that has been highlighted prominently in this chapter. If we take a wider inventory of township belief, the limited and awkward way in which health promotion aligns with this is striking. At worst it stands remote but condemnatory of behaviour; at best it is a partial and compromised ally of certain township factions.[19] Frequently, discussions on AIDS education bemoan how 'more use needs to be made of the churches', which are seen as a potential, but not yet fully tapped, ally. Why they have not been so easy to tap is now, hopefully, clear. Churches are not for hire; they have their own ideas, which only partially overlap with those of most health promotion campaigns.

The account of the women's World AIDS Day event in Butleng illustrates that even within the mainline churches, seen as more reliable allies for health promotion, what is said and believed on the ground may differ from the statements of national church leadership over AIDS. Local spectrums of belief are closer to fundamental readings of the Bible. Religious beliefs in Butleng are far from hostile to the cosmology of the Living Waters Church that Neo embraced.

The end of days

It is not uncommon for comparisons to be made between religious experiences and aspects of the AIDS epidemic. Peer educators are asked to 'preach the gospel of AIDS', and antiretroviral drugs may be likened to new life granted after conversion to a belief in the power of Western medicine. Religious metaphors clearly can be useful to describe phenomena within the epidemic, but the value of metaphor can be over-reached.

Corinne Squire, in her book *HIV in South Africa: Talking About the Big Thing*,[20] explores how people are talking about HIV infection, but her chapter on the religious and moral narratives of HIV is less about religious content and more about how people's narratives mirror religious processes of conversion and testimony. The role of religion within the epidemic painted by Squire is optimistic, but it is narrow. Churches are praised for campaigning on the rights of HIV-positive people, as well as those of gay men and lesbians and, we are reassured, religious discourse in South Africa has 'in general, moved from "othering" to "owning" the virus'.[21] Such approaches run the risk of missing the essence of South Africa's religious culture. They optimistically bolt the (public) stance of (some) churches onto a comfortable conceptual model: a human rights-based, gender-equal and essentially secular framework of how we should respond to HIV/ AIDS. But it's not the word on the street, or in the churches, of South Africa's townships.

We need to contrast this 'township-talk' with the glutinous slogans and mantras of 'AIDS-speak': the global expert consensus over AIDS messages. Within competing agencies of the global AIDS industry, differences may appear huge, for example whether gender is emphasised sufficiently, or whether abstinence is a credible option. But between AIDS-speak and township-talk there is a much more dramatic divergence, such as, for example, miracle cures or whether we live in the Last Days. Whatever we might think, this strand of township-talk cannot be dismissed if we seek to understand how people make sense of AIDS. Claims that the end of the world is nigh have been made for a long time. The list of predictions that have passed without eschatological incident continues to grow. However, if we are to understand the beliefs of others, such as the residents of Potlakong and Butleng, rather than project our beliefs onto them, we cannot merely *liken* aspects of the epidemic to religion. We have to go further. *Moruti* Mofokeng and Neo do not think it is *like* the Last Days. They *live* in the Last Days.

Outside the Pakwes' kitchen it was still light, but the cold of a Butleng winter's night was already upon us and, inside, the stove had been lit. The curtains were drawn and the setting sun, shining directly onto the window, created a yellow gloom in the room. That morning I had driven Neo and her younger sister to Wittenburg. Holekane's health had been deteriorating for weeks and Neo had finally persuaded her to test for HIV. We had all known what the result would be. It was now a race against time to get her onto treatment. A file had been opened at the ARV clinic, but she had come away with only a tin of vitamin-fortified *pap*. First she would have to attend treatment-literacy training sessions. Up till a week ago Holkane had denied that the diarrhoea, weight loss, chronic tiredness and sores pointed to AIDS. Now she was sitting listlessly next to the stove, exhausted after a long day. What those of us in the room now knew was that the HIV tally for Mathabiso's surviving children was two out of three.

There had been a knock on the door and Solly, a neighbour, had come into the kitchen with the news that Tsidiso had departed. Everybody knew Tsidiso. Still in his 30s, he was chair of the ANC Youth League. He was always, as the more cynical township residents put it, travelling to meetings across the Free State so that he would 'know their rights'. That was when he was not hospitalised. The last time I had seen him was several months earlier, slowly making his way up a dirt street in the township. He had accepted a lift and lowered himself into the front seat with a quart bottle of Castle beer. We hadn't seen each other for a while. He looked terrible, he was gaunt and one corner of his mouth was eroded by an ulcer. When he drank, he held the bottle at an angle, keeping it to the good side of his mouth.

Now he was dead, he would be buried the following Saturday. Around the township it was the same story – he had been ill for a while and had been in and out of hospital. This was more than enough to tip the wise. Solly had started with the lines that I was to hear repeated elsewhere as people shared the news. Tsidiso was always travelling, he had many girlfriends. In many other Butleng kitchens this topic would have been enthusiastically taken up in a shared gossip of knowing without quite saying, but on that day in the Pakwes' kitchen, Mathabiso had cut Solly off abruptly before he was even half finished. There had been an uncomfortable silence in the room. Who was next to die? We were silent and still; AIDS was stalking. Mathabiso had had five children: two were now dead, two of those surviving were positive. There were less grandchildren alive than children. The Pakwe line was running out. Time was coming to an end.

I am not suggesting that all township residences believe they live in the Last Days. Some do, many don't, some are not sure, some change their minds, and some scoff at the very idea. But there is fertile terrain for the concept of the Last Days; it does not have to be explained and new signs and suggestions can rapidly spread. In early 2011 there were several weeks of heavy rain. Across South Africa there were floods, bridges were swept away, villages were cut off, informal settlements flooded. For a day or two the headline news in South Africa was the opening of the Vaal River floodgates and the surge of water that went downstream to avoid endangering the dam. On the television news there were reports of flooding in Australia, Pakistan and South America. In the townships talk of the Last Days surfaced The rumour ran that the rain would not stop and the earth was to be washed clean. How many people gave the prophecy any credence is impossible to say; for many people the more pressing problem was drying laundry and, when the rain eventually stopped and the sun shone, there was ridicule of those who had spread this interpretation of events. The point, however, is that the idea was entertained.

That heavy rain, and reports of flooding elsewhere around the world, were transformed into impeding catastrophe so easily was because the end of the world is believed, by at least some, to be around the corner. The rain was not explained through a belief in the Last Days; the rain was one more proof that we were already in the Last Days. AIDS is not dissimilar. It is not as though *Moruti* Mofokeng, worried about AIDS, searched the Bible for an explanation and deduced that we were in the Last Days. *Moruti* Mofokeng already knew that we were living in the Last Days. AIDS was but confirmation of what the Bible says is to come. There is, viewed from this perspective, nothing we should be surprised about other than that God has allowed this sinful world to endure for so long. If there is advice to be given, the priority is not to stop AIDS, but to prepare to meet your Maker.

Reading the small print

Neo believed her HIV infection was a punishment for having sex outside marriage, a contravention of God's law. HIV was not, in her view, something sent by God. Rather, it was a thing of the Devil that she had exposed herself to when she disobeyed the commandment *o se ke wa feba*. That it was Kenny, her partner, who had infected her, while she had been faithful to him, did not mitigate the sin that she had committed: sex outside marriage. However, in believing that her infection was the wages of sin, she also believed that she could be cured, that her HIV status could be changed from positive to negative. God could take HIV from her.

This was, however, the bold-print headline advertising of the religious system of sin and salvation to which she cleaved. Dramatic claims could be supported by selected showpiece miracles, such as respondents to an altar call fainting at the front of the church or headaches being instantaneously banished.[22] But, beyond such attractive promotions was the small print specifying what must be done for an individual's request to be granted.[23] The Living Waters Church's small print was demanding. Miracles do happen, everybody could point to them, but they were not to be taken for granted; salvation had conditions.

Neo was committed to following the path of salvation that her church offered. But it was not easy. There was the danger of being led astray. Just as Western medical professionals are imitated by quacks and fakes, so there is a question of reliability within religious systems of faith and healing. The *bontate* of the Living Waters Church had their concerns about false prophets. Neo had her own concerns. 'Prayers could', she explained to me, 'be "intercepted" by the Devil and used by him to confuse people.'[24] Staying virtuous to the path required faith in a world in which falsehood could masquerade as truth.

Neo had no intention of being misled. But even without the deceptions that the Devil could spin, the true path was not straightforward. One could pray to be healed, but the conditions for this appeal to be granted went beyond simply requesting a miracle. When I asked Neo what she prayed for, she did not, as I had assumed, pray to be cured of HIV/AIDS. Rather, she told me that she prayed to be forgiven for what she had done. If she was forgiven she would be healed. Forgiveness was her priority. But to be forgiven she had to believe that God could and would heal her – without faith nothing was possible. And if she believed in God, then she must be grateful for what she had in life, for what God had already given her.

Neo laid great stress on thanking God for what she had. To be ungrateful would be tantamount to complaining. And, clearly, if you are complaining, you have doubts or suspicions about God. You would, in fact, be demonstrating that you do not really believe in him.[25] You must, then, be grateful even for the sickness that you were asking to be taken from you. Sickness may be sent to test you, to bring you closer to God – for all of these possibilities one must be grateful. And, finally, to be grateful for what you have means that you must forgive others. You cannot be genuinely thanking God if you are angry with others. This presented a particularly difficult problem for Neo as she had not been truly able to forgive Kenny for infecting her. Not just say she forgave him for infecting her, which she had done many times, but really, really forgive him. There was no way of faking it because God could see into her heart. Every time there was a flash of anger at Kenny, she was back to square one.

Over the course of our discussions I realised that Neo's hope for her HIV status to be reversed waxed and waned. Her faith remained strong, but the long and difficult road of salvation from AIDS was sometimes dauntingly difficult. On occasions she was confident that she would be cured. *Modimo o ka etsa tsohle* (God can do all things) was all that needed to be said to support her faith. On other occasions, as when she explained to me the details of what her salvation entailed, it seemed far away.

Separation from *setso*

When our interviews turned into opportunities for Neo to evangelise, as they did on several occasions, she assured me that those who believed in God would, among other benefits, see their CVs prioritised within a pile of applications. Those who believed in God would be protected should they be involved in a road accident; they would even, inexplicably, turn back at the gate when about to set off on a journey. God would be saving them from danger that would otherwise befall them on the road. In making these claims of God's power, Neo was doing what she believed she was commanded to do: to tell others the good news of salvation. I was far from the only person whom she had attempted to convince, though I was the first humanist academic.

Neo's promotion of the benefits of faith missed the mark. I was not unemployed, or looking for a job and, although I do believe that the most likely cause of injury or death for me is on South Africa's roads, I have always approached this hazard with a secular resolve to keep the car roadworthy, drive defensively and drop my speed on potholed roads. Neo would not, however, be off the mark if she were talking to residents of Bulteng or Potlakong where jobs are few and road accidents in the taxis they *palama* (board) are beyond their control.[26]

However, the more significant rival to Neo's beliefs than my secular humanism was that of *setso*. *Setso* is the Sesotho word for tradition and therefore captures African cultural practices and values interpreted to have been inherited from the past. In reality, as with all culture, what is believed and practised is malleable and diffuse, and is fused with other influences. *Setso* is publicly wheeled out and celebrated at social events in the township, but it also retains an ongoing presence in the life of many township residents as a cosmology of values and explanations that can be drawn upon. In competing with traditional explanations of the hazards and hopes of life, Neo took an extreme position: that the *badimo* (ancestors) did not exist. Such a stand made no attempt to accommodate the widespread belief in *badimo*. In this she set herself up as an implacable opponent of *setso*. Traditional healers claim to be the custodians of tradition, but the heart of that tradition, and their key source of power, is the collective belief in *badimo*. Remove this and healers would be left with little other than colourful beads.[27]

In a similar way to how Grace Dlamini's *moruti* dismissed the idea of *badimo*, using the analogy of a tin of fish that when emptied of its contents is nothing but an empty can, so Neo talked about the coldness of cadavers that indicated they were lifeless and no longer of this world.[28] At one of the Living Waters Church's Bible classes, *Moruti* Mofokeng was asked whether it was right for church members to eat food prepared at funerals. The point being raised was that the beast would have been slaughtered in honour of the ancestors and to introduce the departed to the spirit world. *Moruti* Mofokeng gave his audience some room for manoeuvre; eating slaughtered animals might be OK if a point was not being made about the ancestors, but it wasn't something he recommended. He made it clear that he preferred to buy meat *slaheng* (at the butchery) and went on to josh, through one of his many entertaining sketches, those claiming that the *badimo* had drunk from the pot of *jwala* (sorghum beer) offered at a *mosebetsi* (ceremony) when the decreased volume was nothing more than 'evaporation'. More seriously, he warned church members that those who went to traditional healers opened themselves up to attack by *madimone*.

Spirit and *setso*

Much as I have painted a picture of Neo's beliefs about sin and salvation as differing from the perspective of medical science, the more significant tension for her was not between the power of the Holy Spirit and science, but the Spirit and *setso*. We need to comprehend this if we are to grasp that competition between rival healing systems within African townships is genuinely plural. It is not one system versus the rest.

Neo was able to juggle her practical commitment to science, in the form of antiretroviral drugs, with her belief in salvation, with ease. She was quite clear that she would continue to take antiretroviral drugs until she tested negative. Medicine made no claim that it could cure her and she was happy to accept this assistance in keeping the disease at bay while she strove towards the goal of salvation and cure.

By contrast, the conflict between the Spirit and *setso* was much more disruptive. Neo was the only Pakwe to attend the Living Waters Church. Everybody else was, at least nominally, a member of a mainstream church, which left plenty of space for the Pakwes to continue with *setso*. When Neo's father died and a bull was slaughtered, there had been criticism among the assembled men when the man responsible for killing the beast failed to talk loudly enough as he hacked open the animal's neck. Their concern was that the *badimo* needed to be alerted to the blood that was being shed in their honour. The next day we had walked behind *Ntate* Pakwe's coffin to the church for a service before proceeding to the *mabitleng* (graveyard), where, after a prayer from the minister, the wet hide of the slaughtered beast was draped over the coffin before we filled the grave. When this was done, the printed orders of service had been collected and burned to prevent this artefact of the deceased being used for witchcraft. Early the next morning family members had gathered at the house and had shaved their heads in a traditional sign of mourning that respects the deceased.

Neo, who criticised such adherence to tradition that could not be justified by biblical text, also had her head shaved. She dismissed this apparent contradiction with the excuse that her hair had needed cutting. I doubted her, but did not press the point, reckoning that she had buckled to pressure so as to maintain social harmony. But having stumbled, she would have been a step back from salvation.

Conclusion: Neo's salvation

It may be convenient to dismiss Neo's beliefs as nonsense. But her beliefs must be reckoned with if we are to understand the AIDS epidemic. That can only begin if we stop dismissing others' understandings of their world and, rather, engage them with respect. If Neo thought that the most important part of our discussions was the opportunity for her to evangelise, I could not dismiss that and yet expect her to take my questions seriously.

Generally, those who assume a worldview in which the value of medical science is unquestioned do so with an emic understanding of the world that is materially comfortable and procedurally predictable – circumstances that the vast majority of township residents are unfamiliar with. The hope promoted by the Living Waters Church was rooted in a fundamental interpretation of the Bible, gendered family roles, conservative social values, and an emic understanding of the world characterised by material hunger and uncertainty. The Living Waters Church was far from the only contender in Butleng for hearts and minds, but in drawing deeply on resources that the AIDS establishment eschew, it offered Neo salvation.

PART III

Denial Above,
Dissent Below

10

An elite dispute

A hard run

In Herman Melville's *Moby-Dick* the true mission of the *Pequod* is revealed to the crew only when the ship is far from its home port of Nantucket, and the reader a third of the way through this leviathan of a novel. Before Captain Ahab nails a gold coin to the main mast, a reward for whoever first sights the whale that severed his leg, there have been only hints and suspicion that not all is as it appears. Now it is revealed that Ahab is set firm on settling his score with Moby-Dick and this mission will be their lodestar.

Ahab's rousing address swings the crew behind his obsession, but the *Pequod*'s first mate, Starbuck, objects, asking, 'How many barrels [of whale oil] will thy vengeance yield thee?' And answering his own rhetorical question he states, 'It will not fetch thee much in our Nantucket market.' Captain Ahab's response is defiant of Starbuck, the ship's shareholders, and the accounting of profit as the reason for their voyage, 'Nantucket market! Hoot! ... let me tell thee, that my vengeance will fetch a great premium *here*!'[1] From this point in the novel, the crew of the *Pequod* follow Ahab's vengeance to its tragic climax, their mission re-framed to the logic of pursuit, not profit.

Moby-Dick is a story. The AIDS epidemic is not. But similarly, not all is as it appears. Despite hints, signs and suggestions that the medical explanation of HIV/AIDS is being run hard by alternative accounts, there has been a refusal to contemplate that these alternatives are more than ignorance. We have failed to appreciate the agency of others.

An embarrassing chapter

Breakthroughs in the fight against AIDS are regularly announced. Closer inspection reveals that they represent progress in the medical response to the epidemic, but are not *the* step that will end the epidemic. Eventually, we hope a cure or vaccine for HIV/AIDS, or more likely an accumulation of medical developments, will curb the epidemic. It will also close an embarrassing chapter in the history of medicine. There have been 30 frustrating years in which the limits of medical power have been apparent, if not acknowledged.

Each announcement not only signals hope to those infected and affected by the disease, but also shores up confidence in medical science. 'Hold fast; stay with us, we are getting there' is the message. And, probably, we *will* get there, at some point. Then, what people think about AIDS won't matter as much. If their understanding of the disease differs from that of medical science, it will be little more than quaint, as long as they go along with what the doctors prescribe, which they will, if what is prescribed is easy to swallow and quick to cure.

But until then, what people think about AIDS matters because the major weapons in our current armoury involve behavioural change: limiting sexual partners, wearing condoms, complying with indefinite drug regimes and so on. It also matters because if we don't know what people think, then we can't even begin to grasp what the problem is and, somewhat embarrassingly in the 'new' South Africa with its Constitution foundations of equality, it reveals that we do not know one another.

Denial from above

It wasn't clear to begin with whether South African President Thabo Mbeki was, in fact, denying the link between HIV and AIDS. This was partly because complex arguments, often dressed in flowery language and sometimes vaguely put, were advanced, and partly because the idea that politicians might differ from the expert advice over health was not expected. As Helen Schneider outlined, there was initial shock that the medical establishment was being challenged by powerful forces in its own area of expertise. The relationship between state and science over health had been longstanding, and had largely transitioned from Apartheid to democracy, but with AIDS it unravelled. What erupted was a conflict over 'who has the right to speak about AIDS, to determine the response to AIDS, and even to define the problem itself'.[2] People found themselves in very uncomfortable situations, with loyalties stretched between support for the still-new ANC government, with Mbeki at its head, and the scientific consensus over AIDS.

Nathan Geffen has defined AIDS denialism as a belief in 'one or more of three views: that HIV does not cause AIDS; that there is not a large AIDS epidemic in sub-Saharan Africa; and that antiretrovirals cause more harm than good'.[3] Geffen concludes that Mbeki held all three views at some time or another. What this definition of AIDS dissidence does not capture, however, is the motivations that underlie why people support such views, even when, like Mbeki, they know they are swimming against the tide.

The publication *Castro Hlongwane, Caravans, Cats, Geese, Foot & Mouth and Statistics*[4], is a key dissident document that Mbeki regarded as an accurate reflection of his views;[5] it is to him that I attribute authorship.[6] Mbeki's stance has often been portrayed as a rejection of science, but the document indicates otherwise. It cites scientists[7] who make various points and there is clearly a sincere belief in science.[8] The doubt raised is not about science, but about the honesty of scientists; the document argues that we need to be sceptical of 'conformist' AIDS science.

> The question that faces any honest person, having been exposed to the reality that there are many outstanding questions [about AIDS] that require scientific answers, is whether it is possible both to be [an AIDS] conformist and retain one's sense of personal integrity! Is it possible for us to be conformist and actually defeat the AIDS threat that faces our people! The 'scientific proofs' adduced to convince us about the various facets of the HIV/AIDS question rest on very tenuous grounds.[9]

The document appeals for 'honest science' unconstrained by vested interests and concerned rather with people's wellbeing. It asserted that

'Honest medical science recognises the disastrous impact of malnutrition on us as Africans and the rest of the developing countries.'[10] As Anthony Butler[11] has pointed out, what was being put forward was an argument drawing attention to the social determinants of health in which people's environment determines their vulnerability to disease. Instead of the questions of poverty being addressed, Africans' supposed sexual promiscuity was being touted as the cause of the epidemic and expensive drugs proposed as the solution. Mbeki saw this as a deeply rooted racist discourse that threatened to again enslave Africans.[12]

Turning on his tormentors, Mbeki bests the question with which AIDS conformists assign people into the camp of science and rationality on the one side, or the camp of quacks, charlatans and eccentrics on the other: 'yes' or 'no' to the question whether HIV causes AIDS.

> ... to establish his or her credentials, everybody must answer the ballad question – do you believe that HIV causes AIDS! Belief about a scientific matter, and not empirical evidence, thus becomes the criterion of truth.[13]

That a scientific postulate becomes a matter of belief does not make the arguments put forward in the publication *Castro Hlongwane* any more or less valid, but it should make us question how sensitive an analysis of AIDS denial can be if we start with a statement of belief in HIV as the cause of AIDS, as do many who have written about Mbeki and AIDS.[14] No doubt these authors would brush this caution aside. It is not nuances that were called for by protagonists in the Great AIDS Debate. Those on the front lines of the AIDS establishment – doctors, scientists and human rights activists – came to the conclusion that the priority was for AIDS dissidents to be swept aside, drugs prescribed and lives saved.[15] Other concerns were ignored. It was about power and who was in charge of policy-making. What raised the temperature so much in the Great AIDS Debate was that Mbeki's stubborn position was seen as a betrayal of the previous medical–state alliance. For a while, it appeared that the enemies of reason were through the gates.

Science's scapegoats

In the rough and tumble of AIDS politics, it has been easy to blame Mbeki for the notions in people's heads that skew the pitch for scientifically based AIDS education. However, we need to be cautious in seeing Mbeki's role in the epidemic as being central. There were already an estimated 3.5 million people infected with HIV in South Africa when Mbeki became president in 1999; his views can't be held accountable for the magnitude of the epidemic.[16] Alternatively, we can look to neighbouring countries, such as Botswana, whose political elites proactively confronted AIDS with the messages of medical science, but which have HIV prevalence rates similar to or worse than South Africa.

There are a number of reasons why this argument oversteps what blame can be laid on Mbeki.[17] Our Bafana Radebe emerged as a home-grown dissident who never once mentioned Mbeki or drew on the specifics of Mbeki's arguments. Indeed, Bafana rejected outright some ideas, such as AIDS being racial genocide, which can tentatively be linked to Mbeki's thinking. Nor did the peer educators at the mining company Digco turn up much that could be linked directly to Mbeki among the profusion of AIDS myths that they reported. That is not to say that Mbeki's denialism was not raised during the research at Digco. It was. If you want to open a discussion quickly with a group of peer educators, then just unzip the Mbeki controversy. There will be derision and condemnation, and then, if the atmosphere is relaxed, more nuanced discussions that mirror some of the issues raised in this chapter. But, like the virgin rape myth as a cure for AIDS, there is a disjunction, at least of scale or frequency, between professional concerns about grassroots beliefs and actual grassroots conversations.[18]

Attempting to get to the fount of denialism, Seth Kalichman links Mbeki's views to those of Peter Duesberg, perhaps the leading dissident AIDS scientist. For Kalichman, all knowledge, correct or false, must be credited to science. 'Ultimately it [what you believe over AIDS] comes down to trust. Trusting what you hear. Trusting what you read. Trusting what one world-acclaimed scientist says over another.'[19] From this perspective, even the erudite Mbeki was not able to err without the assistance of world-acclaimed scientists.[20] If, Kalichman argues, denialism did not have a scientifically credible proponent, it would never have been considered worthy of attention. He describes how denialism forms a three-tiered pyramid scheme, with the top occupied by dissident scientists who propagate AIDS myths which are transmitted, via 'suspicious-minded persons who gravitate towards conspiracy theories', to the third and largest tier, people 'most likely affected by AIDS, often having tested positive themselves or having a loved one who has tested HIV-positive'.[21] Kalichman articulates, more clearly than most, that the AIDS establishment views people in this third tier as lacking the capacity to think.

An elite debate

Jonny Steinberg has argued that Mbeki brought to the surface South Africa's social fears, particularly the deep divide between races.[22] Yes, but racial theories of AIDS predate Mbeki's AIDS denialism. Mbeki's stand paralleled already existing racial explanations of AIDS. Arguably, Mbeki's view on how Africans were being portrayed helped fertilise the ground for racial conspiracy theories, but the *Castro Hlongwane* document never articulates, or suggests, what these racial folk theories propose – that the virus was created and/or spread by Whites to eliminate Africans. Castro Hlongwane, the 17-year-old African whose name appeared in the document's title, was a victim – but not of AIDS. Rather, he was subjected to racist discrimination by Whites who presumed, on account of his Blackness, that he had AIDS.[23] Further, *Castro Hlongwane*, the document, is silent over traditional beliefs and religion[24] and any relationship these might have to HIV/AIDS. This is not surprising: nobody has ever accused Mbeki of being a 'man of the people'. As he made his stand on AIDS, he neither reflected nor engaged with popular beliefs.

Rather, the Great AIDS Debate was a dispute between elite groups. Scholars documenting this conflict put considerable effort into defining denialism and documenting evidence for charging the government of the time, or at least significant parts of it, with the denialism that they defined. With the entrance of the Treatment Action Campaign

(TAC) into this arena, the scope of commentary expanded to detail the campaigns and court battles waged by this high-profile segment of civil society that challenged government's AIDS policy.

Kerry Cullinan and Anso Thom introduce their book on AIDS denialism, *The Virus, Vitamins and Vegetables,* with the idea that 'The main characters [in this story] were obvious – Thabo Mbeki, Manto Tshabalala-Msimang [South Africa's ex-Minister of Health], Anthony Brink, Tine van der Maas and Matthias Rath [three prominent South African-based AIDS denialists]. Then there were those on the other side of the fence – health workers and AIDS activists.'[25] This folksy portrayal of those campaigning for treatment is overdone. Alongside the TAC stood scientists, academics, journalists and lawyers, many with international connections – what Pieter Fourie and Melissa Meyer refer to as the 'AIDS Community,'[26] which I suggest is better seen as the 'AIDS Establishment', given that it is circumscribed by carefully guarded boundaries of belief about AIDS. What is being projected with the image of an 'AIDS Community' is, however, a principled band of campaigners, armed with truth and reason up against a small cast of deluded but powerful miscreants. Yet, strip away the moral labelling and what remains is the clash of elites over the control of policy.

With Mbeki's dissidence taken mistakenly to heart by South Africans, the argument goes, the epidemic ripped through the population, as public health messages were ignored. Winning the battle against denialists would, it was suggested, win the war against AIDS. The problem for both elites, beyond defeating the other, was to get people to co-operate with the salvation from AIDS that they each differently proposed to implement on the population.

With Mbeki pushed aside and after so much time, money and effort has been spent in teaching people about HIV and AIDS, we still know precariously little about what is believed about the disease. This stems from three interlinked problems: the failure of medical science to discover a decisive response to the disease; the slow and limited impact of behavioural change theory and practice; and the failure of social science to dig deeply into the reasons why behaviours have changed so slowly.

These three connected failures have allowed us to sleepwalk through the epidemic even as we have raged against the suffering that it has brought. We have lazily gone along with the view that the epidemic is driven by insufficient information. And we have gone along with the assumption that people are 'empty vessels' into which the correct information can be deposited. There have been voices arguing otherwise, but they have been ineffectual against the AIDS Establishment's juggernaut. The response to the epidemic has been narrowly framed by medical science articulated with a human rights focus on treatment access, which lost sight of people's ability to think for themselves.

Mbeki and the people

Within the Great AIDS Debate, policy questions, particularly over the provision of antiretroviral drugs, received most attention. By contrast, our focus is on people's responses to AIDS. We should be careful about the easy argument that Mbeki's denialism confused people – there is no clear or direct link between the former president's quixotic stand and people's alternative explanations of AIDS.

To argue that people believed Mbeki, rather than public health messages, is easy, but wrong. It proposes that information from the top cascades down to the population below. If only Mbeki had followed the doctors' advice and supported public health messages, people would have put on condoms and taken their pills. Alternatively, and more plausibly, it could be argued that Mbeki's pronouncements sowed doubt over doctors' infallibility. He did not convince the population of his own perspective, but he gave popular explanations of HIV/AIDS some relief from public health hectoring.[27] This approach allows us to recognise the limited purchase medical science has on the minds of many *and* allows us to credit people with the ability to do their own thinking. It also cautions us not to be overconfident about tackling AIDS, especially prevention, with presidential denialism departed.

Anso Thom describes how the Treatment Action Campaign (TAC) used the courts to close down Matthias Rath's vitamin-cure-for-AIDS business, an operation supported by the then health minister of South

Africa, Tshabalala-Msimang.[28] But a visit to any health store will turn up a range of immune-boosters (code for AIDS treatments) for sale. In 2011, the TAC appealed to the Advertising Standards Authority of South Africa and forced the Christ Embassy church to withdraw its 24-minute faith-healing programme which claimed people could be cured of AIDS.[29] In November 2013, the TAC organised a march in Durban to expose a 'priest's phoney HIV cure' and threatened to prosecute him if the holy water he was administrating failed clinical trials.[30]

If popular defiance of the medical explanation of AIDS was the product of Mbeki's denial, the need for such treatment activism would fade away. It doesn't look like that. Laudable as these actions to close down quackery may be, the endeavours appear as vain as cutting the heads off the mythical Hydra.[31]

11

Agency from below

Nicoli Nattrass has described the legacy of AIDS denialism as the 'tragic undermining of public trust in science'.[1] Clearly, science was challenged, but to assume that the public previously trusted science is to overlook the much more complex world of beliefs present in the South African population that is generated from below, not controlled from above.[2]

Folk and lay theories of AIDS are not based on science. They may adopt elements of medical science, but they never systematically adopt scientific method. This distinction must logically hold; if alternative theories used science systematically, they'd no longer be alternative. The accounts outlined in this book show that township residents think for themselves over AIDS. We might not like what they come up with, but we need to recognise this dissent from below. As Elizabeth Fee describes, people engage with the 'social reality in which disease is produced, experienced and reproduced, and in which the cultural meanings of the experience are defined and struggled over'.[3]

We have met three HIV-positive township residents in this book: Bafana, Grace and Neo, along with Paseka, Bafana's primary support during his health crisis. All are firmly in Kalichman's third tier. Additionally, all four are Africans, are poorly educated and are poor. Bafana, Grace and Neo are dirt poor, surviving on causal jobs, stipends, donations, hawking, social security payments and whatever else they can muster. Paseka is better off with regular domestic work and a sober husband who brings his pay packet home each month.[4]

But, whatever the balance of circumstances, these four lives have been fought on the back foot. No silver spoons and few lucky breaks. Rather, their lives are stamped with setbacks, struggle and suffering. Yet, it is impossible to view these four individuals as passive recipients of AIDS explanations. They have demonstrated remarkable agency in constructing understandings of HIV and AIDS.

That agency cannot reconstruct the biological nature of HIV/AIDS. But we need to recognise how they, and many others, have reached their own understandings of the disease. Sometimes this is in defiance of medical science, more often it is on the sly as parallel understandings of the disease are constructed and direct conflict avoided.[5]

The agency used in the construction of AIDS from below is demonstrated by the complexity, and often coherence, of these alternative theories. The agency of those whom I talked to has also been demonstrated by the relationships that emerged. One of the greatest concerns of university ethics committees is that research is not exploitative. It's an appropriate concern, albeit not one easily adjudicated in the field. But we should not think that because there is an unequal power relationship between a university professor and a township resident that this excludes agency on the part of the latter. Bafana used me to transform his HIV away, even as our interviews progressed. Grace, positive on a public stage, used me to wash her dirty laundry in private. Paseka used me to speak her piece and tell a version of Bafana's illness through the lens of family tensions. Neo used the research relationship to evangelise. Such actions undertaken by supposed 'subjects' complicate research relationships (though they also build friendships). But this also illustrates a much larger point: Bafana, Grace, Paseka and Neo were nobody's puppets, either within the research project or in their understanding of HIV and AIDS. It is their agency, along with that of millions of other South Africans, that we need to engage.

Seeing AIDS differently

The sociologist Erving Goffman grappled with how experience is organised, in his book *Frame Analysis*.[6] As a symbolic interactionist,

Goffman was concerned with how events are psychologically framed by individuals in ways that provide a schema of meaning. Goffman's book is almost as long as Melville's *Moby-Dick*, and over the course of 500 pages the complexity of such psychological framing of experience is explored. A key concept Goffman uses is that of 'keying', how a set of events are psychologically organised in a particular way, and how one set of events can be 're-keyed' differently, resulting in multiple, sometimes overlapping frames that organise the understanding of the same events in alternative ways. We are concerned with how HIV/AIDS is framed. Such framing, in Goffman's schema, is a collective process; an individual can only meaningfully key or re-key an event if the desired frame is mutually credible and acceptable.[7]

Goffman's frame analysis enables us to see how HIV/AIDS is being keyed and re-keyed by actors to construct different frames of understanding: a biomedical disease, a punishment from God, a racial weapon or the consequence of breaking traditional sexual taboos. Each of these frames allows for an almost infinite number of sub-framings. *Moruti* Puleng, whose Apostolic church Grace attended, thought that AIDS, like all illnesses, was a message from God designed to bring back those who had strayed from Him. By contrast, *Ntate* Mofokeng, preacher of the Pentecostal Holy Spirit Church which Neo attended was emphatic that AIDS was an evil spirit or demon and therefore a thing of the Devil. Sister Irene, who attended a Pentecostal church, debated whether AIDS was a thing of God or the Devil, given its multiple effects, some of which were ultimately beneficial, while others impossibly evil. *Ntate* Mofokeng thought that going to a traditional healer could open a portal through which a demon could enter and that witchcraft was real in its effects. *Moruti* Puleng believed there were no such things as witches. Paseka, attending a church, which synchronised belief in God and the ancestors, played down God's role in the epidemic.[8] Rather, she was convinced that Bafana had opened himself up to infection by neglecting his ancestors.

What is needed for multiple framings of HIV/AIDS is individuals willing to key, or interpret, the sickness and its symptoms in a particular way and for others to accept such frameworks as credible. Thus, the major systematic framings of HIV/AIDS, outside the allopathic explanation, are those that draw on psychological resources with wide currency. Within African townships this includes traditional belief, Christianity and the experiences of racism.

I have puzzled as to how the Digco peer educators explained HIV/AIDS in different ways, depending on whether the starting point of a conversation was their peer educator training or a conversation about their varied personal beliefs. What was happening was that two different keying systems were taking place: one leading to a biomedical framing of HIV/AIDS, the other leading to an alternative framing. The reason for my puzzlement was, really, that I'd developed enought rapport to allow keying into two different framings of HIV/AIDS with the peer educators. My ongoing discussions with Bafana about what ailed him can also be seen as his framing his own illness as a unique form of TB that mimicked symptoms of AIDS, not the result of HIV infection. In this he sought to key events in a way that I, and others whom he engaged, would accept.

If the same event can be keyed in different ways, then the frustrating and costly treatment odysseys undertaken by many individuals infected with HIV are not surprising. Sickness, or simply an HIV-positive diagnosis, can be keyed one way, then another, then another, all offering hope for a while and most offering a more attractive alternative than the biomedical framing of the disease that health professionals and peer educators are charged with keying.[9]

Recognising our limits and others' agency

Goffman's frame analysis provides us with a way to explain how plural understandings are generated from one set of events, but it offers cold comfort for what can be done about HIV/AIDS. A grasp of these alternative explanations of HIV/AIDS will not provide a quick fix that renders frictionless resistance to behavioural change messages. The manifold beliefs about HIV/AIDS within South African townships mean that there is no magic bullet to be found in translation. We cannot sketch a few clear alternative explanations of AIDS and give them to health educationalists who could engineer prevention and treatment messages that would directly tackle these alternative perspectives.

What this exploration of the alternative explanations of AIDS suggests is that an effective response will have to work with alternative frames that are not seen as strange but perfectly sound accounts. Only such engagement will allow us to understand what people really know about AIDS. But engagement is impossible without respect. What we have uncovered is the agency of those grappling with the disease. To respect what they are doing, we need to understand why HIV/AIDS is being keyed and re-keyed in these different ways.

Agency in an insecure world

When multiple keyings of a problem are present, it indicates an insecure world. The typical reader of this book is likely to have a clear sense of how they can progress. While things do not always go our own way, we trust, by and large, in the steps that are necessary to achieve a particular outcome. We operate in structures in which the outcomes are largely guaranteed as long as we provide the necessary inputs: passing exams, advancing a career, enforcing our rights, buying a house, maintaining insurance cover, investing for retirement, and so on. As Michel de Certeau outlines, we are able to operate *strategically* to confidently accumulate educational, physical, social and financial resources.[10] Each step or achievement can be realised and held. Excepting unexpected calamities, we inhabit a secure world in which there is alignment between action and outcome.[11]

By contrast, most of the residents of South African townships live with diluted and erratic versions of these systems of certainty and trust. Bafana, Grace, Paseka and Neo operate in often uncertain terrain in which advantage must be snatched when the opportunity arises, knowing that such gains cannot be taken for granted, or necessarily held securely. They must, in De Certeau's terms, act *tactically*. Paseka was at the municipal offices before dawn to force officials' hands and get the housing stand she needed. Grace hoarded treatment in anticipation of another stock-out of drugs in the public health system. Neo lived with two surnames. Bafana eventually abandoned the money owed to him by Firstjob. These are all minor examples of a massive problem. For many people life is a battle lived with only weak rules. Completing education, getting decent work and establishing financial security are all uphill struggles. These things are not impossible, but the odds are stacked against them.

Hardly surprisingly, different sources of advice are approached. Traditional healers, preachers and prophets are called in to help pass exams, recall lovers, inflict revenge on enemies, find work and protect what has been accumulated. Neo was quite adamant that faith in God would, with prayer, see her CV picked out from the tall pile of hopefuls. Similarly, clients' CVs are 'treated' by traditional healers to ensure their success. If proof is needed of the values of these alternative ways to progress, testimonials can be found with little need for fabrication. Neo's church services involved members of the church witnessing how God had helped them – not to find salvation in heaven, but to pass their exams, get to college, find a job, avoid a road accident or be promoted.

It is not that alternative systems are automatically believed, as preachers, prophets and healers are not necessarily trusted. The widespread view that traditional healers from far away or from long ago have genuine and greater powers than those who can be turned to within local neighbourhoods illustrates a belief in the cosmology of traditional belief surpassing faith in individual practitioners.[12]

But even when it is believed that a traditional healer with genuine powers can be found, one had to be careful as, like anybody else, they cannot be fully trusted. One Digco peer educator, in illustrating her general distrust of traditional healers, recounted the story of her aunt. A successful shebeen queen, she had employed traditional healers to protect her business. For a fee, they would bury doctored stakes around the perimeter of the property. Notwithstanding that she went far and wide to Lesotho, Mozambique, and Swaziland to employ a different traditional healer each year, her business had gone downhill and she had started to be assaulted, in her dreams, by snakes and wild animals. The peer educator was in no doubt that these originated from one of the traditional healers who, instead of protecting her aunt, had introduced these malevolent forces.[13]

Adam Ashforth addresses the insecurity of Soweto township residents resulting from witchcraft in which, '[t]he abiding presence of occult assault in a world of witches arouses a pervasive sense of insecurity and injustice resulting from the experience of suffering as harm.'[14] Ashforth describes a world of insecurity; a world in which people suffer beyond what they can account for and must resort to supernatural beliefs. Once these supernatural beliefs become explanations for outcomes, then there exists 'spiritual insecurity'. Such spiritual insecurity extends far beyond the belief in witchcraft, to the gamut of concerns over physical and psychological security raised by a litany of ills: inequality, crime, sexual abuse, absent fathers, corruption, fraud, unemployment, addictions, poverty, want and sickness. Within all this the typical township resident must find ways of making sense and ways of moving forward.

AIDS speakeasies

Making sense and making headway are not things that individuals can pursue in isolation; they take place within social contexts and shared psychological framings. Alternative theories of HIV/AIDS provide attractive explanations, compared to that of medical science, based on their plausibility and palatability. Linking these beliefs and their benefits is of value, but there is a danger that in extracting the core essence of the different theories of HIV/AIDS and chalking up their relative merits we strip them from their social and psychological context. It is useful to identify the various constellations of belief over HIV/AIDS and these different theories' relative strengths, but only if we root this analysis within the same context in which these beliefs reside.

Even lay theories of HIV/AIDS that originate from the cunning and creativity of an individual mind must be shared with others if they are to successfully key the disease into a particular frame. Bafana's efforts to carry me and his neighbours, along with his particular explanation of HIV/AIDS, illustrate this well. But it is the folk theories of HIV/AIDS where the collective nature of knowledge is really underscored. The three major folk explanations of the disease are not only constructed arguments but also tenets of belief within different communities. These have widely ranging boundaries and very different membership criteria, but they constitute communities of belief within which alternative framings of AIDS are shared. Racial explanations of the disease can find a foothold among those who share experiences of racial oppression; traditional explanations among those who hold to ancestral, pollution and witchcraft beliefs; and religious explanations among church congregants.

Membership of these communities does not determine belief in these alternative explanations, but it makes it more likely. Racial understanding of the disease is far more likely to be considered when Whites are absent – as they are almost completely so from South African townships. Within the townships, communities of belief, say church congregations, mean that an individual's perspective is shared and supported by others. Occasionally, these alternative explanations surface into view, such as the healing messages of the Christ Embassy Church being aired on television. At this point the message proponents are vulnerable to scientific criticism and censure through the courts.[15] For the most part, however, alternative accounts of HIV/AIDS lie below national public discourse. In the township, there are many public spaces free from censorship, litigation or ridicule of the medical profession and AIDS NGOs. These AIDS speakeasies include churches, sangomas' *ndumba* (consultation rooms), street corners, yards, kitchens, and the relaxed talk at *mesebetsi* (ceremonies) and other township gatherings or get-togethers.[16] Here, alternative framings of AIDS are openly expressed, affirmed and refined.

A stupid conflict

Responding to the AIDS epidemic is an army of professional health care workers, lay assistants, volunteer peer educators and concerned citizens playing their part. Many of those in the lower ranks of this army have a foot in both the AIDS speakeasies of the township and the clinics and hospitals of the government. Grace Dlamini was on the front line in Bophelo Clinic, counselling those tested, squashing waiting room dissent, and spinning lies about treatment to allay people's fears.

But she sometimes doubted what she preached and always hoped for something better. Grace illustrates that there is doubt in the ranks of the army against AIDS. And if Grace was a foot soldier, then Sister Irene was a sergeant in charge of the clinic's HIV/AIDS programme. She too held other framings of AIDS, even as she rolled out antiretroviral treatment.

Kabelo and Bernard, who sparred with each other in the shade of a township tree, illustrated the value of peer status for effective communication. Their competitive advice over girlfriends, *spares* and safe sex illustrates that township residents engage with and criticise official health promotion messages over AIDS. Indeed, the Kabelos and Bernards of the township can beat peer educators back into retreat. If they are the adversary in a war that we have chosen to wage over the meaning of AIDS, then the enemy is legion and our own forces less than reliable.

More than a decade ago Quentin Gausset made the point that we need to avoid a fight between cultures.[17] But we have been waging such a war, stupidly, without understanding the balance of forces or the lie of the land on which combat is taking place. The resistance has been guerrilla-like, stubborn and sullen. Our victories have been Pyrrhic. We have been waging a war on those we sought to help.

How did we get ourselves into this position? Because we have refused to accept that people think, over matters of importance, differently from us. Our dogged determination to instill into the population a scientific understanding of HIV/AIDS, in the face of dismal results, bears testament to this refusal. It is not only over sickness that people have parallel belief structures to those of experts. Away from the controversy and tragedy of AIDS, it may be easy for us to see how people think differently, and are yet able to manage. Willett Kempton studied how individuals understood their home heating systems and used them to achieve desired temperatures. He found two predominating theories of how a thermostat regulated temperature, neither corresponding to how an engineer would understand its operation. These theories were based on everyday experience, they varied between individuals but had elements that were shared, and they were inconsistent with expert understandings.[18] Kempton stresses that they did indeed solve the problem, in this case of how to keep a house at a desired temperature, and he argues that their practical value did not relate to how closely they approximated experts' understandings. Further, because they are not acknowledged as *theories*, but as descriptions of reality, they are difficult to change.[19] The robustness of lay or folk theories is supported by Dorothy Holland and Naomi Quinn, who point to the ability of individuals to incorporate new components, including information provided by experts, into their own models, rather than change them (to that of the experts).[20] In addition to incorporating new information or ideas, individuals do not find it hard to hold different theories of explanation simultaneously.[21]

Neo Pakwe made sense of her HIV infection through her religious faith, which provided a foundational account and hope for the future. Her belief, that she could be unburdened of her status if saved from sin, is incompatible with the medical model of HIV/AIDS. Yet, she juggled her faith and medical treatment, even championing the latter as she got her sister onto treatment at the eleventh hour. Separating the biological process of viral infection from a moral framework, and separating the therapeutic value of medication from the prospect of a faith-based cure, allowed Neo to manage medical treatment and her faith.

Measured by emotional commitment, the medical treatment that was keeping Neo alive was strikingly peripheral.[22] By contrast, Neo's religious cosmology was nurtured with intensity. Its internal logic and the implication for her behaviour and her thoughts were constantly on her mind. She was determined to stay the course. Other HIV-positive individuals shop around the multitude of alternatives on offer. The case of Neo shows that managing one's alternative framing of AIDS, different from that of medical science, with a commitment to its small print, is more conducive to accommodation of antiretroviral drugs than an oscillation between different belief systems.

We are, then, back to the wisdom of the Digco peer educators. Despite their limitations, as measured by their medical knowledge, what they did understand is that there had to be compromises between the medical treatment of HIV and people's beliefs. Some of those beliefs are easier to work with, however their importance is not measured by their compatibility with medical science but by their hold on people.

To fight or talk?

I have made use of the mythological Hydra as a metaphor for the alternative explanation of HIV/AIDS in South African townships. It was a valuable metaphor in capturing both the multiplicity of accounts and their ability to mutate and regenerate. But it is a comparison that we should abandon if it frames our relationship with the alternative explanations of HIV/AIDS as combat. If we take on the role of Hercules and seek to slay the monster, we set ourselves in opposition to large sections of the population. The heads of the Hydra we seek to conquer are the beliefs of the people we are seeking to save. We may convince ourselves that we are fighting the good fight, but we are failing to see that township residents are not the enemy and we must find more respectful ways to engage with them, and their beliefs, over HIV/AIDS.

That does not provide an easy answer. In addressing the alternative explanations of HIV/AIDS, we still encounter a hydra, a persistent or many-sided problem that presents new obstacles as soon as one aspect is solved,[23] but we must rid ourselves of the idea that we confront a monster.

Within African culture there is a strong emphasis on discussion and consensus. The often vicious social conditions of township life provide room for scepticism over what this means and what it can achieve, but it is an important principle of our shared humanity: that there are many opinions when people meet, but if they talk together, these differences diminish and people become one in purpose.

That this has not happened over HIV/AIDS is a reflection of the much wider gulf that characterises South African society. The economic inequality in South Africa is relatively easy to measure, even if it is stubbornly difficult to address, but the gap in beliefs is something we have given less attention. For all the stress on human rights in the fight against AIDS, we have ended up de-humanising others.[24] We have failed to grasp how alternative theories of the disease represent agency on the part of those whom we are trying to instruct. Viewed from the perspective of a scientifically valid explanation of HIV/AIDS, we have dismissed alternative explanations of the disease as ignorance or mischief. In doing so, we have failed to understand why HIV/AIDS health promotion has been so ineffective and we have failed to understand the subjects of our endeavours. These two failures are interlinked: we cannot help those whom we do not understand and we cannot understand those we infantilise because they believe differently from ourselves.

APPENDIX 1

The unwritten language of the kasi

South Africa is a polyglot society, but not multi-lingual in the way suggested by the hackneyed mantra of there being 11 official languages. In fact, a lot of bunk is talked about languages in South Africa. I challenge this chatter with some trepidation – I am a terrible linguist and was glad to abandon language studies at school with a scraped pass in French. In South Africa, and after a couple of false starts, I started to learn Sesotho. With dogged determination I have been inflicting it on Sesotho speakers ever since. By and large, they have borne with me, and what linguistic ability I have is thanks to them. They know my true linguistic competence and, kindly, make allowances. After all, communication is a joint endeavour and much can be achieved with good will. But, even for an amateur linguist, it is obvious that the comfortable picture of 11 official languages does not correspond to the reality of South Africa.

But, to start, let's summarise what an analysis of these 11 official languages does tell us. Two are European in origin: English and Afrikaans. Nine are African and all of these belong to the Bantu language family. Four can be grouped together as Nguni languages: isiZulu, isiXhosa, siSwati and isiNdebele. Three can be grouped as Sesotho languages: Sesotho (or Southern Sotho), Sepedi (or Nothern Sotho) and Setswana. The two remaining are Tshivenda and Xitsonga (often, wrongly, called Shangaan). The Nguni and Sesotho language groups are each, to different degrees, mutually intelligible and, arguably, represent just two languages with distinct dialects. Conversely, each of the nine recognised African languages is not homogeneous – there are dialects and variations within them, again to different degrees.

Statistics South Africa asks in its censuses the first language of individuals. That question possibly hides more than it reveals, but what it does tell us is that in the 2011 Census:[1] 43.4 per cent reported their first language being Nguni (the vast majority of these being isiZulu and isiXhosa); 24.7 per cent a Sesotho language (fairly evenly divided between the three sub-languages); 13.5 per cent Afrikaans; 9.6 per cent English; 4.6 per cent Xitsonga; and 2.4 per cent Tshivenda. Additionally, the census recorded 0.5 per cent reporting Signing as their primary language and 1.6 per cent another language altogether.

The distribution of first languages recorded by the census has some relationship to South Africa's provincial boundaries and geography.[2] The predominant language in KwaZulu-Natal is isiZulu; in the Eastern Cape, isiXhosa; in the Free State, Sesotho; in the North West Province, Setswana; and in Limpopo, Sepedi (though Limpopo is also home to the largest concentrations of South Africa's Tshivenda and Xitsonga speakers). The Western Cape's most common first language is Afrikaans (spoken by both Whites and Coloureds), but with English and isiXhosa both being important. The Northern Cape's most common language is Afrikaans, followed by Setswana. Mpumalanga is linguistically diverse, but with isiZulu and siSwati between them accounting for over 50 per cent. Gauteng is the most linguistically mixed, with five languages (Afrikaans, English, isiZulu, Sepedi and Sesotho), making it into double-digit percentages.

Of course the country's provincial geography, while important, represents a somewhat antiseptic account of linguistic distribution. More telling, historically and sociologically, is that the vast majority of those whose first language is African live either in a township or 'rural area',[3] overwhelmingly the poorer parts of the country.

In those geographical spaces where European languages dominate, including the traditionally White universities, being able to speak a little of any African language can be interpreted as fluency, but that's only because in the land of the blind the one-eyed man is king. Or, in other words, the vast majority of White South Africans speak hardly a word of any African language. This situation is not always very different for the increasing African middle class for whom, educated in private or semi-private Model C schools, English is also their first language. There is an aspect of class-based, cross-cultural collaboration in this situation; crudely put, Whites are relieved of the tiresome burden of learning an unfamiliar language for which they see little use, and Africans seeking to get ahead welcome abandoning the social shackles of parochial tongues. This reflects the *realpolitik* of language.

The brutal reality of language in South Africa is that 9 of the 11 official tongues, which are all nominally equal, are dying. The guardians of Afrikaans periodically rail against its marginalisation, and in historical context they make a valid observation, but it is the nine African languages that are disappearing *ka pele* (at speed). They are being abandoned by those who seek to get ahead. To get ahead means immersion in a world that communicates in English, the language of the university, the language of science, the language of business, the language of law, the language of diplomacy, the language of the future.[4] To be abandoned by the educated is the death knell for any language. It is left defenceless with no dictionaries, no grammars, no literature, no translations, no custodians, no champions.[5]

This extinction will take time as there still remain pockets of linguistic vibrancy: isiZulu newspapers, Sesotho radio stations and so on. But the writing is on the wall.

What will endure much longer is written nowhere: Sekasi, the *lingua franca*, or common language, of the township that mixes any and all vocabularies and grammars as well as coining its own lexicon. Precisely because it is unwritten, there is not even a single name for this language. Sekasi is the Sesotho name; literally it means the language of the *kasi*[6] (township). But there are other names: Isicamtho (of Nguni origin), Tsotsitaal (of Afrikaans origin) and simply Kasi Lingo. It is this language that you will encounter on the streets of South Africa's townships, not isiZulu, not Sesotho, nor any other of the nine official African languages. The so-called rural areas are often cited as the repositories of the true tongue, but that's only correct to a degree. In Gauteng townships, you will be told, for example, that in the Free State they speak Sesotho *sa sebele* (true Sesotho) or Sesotho *se tebileng* (deep Sesotho). The Sesotho spoken there *is* closer to the Sesotho captured by RA Paroz,[7] CM Doke and SM Mofokeng[8] more than 50 years ago[9] than that on township streets of Gauteng. But it's rarely 'Sesotho A' (formal or high Sesotho). Rather, you will be told that it is across the border, in Lesotho, where they truly speak Sesotho *se tebileng*. Again, this is only partly true. Even in a remote Lesotho village in the Maloti Mountains you'll hear plenty of words and phrases that have washed back from Gauteng and elsewhere.

Put the census aside! The most widely spoken language in South Africa is not one of the 11. Nor does it have a single name. Nor is it written anywhere. It's Sekasi/Isicamtho/Tsotsitaal/Kasi Lingo ...

It is worth making this point to shake up the complacency around languages in South Africa. However, it would be wrong to suggest that Sekasi represents a single spoken tongue. It varies widely across time and space. Tsotsitaal is an earlier, Afrikaans-heavy version of Sekasi, still spoken by older township residents. The Sekasi of one township differs from that of another. In some cases, this is informally recognised, as in Pretoriataal, the Sekasi dialect spoken in townships around Pretoria, which is distinct from that spoken in other Gauteng townships. Like all languages Sekasi is constantly under construction. The vibrant street scene of South African townships, particularly youth cultures that also spill into social media and musical arenas, makes Sekasi a fast-responding language that picks up words and phrases *ka speed*.

Sekasi is also a language of resistance, the language owned by those without power in South African society.[10] Those seeking to understand township life, and particularly the lives of the township underclasses (the youth, unemployed, casual workers, backyard dwellers, street hawkers and others), should recognise that it is this diverse, unwritten and fast-changing language through which meaning is constructed, jokes told, hopes articulated, gossip traded and dissent expressed.

APPENDIX 2

Glossary of South African & township words and phrases

Introduction

The following is a list of words and phrases that appear in the book. Most form part of the Sesotho-heavy Sekasi that I worked in, along with English, in conducting research for this book.

Nouns are ordered by their singular format (unless the noun is collective); the plural is indicated in the left-hand column after the slash sign (/), for example:

Kereke/dikereke   Church(es) (Sesotho)

To find a noun used in its plural form requires knowing the noun class to which it belongs (as plurals are formed using prefixes in Sesotho). Following Paroz ([1961] 1988):

Noun class	Singular prefix	Plural prefix
1	Mo-	Ba-
2	Mo-	Me-
3	Le-	Ma-
4	Se-	Di-
5	(N)-	Di-
6	Bo-	Ma-
7		Ho-

After the description, the language(s) in which the word is used is indicated. Within Sesotho-heavy Sekasi, words and phrases can form 'good' Sesotho, 'good' Nguni (the generic term for the four Nguni languages in South Africa), 'good' English, etc., as well as being words within Sekasi (which has no standard lexicography and so can't be 'good' – outside the context of its actual use). The location within different language vocabularies is indicated by separation with a slash sign (/), for example:

Kuku/dikuku   Cake(s), also slang for vagina (Sekasi/Sesotho)

and

Kwaal   Envy, jealousy (Sekasi/Afrikaans)

Words can originate from one language (and phases from more than one) but with grammatical rules from a different language applied, for example the 'Sesothoisation' of the English verb 'to enjoy', making the Sekasi verb *enjoya* (and *enjoyile* in the past form). Where this is the case, the likely origin of a Sekasi word is indicated after the | sign, for example:

Enjoya (verb)   To enjoy (Sekasi | English)

Beyond adoption within Sekasi there are words that are loaned widely by different language speakers in South Africa, for example *sangoma,* a traditional healer (specifically diviner) in Nguni, which is widely used among speakers of English, Afrikaans and other African languages. This is noted as the word being a 'common South African loan word'.

Glossary

Amper	Nearly (Afrikaans/Sekasi)
Apara (verb)	To wear (Sesotho)
Ba papala ka batho	They play/mistreat people (Sesotho)
Badimo	Ancestors (Sesotho)
Bala (verb)	To study, to read (Sesotho
Bana ba motho	Children (descendants) of one person; applies to cousins as well as siblings (Sesotho)
Bapala (verb)	To play (Sesotho)
Batjha	Youth (Sesotho)
Batla (verb)	To want, to need (Sesotho)
Beemer	BMW car (English/Sekasi)
Belaela (verb)	To suspect, doubt (Sesotho)
Bibele	Bible (Sesotho I English)
Bioscope	Cinema (Sekasi/South African English)
Biri	Beer (Sekasi I English)
Black Diamond	Marketing speak for the emerging Black middle-class in South Africa (English)
Bodutu	Boredom (Sesotho)
Boemo/maemo	Situation, status (Sesotho)
Bohale	Angry (a person), strong (alcohol), sharp (a knife) (Sesotho)
Boladu	Pus (Sesotho)
Bolla (verb)	To circumcise; also refers to traditional initiation processes in which young people graduate into adulthood (Sesotho)
Boloyi	Witchcraft (Sesotho)
Bona (verb)	To look, to see (Sesotho)
Bonang! (verb)	Look! (command, addressing more than one person) (Sesotho)
Bontate	Senior men (Sesotho)
Bontsha (verb)	To show (Sesotho)
Bopilwe (verb)	To have been created (Sesotho)
Born Frees	Children, particularly Black, born after the 1994 advent of democracy (English)
Botho	Shared humanity (Sesotho); interchangeable with *ubuntu* (Nguni)

310

Botsotsi	Crime (Sekasi)
Bua (verb)	To speak (Sesotho)
Chaf pozi	Informal bar or pub; often a room in a house (Sekasi/Nguni); also called a shebeen
Cheri	Girlfriend (Sekasi)
Clipper	One hundred rands (Sekasi | English – notes that will be clipped together)
Cucumberi/Dicucumberi	Cucumber (Sesotho/Sekasi | English)
Daka boy	Builders' labour, especially employed to mix cement; can be used derogatorily (Sekasi | Nguni and English)
Di batla di tshwana	They're almost the same (Sesotho)
Di haufinyane	They're really close together (Sesotho)
Dihlong	Shame (Sesotho)
Dikwankwara	Hard biscuits; often sold from *spaza* shops and street-side stalls (Sekasi)
Dikupu	Drums (Sekasi)
Dipatlisiso	Research, enquiries (Sesotho)
Dipatsi	Firewood (Sesotho)
(Di)pilisi ho sebedisa mala	Literally: pills that work the bowels; laxative pills (Sesotho)
Dipompong	Sweets (Sesotho | French)
Disiki tsa tlhahlo	Natural illnesses (Sekasi | Sesotho and English)
Diso	Sores, ulcers (Sesotho)
Ditaola	Divining bones of a healer (Sesotho)
Ditshila	Dirt (Sesotho)
Docteng	At the (Western-trained) doctor's surgery (Sekasi | English/Sesotho)
Dorp	Small town (Afrikaans, common South African loan word)
Dos	Light, match (Sekasi)
Drop	Sexually transmitted infection (English/Sekasi)
Efankgedi	Gospel, evangelist (Sekasi | English)
Empa	But (Sesotho)
Eng?	What? (Sesotho)
Enjoya (verb)	To enjoy (Sekasi | English)
Entshe!	Take it off! (Sesotho, formally *e ntshe*, but pronounced as one word)

Ethnobongo	Ethnic nonsense-speak (English)
Etsa (verb)	To do, to make (Sesotho)
Fapane	Different (Sesotho)
Fatcakes	Deep-fried dough balls, often eaten with achaar or polony (English); also known as *makwena* (Sesotho/Sekasi) and *vetkoek* (Afrikaans)
Feba (verb)	To commit adultery (Sesotho)
Feela	Only (Sesotho)
Femeng	In the company, factory work (Sekasi I English)
Fokotsa (verb)	To reduce or to decrease (Sesotho)
Futha (verb)	To steam (Sesotho)
Garden boy	Demeaning term for an African gardener or outdoor assistant (English)
Ghosts	Corn-puff snack (Sekasi)
Grey area	Residential areas that have become racially mixed (English)
Ha di fapane haholo	They're not very different (Sesotho)
Ha e yo	There isn't any/I don't have; a polite way to refuse requests (Sesotho)
Habo	The (birth) home of (third person) (Sesotho)
Haholo	A lot, very, much (Sesotho)
Hang hang	All at once (Sesotho)
Hape	Again (Sesotho)
Hlaba sepeite	To cleanse by injection (Sesotho/Sekasi)
Hlahloba (verb)	To examine (Sesotho)
Hlapa (verb)	To wash oneself (Sesotho)
Hlokahala (verb)	To die, to pass away (Sesotho)
Hlompisa (verb)	To respect somebody/something (Sesotho)
Ho a bata!	It's cold! (Sesotho)
Ho tla loka	It will be OK (Sesotho)
Hopola (verb)	To remember, to miss, to think of (Sesotho)
Hukung	Literally: on the corner; used for street-side stall or hawker's stand
Imbiza	Traditional medicine (Nguni)
Inehela (verb)	To surrender oneself to (Sesotho)
Inyoga/Izinyoga	Literally: snake(s) (Nguni); the Eskom electricity company attempted to coin it as

	a pejorative loan word for electricity and cable thieves, but it's used in Sekasi in a less pejorative way
Ithabisa (verb)	To enjoy oneself (Sesotho)
Isidliso	Traditional wasting disease, sometimes translated as TB (Nguni)
Jesu	Jesus (Sesotho | English)
Jumpa (verb)	To jump, to skip (Sekasi | English)
Jwala	Traditional sorghum beer (especially when specified as *jwala ba bosotho*), beer, alcohol (Sesotho)
Jwalo	Like, in the manner of (Sesotho)
Jwang?	How? (Sesotho)
Ka pele	With speed, speedily (Sesotho)
Ka speed	With speed, speedily (Sekasi | Sesotho and English)
Kakamelo	Curiosity, interest in other people's business (Sesotho)
Kankere	Cancer (Sesotho | English)
Kaofela	Everything (Sesotho)
Kapa (verb)	To vomit, to induce vomiting using warm water usually laced with vinegar, salt or herbs (Sesotho/Sekasi)
Kasi, kasie or ekasi	Township, location (Sekasi | Afrikaans)
Kellelo	Intelligence (Sesotho)
Kereke/dikereke	Church(es) (Sesotho)
Kereke ya Fora	Literally: French Church, i.e. Lutheran Church (Sesotho)
Kereke ya Roma	Catholic Church (Sesotho | Latin)
Kereke ya Tjhatjhe	Anglican Church (Sesotho)
Kereke ya Wesele	Methodist Church (Sesotho | English – Charles Wesley)
Kerekeng	At or in a church (Sesotho)
Kgarebe	Formal girlfriend (Sesotho)
Kgemere	Homemade ginger-flavoured cool drink (Sesotho | Afrikaans)
Kgohlela (verb)	To cough (Sesotho)
Kgubedu	Red (Sesotho)

Kguthswane	Short (Sesotho)
Khabetjhe/dikhabetjhe	Cabbage (Sesotho/Sekasi I English)
Kick 'n bhoboza	Literally: kick and puncture, i.e. sharply pointed footwear (Sekasi I English and Nguni)
Kitjhining	Literally: in the kitchen; denotes domestic work (Sekasi I English)
Klim	Milk powder; a brand made by Nestlé, common in South Africa ('milk' spelt backwards, used in township as a generic name for milk powder)
Kobela	Instructor and mentor of a traditional healer initiate; a supportive relationship is ideally maintained once the graduate has become a fully fledged healer themselves (Sesotho, from the verb 'to kneel')
Kodi/dikodi	Blemish(es), small sin(s) (Sesotho)
Koko koko	'Knock knock', used before entering a house (Sesotho)
Koloi/dikoloi	Car(s) (Sesotho)
Kontane	Cash (Sekasi)
Konyana	Lamb (Sesotho)
Kopa (verb)	To ask, to plead (Sesotho)
Kos	Food (Afrikaans/Sekasi); see also Sunday *kos*
Kota/dikota	Township fast food; chips and fried food in a quarter loaf of bread (Sekasi I English)
Kotla	Blow or punishment, including from the ancestors (Sesotho)
Kuku/dikuku	Cake(s); also slang for vagina (Sekasi/Sesotho)
Kula (verb)	To be ill (Sesotho)
Kwaal	Envy, jealousy (Sekasi/Afrikaans)
Kwae	Cigarettes, tobacco; also slang for penis (Sesotho/Sekasi)
Kwetse (verb)	To be closed (Sesotho)
Leano/maano	Trick(s), scam(s) (Sesotho)
(Le)baka/mabaka	Reason(s), excuse(s) (Sesotho)
Lebala/mabala	Dirt yard(s) (Sesotho)
Lebese	Milk (Sesotho)

Lebollong	Literally: the place of circumcision, i.e. initiation school (Sesotho)
Lefatse	Earth (Sesotho)
Lefifi	Darkness (Sesotho)
Lefu/mafu	Sickness(es), disease(s), death (Sesotho)
Lefuba	TB, though the term is rarely used outside translated information sheets (Sesotho)
Lefung	Funeral (Sesotho)
Lefusto	Hereditary (Sesotho)
Lehae/mahae	Original 'real' homes or places of origin (Sesotho)
Lekgowa/makgowa	White person/people (mildly derogatory), boss (Sesotho/Sekasi)
Lekker	Good (Afrikaans, common South African loan word)
Lesaka/masaka	Kraal(s) (Sesotho)
Letho	Nothing (Sesotho)
Lethopa/mathopa	Boil(s), swelling(s) (Sesotho)
Lethwasong	The location where a traditional healer is trained (see *thwasitse*) (Nguni/Sesotho grammar)
Letjhoba/matjhoba	Fly whisk(s) made from cows' tails and symbols of traditional authority (Sesotho)
Letsatsi	Day, sun, light (Sesotho)
Letsoho/matsoho	Hand(s) (Sesotho)
Lobola	Bride wealth to be paid by potential husband's family before marriage (Nguni, common South African loan word)
Loka (verb)	To be right, to be good, to be OK (*Ho tla loka*: it will be OK. *Ho lokile*: OK) (Sesotho)
Loose draw	A single cigarette, typically sold from *spaza* shops and street-side stalls (English/Sekasi)
Loxion manager	Location manager; an ironic term for young men hanging around the township or location (Sekasi I English)
Mabitleng	Graveyard; also, at the graveyard (Sesotho)
Madam	White woman in authority (Common South African loan word I English)

Madi	Blood, semen (Sesotho)
Madimabe	Bad luck, misfortune (Sesotho)
Maele	Saying, aphorism (Sesotho)
Mafu a sa foleng	Incurable diseases (Sesotho)
Mageu	Maize-based, non-alcoholic drink (Sesotho)
Maindia	Indian people, but in context the shops owned by Indians; often large, budget supermarkets in town (Sekasi | English)
Majabajaba laonj	A fancy lounge (Sekasi | partly English)
Maka	Fib; respectful way to talk about a lie (Sesotho/Sekasi)
Makgonatshole	Potassium permanganate; literally: 'that which can do anything' (Sesotho)
Makwenya	Deep-fried dough balls, often eaten with achaar or polony (Sekasi/Sesotho); also known as *vetkoek* (Afrikaans) and fatcakes (English)
Makwerekwere	Foreigners (derogatory) (Sekasi)
Mala	Bowels (Sesotho)
Manyano	Church women's guild (Nguni?)
Mara	But (Sekasi | Afrikaans)
Mashonisa	Locally based informal lenders (Sekasi)
Mashwa	Traditional illness; affliction resulting from breaching taboos (Sesotho)
Maslamosa	Magic (Sekasi)
Masole a mmele	The body's immune system; literally: 'soldiers of the body' (Sesotho)
Matekwane	Cannabis (Sesotho)
Mathaka	Age-mates, people of the same age (Sesotho)
Matimona	Demons (Sekasi | English)
Masutsa	Delicious (Sesotho)
Meetlo	Tradition(s) (Sesotho)
Mekgudisana	Revolving credit scheme (Sesotho)
Meroho	Spinach, greens, vegetables in general (Sesotho)
Metsi	Water (Sesotho)
Meya e ditshila	Evil spirits (Sesotho)
Mielies	Maize cobs (Afrikaans/Sekasi)
Mme/bomme	Lady/ladies, mother(s) (Sesotho)

Mo	He or she (when the object of a sentence) (Sesotho)
Model C School	A semi-private school, based on the now defunct Model C format (English)
Modimo	God (Sesotho)
Modisa/badisa	Shepherd(s) (Sesotho)
Moetsi	The doer of something, actor (Sesotho)
Moetsuwa	The person on whom something is done, victim, recipient (Sesotho)
Mofumahadi	Wife, queen (Sesotho)
Mofutsana/bafutsana	Poor person, people (Sesotho)
Mohlomong	Perhaps (Sesotho)
Mokete	Function (Sesotho)
Mokgodisano/mekgodisano	Revolving credit scheme(s) (Sekasi)
Mokhukhu/mekhukuhu	Shack(s) (usually made from corrugated iron) (Sekasi/Sesotho)
Mokopi/bakopi	Someone asking for something, supplicant(s) (Sesotho)
Mokudi	Patient, sick person (Sesotho)
Molato/melato	Sin(s), fault(s) (Sesotho)
Moletelo	A night vigil on the eve of a funeral (Sesotho)
Monga	Owner (Sesotho)
Monko	Smell (Seotho)
Monna/banna	Man/men (Sesotho)
Monyetla/menyetla	Opportunity/opportunities (Sesotho)
Moputso	Wage, reward
Moqwenati	Counterfeit (Sekasi)
Morekisi/barekisi	Seller(s) (Sesotho)
Moriana	Medicine (Sesotho)
Moriana wa ho hlatswa madi	Medicine that cleans the blood (Sesotho)
Moriana wa sekgowa	Western medicine; literally: medicine of the Whites (Sesotho)
Moriana wa setso	Traditional medicine (Sesotho)
Moroho/meroho	Vegetables, greens, spinach (Sesotho)
Moruti/baruti	Preacher(s) (Sesotho)
Mosadi/basadi	Woman/women (Sesotho)
Mosebetsi	A traditional gathering, usually linked to the ancestors, also work (Sesotho)

Mosebetsi wa badimo	A ceremony for the ancestors, often to give thanks or make a request
Moswang	Chime (Sesotho)
Mothapo/methapo	Blood vessel, root (Sesotho)
Motoho	Thin, slightly fermented sorghum porridge (Sesotho)
Motomboti	Traditional sorghum beer (Nguni/Sekasi)
Motswakantle/batswakantle	Literally: those that come from outside, foreigners (polite) (Sesotho)
Moya/meya	Air, wind, spirit (Sesotho)
Moya o ditshila	Evil spirit, demon (Sesotho)
Moya o Halelelang	Holy Spirit (Sesotho)
Moya wa badimo	Spirit of the ancestors or calling to be a healer (Sesotho)
Muthi	Traditional medicine, traditional magic (Nguni, a common South African loan word)
Mzanzi fosho	South African nickname for government-issued condoms (Sekasi | Nguni)
Nama	Meat, flesh (Sesotho)
Ngaka	Doctor (Sesotho)
Ngaka ya sekgowa	Western doctor (Sesotho)
Ngaka ya setso	Traditional healer (Sesotho)
Ngwana/bana	Child/children (Sesotho)
Ngwaneso	Child within a family; often used for adults within the context of extended families and long-term household members (Sesotho)
Ntate	Father, Mister, Sir (Sesotho)
Ntho/dintho	Thing(s) (Sesotho)
Ntlwana ya mokoti	A long-drop toilet (Sesotho)
Nwa (verb)	To drink, to swallow pills (Sesotho)
Nyala o nyele	A saying (*maele*): Marriage is like shitting in your pants
Nyanga	Zulu medicine man (Nguni)
Nyatsi/dinyatsi	Clandestine girlfriend(s), mistress (Sesotho/Sekasi)
Nyoko	Bile or gall, an ethnoecological condition among Africans believed to be caused by too much sugar; accumulated *nyoko* must be

	regularly purged if it is not to build up with harmful effects (Sesotho/Sekasi)
O se ke wa feba	Thou shall not commit adultery (Sesotho)
Otile (verb)	To have become thin (Sesotho)
Pae	Social security payment (pension, child benefit, disability allowance) (Sekasi | English)
Palama (verb)	To board and travel in a vehicle or on a horse (Sesotho)
Palama habedi	To board twice or change transport during a journey
Paola/dipaola	A brazier, typically made from a steel drum with holes punched into the side (Sesotho/Sekasi)
Pap	Stiff maize porridge/starch (Afrikaans, common South African loan word)
Pap 'n lebese	Maize starch and milk; a staple, cheap meal (Afrikaans/Sesotho/English grammar)
Pap 'n vleis	Maize starch and (grilled) meat (Afrikaans/English grammar, a common South African loan phrase)
Patala (verb)	To pay (Sesotho/English)
Pele	Before, in front (Sesotho)
Pere/dipere	Horse(s) (Sesotho)
Phahamisetsa (verb)	To raise up one's hands, to surrender (Sesotho)
Phahla (verb)	To communicate with one's ancestors (Sesotho)
Phamokate	AIDS (Sesotho)
Pheha (verb)	To cook (Sesotho)
Phela (verb)	To live or to be healthy (Sesotho)
Phio/diphio	Kidney(s) (Sesotho)
Phofo ya poone	Maize meal (Sesotho)
Pholosa (verb)	To save (especially in a religious sense) (Sesotho/Sekasi)
Pholosong	Literally: place of salvation, meaning a Pentecostal/Charismatic township church (Sesotho/Sekasi)
Phoso/diphoso	Mistake(s) (Sesotho)
Pilisi/dipilisi	Pill(s) (Sesotho/Sekasi | English)
Pimpa (verb)	To inform on somebody (Sekasi)

Pitsa/dipitsa	Cooking pot(s); also indicates traditional medicine (Sesotho)
Ponto	Two rands (Sesotho/Sekasi I English – from pound sterling)
Pontsho	Signifier, sign (Sesotho)
Qhoma (verb)	To jump (Sesotho)
Rata (verb)	To like, to love (Sesotho)
Re (verb)	To say (Sesotho)
Reka (verb)	To buy (Sesotho)
Rekisa (verb)	To sell (Seotho)
Rera (verb)	To preach, to prophesy; also to plan (Sesotho)
Rondavel	Traditional round hut (common South African loan word I Afrikaans)
Russian	Type of sausage, often deep-fried and one ingredient for a *kota*; also the name (largely historical) for Basotho-dominated township gangs (Sekasi)
Sangoma	Traditional healer (Nguni, a common South African loan word)
Satane	Satan (Sesotho I English)
Sebe/dibe	Sins(s) (Sesotho)
Sebele	True, truly (Sesotho)
Sebeletsa (verb)	To work for, to serve (Sesotho)
Sebesta (verb)	To work (Sesotho)
Sefuba	Flu, infection; also a common way to answer/deflect enquiries about one's health (Sesotho)
Sejeso	Witchcraft in which a creature is introduced into a person (Sesotho)
Sekasi	Township hybrid language(s) acting as a popular *lingua franca* based on African and European languages, older form known as *tsotsitaal*, varies by township (Sesotho/Sekasi); also known as *isiscamto* (Nguni)
Seketekete/diketekete	Piggy bank(s) (Sekasi I carbide light (Sesotho))
Selemo/dilemo	Year(s) (Sesotho)
Sendau	A possessing spirit from outside the sangoma's family, i.e. not *badimo* (Sekasi I ?)

Seneifi	Snuff (Sesotho/Sekasi | English)
Senyehile (verb)	Spoiled, damaged or rotten (Sesotho)
Sepeiti or s'peiti	Colonic irrigation or the use of laxatives for the purpose of purging the body of impurities; can be used as a verb; also generic for cleansing (see *hlaba sepeite*) (Sesotho/Sekasi)
Sephiri/diphiri	Secret(s) (Sesotho)
Sepoto/dipoto	A 'spot' usually serving *jwala* or *mtombote*; the lowest level of drinking establishment (Sekasi | English)
Seriti	Dignity; also, shadow of a person (Sesotho)
Seshebo	Whatever pap is eaten with, such as meat, gravy or sauce (Sesotho)
Setjhaba	Public, nation, people (Sesotho)
Setlamatlama/ditlamatlama	Hangover(s) (Sekasi)
Setsha/ditsha	Stand plot (for a house) (Sesotho)
Setso	Tradition, traditional ways (Sesotho)
Sharp!	Good! OK! Thumbs up! (Sekasi, common South African loan word)
Sheba nna feela	Magic used to keep somebody faithful; literally: 'look only at me' (Sesotho)
Shebeen	Informal bar or pub, often a room in a house (Sekasi | Irish); also called a *chaf pozi*
Simba/disimba	Crisps (Sekasi – from a common trade name)
Sissy/sissi	Sister (Sekasi | English)
Skaam	Shame (Sekasi | Afrikaans)
Skontiri	Tarred road (Sekasi | Afrikaans)
Slakga	Butchery (Sekasi | Afrikaans)
Slakgeng	At the butchery (Sekasi | Afrikaans)
Slapi	Final cigarette of the day smoked before sleeping (Sekasi | Afrikaans)
Sokola (verb)	To suffer, to lack (Sesotho/Sekasi | Afrikaans)
Spare	A secondary sexual partner, particularly girlfriend (Sekasi | English)
Spaza or *spaza shop*	Small informal convenience store in the township (Sekasi, common South African loan word)

Spiel	Mirror (Sekasi | Afrikaans)
Spruit	Stream (Afrikaans, common South African loan word)
Stoep	Veranda (Afrikaans, common South African loan word)
Sunday *kos*	Sunday lunch, i.e. a full plate of food (Sekasi | English/Afrikaans)
Tabola (verb)	To tear, to rip (Sesotho)
Takkies	Training shoes (South African English)
Tamati/ditamati	Tomato (Sesotho/Sekasi | English)
Tatile (verb)	To be in a hurry (Sesotho)
Tauwe (verb)	To be drunk, to be intoxicated (Sesotho)
Tebileng	Something deep or profound (Sesotho)
Thapo	Mourning clothes (Sesotho)
Thipa/dithipa	Knife (knives) (Sesotho)
Thoba (verb)	To calm, to soothe (Sesotho)
Thobalano	Sex (Sesotho)
Thohako	Curse (Sesotho)
Thoko/mathoko	Side (Sesotho)
Tholwana/ditholwana	Fruit (Sesotho)
Thothomela (verb)	To tremble, to shake (Sesotho)
Thwasitse (verb)	To have trained and graduated as a traditional healer (Nguni)
Tiger	Ten rand note (Sekasi)
Tjhaka (verb)	To visit and socialise with people (Sesotho)
Tjhelete	Money (Sesotho)
Tjhobolo	Long-tailed widow bird [commonly known as '*moruti*' (preacher)], a talkative person (Sesotho)
Tjhonne (verb)	To be broke, have no money (Sekasi)
Tjhova (verb)	To peddle, to shuffle cards (Sesotho)
Tlhaho	Original, natural, birth (Sesotho)
Toyi-toyi	Protest dance, protest (Sekasi, common South African loan word)
Toyi-toying (verb)	To dance when protesting, to protest (Sekasi, common South African loan word)
Trekile (verb)	Literally: to be ironed, meaning to be smartly dressed (Sekasi/Afrikaans)

Tseba (verb)	To know (Sesotho)
Tsela	Road, path, way (Sesotho)
Tshehla	Yellow (Sesotho)
Tshwarelo	Forgiveness (Sesotho)
Tsietsi	Trouble, suffering (Sesotho)
Tsotsi/ditsotsi	Hoodlum(s) (Sekasi)
Tsotsitaal	Older form of Afrikaans-heavy township *lingua franca* (Sekasi | Tsotsitaal/Afrikaans)
Tsuba (verb)	To inhale, to snort, to smoke (Sesotho)
Tswekere	Sugar, sweetness, diabetes (Sesotho)
Two litre	A two-litre bottle of traditional medicine (Sekasi | English)
Ubuntu	Shared humanity (Nguni, but a common loan word in other South African languages)
Udokotela	Doctor (Nguni)
Univesithi	University (Sesotho | English)
Uzifozonke	Literally: cures everything; branded commercial traditional patent medicine (Nguni)
Veld/veldt	Open country, wasteland outside of a township (Afrikaans, common South African loan word)
Waskom	Plastic washbowl, used for bathing as well as washing clothes (Sekasi / Afrikaans)
Waslap/waslaps	Face cloth(s) or flannel(s) (Sekasi / Afrikaans)
Winahela (verb)	To win, to succeed (Sekasi | English)
Yena	He or she (Sesotho)
Zama (verb)	To try, to get by through one's own efforts (Sekasi)
Zamalek	An affectionate name for Black Label lager (Sekasi/English)
Zol	Cannabis, cannabis joint (Sekasi/Afrikaans)

APPENDIX 3

Methodology:
Embedded research

Beyond *pap 'n lebese* research

Methodology is the way in which research is conducted – how research is done, how data is collected. Data can take many forms: recorded statistics, stories told, questions answered, silences noted, pictures taken, gestures observed, almost anything. When reporting research results, the reader needs to know how data was collected. Only then can they assess the credibility of the research.

Part of such an assessment is whether the research methods were appropriate. The *way* in which data is collected determines *what* data can be collected, and *how well* it can be collected. This influences what questions can be successfully asked. Given this, an important principle in designing research is that the selection of methods should follow the choice of questions. It may not always be quite so straightforward as this maxim suggests, but 'method follows question' is a good rule of thumb to follow.

Reported accounts of research methodology often attempt to vouch for the research credibility by recounting the volume of data captured. But documenting how much research was done does not tell us how appropriate the research methods were, nor how skilfully implemented. It is easy to get caught up in such 'numbers games': how many interviews conducted, the hours of taped recordings, the pages of written notes; but these statistics are not the most important thing by which the methodology, and the research itself, should be judged.

In this book I have described my methodological choices, and some methodological statistics, in an integrated way. Rather than a stand-alone chapter or section, methodological decisions and outcomes pepper the book right up to the final section. This underlines the point that there is a close relationship between *how* data is collected and *what* data is collected. But it also helps illustrate that this book provides a narrative of my own intellectual journey. As my own understanding of alternative explanations of AIDS changed, so did my questions. And, given this, so did the research methodology. It is necessary for the reader to be aware of these changes and the reasons for them if they are to grasp what I describe and analyse.

Given the integration of research methods within the text, this appendix is not a conventional methodological description. I provide a whistle-stop summary of the research in the next section, but beyond this I strive to provide a few brief 'behind the scenes' reflections on research methods. This is aimed at those curious to know why I researched the way I did. It is also aimed at social science students who might want to up their research with less conventional, but more penetrating, methods. The discipline of anthropology already has much of this ground covered: it specialises (most of the time) in long-term, embedded research relationships employing multiple methods of recording data. What is outlined here is suggestions as to how social scientists, from whatever sub-discipline, might want to think about their research and reflect on the relationship between questions, methods and answers.

Having taught research methodology courses and supervised post-graduate research, I'm aware of how hard it can be to break away from the basic staple *pap 'n lebese* (porridge and milk) of social science research – a series of one-hour interviews with a selection of respondents. Indeed, up to PhD level, the constraints of research reports required for the purposes of degree conferment make it difficult to break from this mould. But it can be done. And it should be considered, taking into account whether different methodologies would better address the research question.

Recapping the research for *A Different Kind of AIDS*

What I sought to answer in this research was, initially: What 'AIDS myths' circulate in African townships? And how best could these be countered? My thesis or idea was that peer educators would be better off using stories or parables to 'bust' these myths rather than repeating medically correct information as they were usually trained. This idea had emerged from earlier research aimed at establishing what peer educators were actually doing.[1]

The participatory action research project[2] that I ran in Digco was designed with two key objectives. The first was to establish the AIDS myths in circulation, through the peer educators recording those they heard, and the second was to then develop stories that the peer educators could use to respond to these myths. Over the six months of the project, the peer educators played different roles: as researchers collecting and reporting AIDS myths; as lay heath educators with their ongoing voluntary peer educator role; as partners in developing stories and parables; and as research subjects when I interviewed them.

What the peer educators reported, as researchers, forced me to revise how I understood AIDS myths and to, rather, view them as folk and lay theories that had meaning and promised hope and comfort. Further, what the peer educators told me as research subjects made me re-evaluate how I saw them – no longer as uncomplicated allies in the medico-human rights response to HIV/AIDS, but as individuals themselves embedded in the cosmologies of folk theories and the construction of lay theories. Seeing this, I revised my interview schedules to explore the complexities of their own beliefs.

I went into the second stage of the research thinking differently. While the repeated interviews with township residents that formed the key methodology of the second research phase could be seen as simply a further angle to view the original problem, I was now thinking differently about alternative explanations of AIDS. I was much more interested in what made these beliefs so resilient within township contexts and was less concerned with finding out a quick route to routing them, something which I no longer thought was possible. As well as interviewing Bafana, Paseka, Grace and Neo, I established a more complete picture of their lives, particularly as they related to HIV. But I also tried to place their HIV in the context of other critical aspects of their lives: Bafana's precarious employment, Paseka's responsibility for family, Grace's struggle for respectability, and Neo's commitment to God. These were all important facets of their lives and researchers should always be willing to follow what matters to those researched.

The importance of reflection

The formula that research students are generally trained to implement consists of identifying a 'gap' or something that remains unknown in the academic literature, developing a research question addressing this gap, the collection of data (through one-off interviews or, alternatively, surveys), and the reporting of results. There is a built-in circularity to this process – the concerns investigated are the concerns identified in academic literature, and new research remains locked within this set of concerns. Yet, academics' concerns are only partially aligned, at best, to the problems people face. Without reflection during research, this may never become apparent. The result is an extensive process of inquiry, but one that fails to address people's lives as they are actually lived and instead fuels a separate, detached process of academic debate and deliberation.

I have recounted how my own reflections during research led me to re-think how I needed to think about AIDS beliefs. The extended nature of the research, and the fact that it involved distinct phases, facilitated this process. However, reflection needs to be undertaken during every step of all research projects. In Chapter 6, I describe my reflections on the discussions I'd had with Bafana on his HIV status and how I decided to pursue a new approach. In grasping what had been happening between us, I was able to re-think my methods, something that turned out to be an important move.

Indeed, reflection should be built into every step of research, particularly fieldwork. Frustratingly, this advice is regularly ignored by many, probably most, of my research students. I tell them to allocate time between each interview and to use these as opportunities to review notes and transcripts, and to reflect on what they have learned. In doing this I suggest that they will deepen their understanding; that they will realise that there may be more to their inquiry than the research question with which they started. One problem is that I am, in effect, proposing more work than is required. In their research proposal, formally approved by Department, School and Faculty authorities, they set out the scope of work; say, for example, one research question and 20 interviews. What I am proposing means that the question may change, or even multiply. The scope of work will expand. The more attractive option is to follow the formula, which has, after all, been sanctioned, and the faster they can clock up 20 interviews, the quicker they can finish. To be fair, students are under pressure to complete their degrees. But the problem should be obvious: if the research question correctly addressed a gap in the academic literature but didn't address problems on the ground, a tally of 20 interviews isn't of any real value. Neatly written up, it is, however, sufficient for the student to pass muster as research competent. In theory and in future, away from degree deadlines, they could take a different tack. But that's unlikely; they've already been taught otherwise and the pressures to quickly churn out research results are intense both inside and outside universities.

Researching across social distance

South Africa is plagued by social distance: the psychological separation of people in different social circumstances created by economic inequality, racial division, spatial segregation and other divisions. Researchers generally stand on the privileged side of society, almost always on the comfortable side of the canyon that separates rich from poor, the great inner-social barrier of South African society. I have used the shorthand of township and suburb to summarise this division. I do not suggest that it completely captures the situation, as townships are not homogeneous and neither are suburbs. But the township–suburb contrast sums up much of what divides us.

Such gaps have implications for research, not least the point I have already stressed: that of asking relevant questions. Social science research involves crossing this divide. Not always, we can and should research the rich and the privileged, but researching in and about the lives of the poor and the marginalised must be a critical component of social science. Research is, however, rarely framed as a crossing of these divides. Rather, it is sanitised as a technical procedure – like a surgeon operating on a patient, it is suggested that the social status or beliefs of the *moetsi* and *moetsuwa* (the doer and the one to whom something is done) do not matter. But these things matter very much.

We should be acutely aware of these issues. Research conducted at a distance – surveys, censuses and the like – avoid this problem. What they attempt to do is extract data, usually in forms that can be counted, and that do not require any real engagement with people. Such research methods – ticking boxes, saying 'yes' or 'no', rating a statement on a five-point scale, and so on – are clearly inappropriate for more complex issues, such as what people believe about HIV/AIDS. My scorn for such attempts has been made clear in Chapter 1. Rather, what is needed is to 'get in close' and to talk to people.

However, getting in close can be done in different ways. Interviews and focus groups get in close when researcher and researched are face to face, but that proximity may be illusionary. A valid critique of social science research is that all too often it is of the 'parachute' variety. The alternative metaphor of 'helicopter research' may be more appropriate, since a helicopter would allow the researcher to ascend from, as well as descend on, the field at speed, while the parachutist can only descend. Nevertheless, quibbling over airborne allusions aside, the point is that engagement while up close may be brief, such as the *pap 'n lebese* research of a series of one-off interviews. Researcher and researched meet for an hour and then part. Like strangers thrown together in a waiting room, both sides are equally free to project the image they judge best, secure that they are not accountable to each other.

This problem is mitigated, to an extent, when the social scientist interviews others in similar class or educational positions: now the two parties have much in common, and the process of question and answer is more straightforward, however sophisticated the content might be. As I outline in the concluding chapter, the poor must construct their beliefs within tight parameters. Many of these constraints will not be apparent to a researcher from the 'other side of the tracks'. Nor will they likely become apparent if each interview is with a different individual, on a different day, in a different place, but asking the same questions. Questions may be answered, but the researcher may find out little of the context that has framed them, or why they have been answered in the way they have. To do this takes time.

The partnerships of embedded research

Embedded research involves not only being there but also being there for long. As to how long there is no real answer, but longer than a one-off, hour-long interview is a start. Extended contact has profound influences on research – most of these are unambiguously good. The establishment of partnerships is one of these. All research should strive to set up partnerships. As Robert Weiss explains, 'What is essential in interviewing is to maintain a working research partnership ... What you can't get away with is failure to work with the respondent as a partner in the production of useful material.'[3] This is good advice, though the extent to which a partnership can be established, over something such as AIDS beliefs in contemporary South Africa, in an hour, should not be overestimated.

Establishing a partnership is not something achieved by a formula. The honesty of the Digco peer educators that I describe in Chapter 3 resulted from our interactions in the project workshops and, among other things, the chance this gave me to show (not just to say) that I valued frank talk and that they would not be put down if they confided something 'wrong' for a peer educator to believe, such as not falling for the explanation that HIV came from monkeys. The partnerships with Bafana, Paseka, Grace and Neo were forged in different, much more individualised, ways. Even if I already knew them, the research was a process of getting to know them better, of understanding them as individuals, not simply as research subjects who could provide me with the material I sought. The truth is that they could not provide me with this information unless I understood them well enough to step, at least for a while, into their shoes.

Understanding a person is not only a process of getting to know them by, for example, spending time listening to their life history. If one is seeking to understand them in context, it is necessary to know some of the people and places that make up their lives. In this regard meeting, visiting and interviewing people who appear significantly in research partners' accounts is important. Not only do they provide different perspectives, but they also build the research relationship.

Establishing strong research partnerships does not mean that things will be explained in a straightforward manner. Working in sensitive areas may involve a range of less than explicit exchanges, even if what is communicated is frank enough: Paseka's view that Bafana's sickness resulted from an ancestral *kotla*; Grace's always-the-last-time, unprotected sex with her latest boyfriend; Bafana's own TB strain that mimicked HIV; and Neo's hope for a cure. None of this was directly, clinically, communicated. Just as it 'takes time to know somebody', so too is this true in research. The researcher must not only ask questions but also observe, watch events, ask for second opinions, interpret, evaluate and ultimately make judgement calls.

Shifting sands

Within embedded research processes, data becomes less categorical, even as a more holistic and more accurate picture comes into focus. The explanations of illness that circulated around Bafana's sickbed were options in play. There was no agreement, within the family, as to what ailed him. To ask one person what the problem was might result in a clear, single answer. Ask around and you would get multiple answers. Over a longer time period, Grace's treatment odyssey similarly illustrates the waxing and waning of competing explanations of AIDS. Should Grace have been interviewed by a series of independent researchers every year from the first time she was diagnosed HIV positive, each one might well have come up with a different take on what Grace thought about her condition. And it is not only issues as complex as AIDS beliefs that can pose such problems for researchers – Grace's relationship with her neighbours would similarly appear in very different guises if we only had snapshot pictures taken at different times.

Data may at any point be still under construction, as for example Paseka's understanding of TB over the interviews that we discussed this. And even when accounts are firmed up, it does not mean that they necessarily correspond with each other. It was, for example, impossible to reconcile how Grace recalled meeting Sister Irene, with how Sister Irene recalled meeting Grace. Indeed, even my own understanding of why I bought KFC chicken for Sister Irene did not correspond with the sincere account she gave an hour or two later. Sometimes these contradictions must be accepted; indeed, the contradiction itself may be useful information.

Pushing limits

Researchers should push the limits of the research relationship. Indeed, it can be argued that this is how relationships are strengthened. I recount, in Chapter 3, how I punctured a peer educator's explanation of the origins of AIDS. What she said, and the way she said it, made it clear that she wasn't saying what she really thought and I called her out. She took it well and we got to a more truthful account. Again, this can be done in one-off interviews, but only to an extent. Without obvious clues, you may not know when you are being given a sanitised account, or even having the wool pulled over your eyes.

That I knew Bafana, Paseka, Grace and Neo before starting the formal interviews gave me an extended period over which to assess their experience and understandings of HIV/AIDS. One benefit of this was that it allowed me to carefully challenge some of the accounts they gave in interviews. The relationship between the researcher and the researched may well be complex once the relative shelter of one-off interviews is abandoned. The firmer the relationship, the more difficult the questions that can be posed: I challenged Grace over selling cigarettes, I pointed to Neo's inconsistency in holding to her beliefs under family pressure. As with all relationships, one must evaluate how far things can be pushed and the value of doing so.

The difficulties and benefits of embedded research

Rewarding as embedded research can be, there are obvious difficulties. Time is one. If you don't have time to hang out with people, then you can't conduct embedded research. Recalling the maxim 'method follows questions', should answering a question require embedded research, then helicoptering in (and out) to conduct interviews may well set back, not advance, what we know.

Distant and helicopter research largely insulates the researcher from confronting the social distance that divides us. That's ironic, because the researcher may well be attempting to find out the situation across the divide with the intention of improving the lot of others. But such research methods reinforce, rather than challenge, divisions. Embedded researchers, by contrast, have to wrestle with the complexities of straddling these divisions, at least for a while. For example, when in the African townships that I have been involved with for over a decade, I remain a White man, I remain a professor, I remain a resident of the suburbs, and I remain, in comparison, rich. Those differences are not forgotten, but they are absorbed into the ongoing tensions of the township that I describe in Chapter 5. For all my differences, I am also an insider, albeit of a special kind.

But such situations, solutions to the problem of how we know the lives of others, are only partial and only temporary. Beyond my circle of friends and acquaintances, beyond the boundaries of my embeddedness, it is different. Should I wander a few streets away, without introduction, my relationship with those I meet starts *de novo*; I am a White man carrying the baggage of South Africa's history.

Living in different worlds involves managing contradictions. Embed yourself firmly enough in one or more research setting and you start to feel like a chameleon, with contradictory, context-determined behaviour that can't be fitted together: a humanist in one context, attending church in another; championing civic responsibility in one context, turning a blind eye to electricity theft in another; directly getting to the point in one context, knowing that this is rude in another; always busy in one context, hanging out in another. Of course everybody's lives are fragmented and separated, but this division can be particularly acute for South African researchers; there are few more divided societies. The privilege of having to juggle these contradictions is the opportunity to learn and to change. Research should not only be about knowing others, but also changing oneself.

Bibliography

Achmat, Z. (2003). Preface. In A. Irwin, J. Millen & D. Fallows (Eds.), *Global AIDS: Myths and Facts: Tools for Fighting the AIDS Pandemic*. Cambridge, MA: South End Pres.

African Bank. (2013). Personal Loans. Retrieved 6/2/2013, from www.africanbank.co.za

Ashforth, A. (2002). An Epidemic of Witchcraft? The Implications of AIDS for the Post-Apartheid State. *African Studies, 61*(1), 121-143.

Ashforth, A. (2005). *Witchcraft, Violence, and Democracy in South Africa*. Chicago: University of Chicago Press.

Bayer, R. (1991). Public health policy and the AIDS epidemic: an end to HIV exceptionalism? Author(s): Bayer, Ronald. Date:1991. Type:Articles Department: Center for the History and Ethics of Public Health. Volume: 324. *324.* doi:http://hdl.handle.net/10022/AC:P:10012.

Bayer, R. (1999). Clinical Progress and the Future of HIV Exceptionalism. *Archives of Internal Medicine, 159*(10), 1042-1048.

Butler, A. (2005). South Africa's HIV/AIDS Policy, 1994-2004: How Can It Be Explained? *African Affairs, 104*(417), 591-614.

Cairns, M., Dickinson, D. & Orr, W. (2006). Wits University's Response to HIV/AIDS: Flagship Programme or 'Tramp Steamer'? *African Journal of AIDS Research, 5*(2), 159-166.

Chambers, R. (1994). Participatory Rural Appraisal (PRA): Analysis of Experience. *World Development, 22*(9), 1253-1268.

Cock, K. D., Mbori-Ngacha, D. & Marum, E. (2002). Shadow on the Continent: Public Health and HIV/AIDS in Africa in the 21st Century. *The Lancet, 360*(9326), 1.

Cohen, S. (2002). *States of Denial: Knowing About Atrocities and Suffering*. Cambridge, UK: Polity Press.

Collins, A. & Gentner, D. (1987). How People Construct Mental Models. In N. Quinn & D. Holland (Eds.), *Cultural Models in Language and Thought*. Cambridge: Cambridge University Press.

Cornwell, J. (1984). *Hard-Earned Lives: Account of Health and Illness from East London*. London: Tavistock.

Crepaz, N., Hart, T. & Marks, G. (2004). Highly Active Antiretroviral Therapy and Sexual Risk Behaviour. *Journal of the American Medical Association, 292*(2), 224-236.

Cu-Uvin, S., DeLong, A., Venkatesh, K., Hogan, J., Ingersoll, J., Kurpewski, J., . . . Caliendo, A. (2010). Genital tract HIV-1 RNA shedding among women with below detectable plasma viral load. *AIDS, 24*(16), 2489–2497. doi: 10.1097/QAD.0b013e32833e5043.

Cullinan, K. & Thom, A. (2009). *The Virus, Vitamins & Vegetables: The South African HIV/AIDS Mystery*. Johannesburg: Jacana Media.

De Certeau, M. (1984). *The Practice of Everyday Life*. Berkeley, CA: University of California Press.

Department of Health. (2011). The 2010 National Antenatal Sentinel HIV & Syphilis Prevalence Survey in South Africa. Pretoria.

Dickinson, D. (2002). Sasol's Response to HIV/AIDS. Johannesburg: Wits Business School, University of the Witwatersrand.

Dickinson, D. (2003). Managing HIV/AIDS in the South African Workplace: Just Another Duty? *South African Journal of Economic and Management Science, 6*(1), 25-49.

Dickinson, D. (2004). The Corporate South Africa's Response to HIV/AIDS: Why So Slow? *Journal of Southern African Studies, 30*(3), 627-650.

Dickinson, D. (2005). AIDS, Order and 'Best Practice' in South African Companies: Managers, Peer Educators, Traditional Healers and Folk Theories. *African Journal of AIDS Research, 4*(1), 11-20.

Dickinson, D. (2007). Talking About AIDS: A Study of Informal Activities Undertaken by Workplace HIV/AIDS Peer Educators in a South African Company. Johannesburg: Wits Business School, University of the Witwatersrand.

Dickinson, D. (2008a). Research is About Changing Lives: Health South Africa. *Research is about Changing Lives.* from http://ns2.ipsnoticias.net/new_focus/changelives/opinion1.asp.

Dickinson, D. (2008b). Traditional Healers and Company HIV/AIDS Programmes. *African Journal of AIDS Research, 7*(3), 281-291.

Dickinson, D. (2009). *Changing the Course of AIDS: Peer Education in South Africa and Its Lessons for the Global Crisis.* Ithaca: Cornell University Press.

Dickinson, D. (2011). Myths, Science and Stories: Working with Peer Educators to Counter AIDS Myths. *African Journal of AIDS Research, 10 Supplement*, 335-344.

Dickinson, D. & Innes, D. (2004). Fronts or Front-lines? HIV/AIDS and Big Business in South Africa. *Transformation, 55*, 28-54.

Dickinson, D. & Stevens, M. (2005). Understanding the Response of Large South African Companies to HIV/AIDS. *Journal of Social Aspects of HIV/AIDS, 2*(2), 286-295.

Digco. (2009). *HIV/AIDS Peer Educator Training Manual.*

Dlamini, B. (2011, 9-16 September). The Necessity of a Rights-based Approach to HIV and AIDS Treament. *The Weekly: Free State,* 12.

Doke, C. M. & Mofokeng, S. M. (1957). *Textbook of Southern Sotho Grammar.* Cape Town: Longman.

Douglas, M. ([1966] 2006). *Purity and Danger.* London: Routledge.

Duncan, J. (2013). *Marikana and the Paradox of Press Transformation.* Paper presented at the University of Johannesburg's Department of Sociology Wednesday Seminar: 5 March 2013, University of Johannesburg, Johannesburg.

Eliade, M. (1964). *Myth and Reality.* Northampton: George Allen and Unwin.

eNCA. (2013). HIV/AIDS Holy Water Cure Put to the Test. Retrieved 7/11/2013, from http://enca.com/south-africa/hivaids-holy-water-cure-put-test.

Epstein, S. (1997). AIDS Activism and the Retreat from the 'Genocide' Frame. *Social Identities, 3*(4), 415-439.

Farmer, P. (1994). AIDS-Talk and the Constitution of Cultural Models. *Social Science & Medicine, 38*(6), 801-809.

Farmer, P. (2003). Introduction *Global AIDS: Myths and Facts.* Cambridge, MA: South End Press.

Fassin, D. (2007). *When Bodies Remember: Experiences and Politics of AIDS in South Africa.* Berkeley, CA: University of California Press.

Fassin, D. & Schneider, H. (2003). The Politics of AIDS in South Africa: Beyond the Controversies. *British Medical Journal, 326*, 495-497.

Fee, E. (1988). Sin Versus Science: Veneral Diseases in Twentieth-Century Baltimore. In E. Fee & D. Fox (Eds.), *AIDS: The Burdens of History.* Berkeley, CA: University of California Press.

Fourie, P. & Meyer, M. (2010). *The Politics of AIDS Denialism: South Africa's Failure to Respond.* Farnham, UK: Ashgate.

Frankham, J. (1998). Peer Education: The Unauthorised Version. *British Educational Research Journal, 24*(2), 179-194.

Frith, A. (2013). Census 2011. Retrieved 7/11/2013, from http://census2011.adrianfrith.com.

Gausset, Q. (2001). AIDS and Cultural Practices in Africa: The Case of the Tonga (Zambia). *Social Science & Medicine, 52*(509-518).

Gay, J. (1993). *Disease in Lesotho: Perception and Prevalence*. Ministry of Health, Government of Lesotho.

Geffen, N. (2010). *Debunking AIDS: The Inside Story of the Treatment Action Campaign*. Johannesburg: Jacana Media.

Gevisser, M. (2007). *Thabo Mbeki: The Dream Deferred*. Johannesburg: Jonathan Ball.

Gilbert, L. (2012). Upstream/downstream – Locating the 'Social' in Health Promotion and HIV/AIDS in South Africa? *South African Review of Sociology, 43*(1), 62-80.

Goffman, E. (1974). *Frame Analysis: An Essay on the Organisation of Experience*. Boston: Northeastern University Press.

Goldstein, D. (2004). *Once Upon a Virus: AIDS Legends and Vernacular Risk Perception*. Logan, UT: Utah State University Press.

Green, E. (1994). *AIDS and STDs in Africa: Bridging the Gap Between Traditional Healing and Modern Medicine*. Boulder, CO: Westview Press.

Haram, L. (1991). Tswana Medicine in Interaction with Biomedicine. *Social Science & Medicine, 33*(2), 167-175.

Heald, S. (2002). It's Never as Easy as ABC: Understandings of AIDS in Botswana. *African Journal of AIDS Research, 1*, 1-10.

Heald, S. (2006). Abstain or Die: The Development of HIV/AIDS Policy in Botswana. *Journal of Biosocial Science, 38*(29-41).

Health & Development Africa. (2009a). Community Study of Merafong City Local Municipality. Retrieved 2/2/2010, from http://www.jhhesa.org.

Health & Development Africa. (2009b). Community Study of eThekwini Municipality. Retrieved 2/2/2010, from http://www.jhhesa.org.

Health & Development Africa. (2009c). Community Study of Madibeng Local Municipality. Retrieved 2/2/2010, from http://www.jhhesa.org.

Health & Development Africa. (2009d). Community Study of Matjhabeng and Masilonyana Municipalities. Retrieved 2/2/2010, from http://www.jhhesa.org.

Helman, C. (1978). 'Feed a Cold, Starve a Fever' – Folk Models of Infection in an English Suburban Community, and Their Relation to Medical Treatement. *Culture, Medicine and Psychiatry, 2*, 107-137.

Holland, D. & Quinn, N. (1987). Introduction. In D. Holland & N. Quin (Eds.), *Cultural Models in Language and Thought*. Cambridge: Cambridge University Press.

Horton, R. (1971). African Traditional Thought and Western Science. In M. Young (Ed.), *Knowledge and Control: New Directions for the Sociology of Education*. London: Collier Macmillan.

Hunter, M. (2010). *Love in the Time of AIDS: Inequality, Gender, and Rights in South Africa*. Bloomington, IN: Indiana University Press.

Illich, I. (1974). *Medical Nemesis: The Limits to Medicine*. London: Calder & Boyars.

Inagaki, N. (2007). Communicating the Impact of Communication for Development: Recent Trends in Empirical Research. *World Bank Working Paper*. Washington, DC: World Bank.

Ingstad, B. (1990). The Cultural Construction of AIDS and its Consequences for Prevention in Botswana. *Medical Anthropology Quarterly, 4*(1), 28-40.

Irwin, A., Millen, J. & Fallows, D. (2003). *Global AIDS: Myths and Facts*. Cambridge, MA: South End Press.

John, V. (2012). 'Alarm' at SA Pupils' Lack of HIV/AIDS Knowledge, *Mail & Guardian*. Retrieved 9/2/2012, from www.mg.co.za.

Johns Hopkins Health and Education in South Africa. (2009). HIV/AIDS Communication Programmes are Getting the Message Across: National Survey Finds. Retrieved 2/2/2010.

Jordanova, L. (1995). The Social Construction of Medical Knowledge. *Social History of Medicine, 8*(3), 361-381.

Kalichman, S. (2009). *Denying AIDS: Conspiracy Theories, Pseudoscience, and Human Tragedy.* New York: Springer.

Kempton, W. (1987). Two Theories of Home Heat Control. In D. Holland & N. Quinn (Eds.), *Cultural Models in Language & Thought.* Cambridge: Cambridge University Press.

Kleinman, A. (1980). *Patients and Healers in the Context of Culture: An Exploration of the Borderland Between Anthropology, Medicine, and Psychiatry.* Berkeley, CA: University of California Press.

Kleinman, A. (1988). *The Illness Narratives: Suffering, Healing and the Human Condition.* USA: Basic Books.

Kleinman, A., Eisenberg, L. & Good, B. (1978). Culture, Illness, and Care: Clinical Lessons from Anthropological and Cross-Cultural Research. *Annals of Internal Medicine, 88*, 251-258.

Kunda, J-E. & Tomaselli, K. (2010). Social Representations of HIV/AIDS in South Africa and Zambia: Lessons for Health Communication. In L. Lagerwerf, H. Boer & H. Wasserman (Eds.), *Health Communication in Southern Africa: Engaging with Social and Cultural Diversity.* Pretoria: UNISA Press.

Lakatos, I. (1978). *The Methodology of Scientific Research Programmes.* Cambridge, UK: Cambridge University Press.

Lalbahadur, Y. (2013). *Influences on People's Choice of Ayurvedic Healing in South Africa.* (Master's in Sociology), University of the Witwatersrand, Johannesburg.

Last, M. (1981). The Importance of Knowing about Not Knowing. *Social Science & Medicine, 15*(3), 387-392.

Lazzarini, Z. (2001). What Lessons Can We Learn from the Exceptionalism Debate (Finally). *Journal of Law, Medicine & Ethics, 29*, 149-151.

Levine, M. & Siegel, K. (1992). Unprotected Sex: Understanding Gay Men's Participation. In J. Huber & B. Schnieder (Eds.), *The Social Context of AIDS* (pp. 47-72). Newbury Park: Sage.

Liddell, C., Barrett, L. & Bydawell, M. (2005). Indigenous Representations of Illness and AIDS in Sub-Saharan Africa. *Social Science & Medicine, 60*, 691-700.

Low-Beer, D. & Stoneburner, R. L. (2003). Behaviour and Communication Change in Reducing HIV: Is Uganda Unique? *African Journal of AIDS Research, 2*(1), 9-21.

Lowy, E. & Ross, M. (1994). 'It'll Never Happen to Me': Gay Men's Beliefs, Perceptions and Folk Construction of Sexual Risk. *AIDS Education and Prevention, 66*(6), 467-482.

Macdonald, D. (1996). Notes on the Socio-Economic and Cultural Factors Influencing the Transmission of HIV In Botswana. *Social Science & Medicine, 42*(9), 1325-1333.

Mackenzie, S. (2011). Dissecting the Social Body: Social Inequality through AIDS Counter-narratives. *Public Understanding of Science, 20*(4), 491-505.

Malinowsk, B. (1984). The Role of Myth in Life. In A. Dundes (Ed.), *Sacred Narrative: Readings in the Theory of Myth* (pp. 193-206). Berkeley, CA: University of California Press.

Marrazzo, J., Ramjee, G., Nair, G., Palanee, T., Mkhize, B., Nakabilto, C., . . . Team, V. S. (2013). *Pre-exposure prophylaxis for HIV in women: daily oral tenofovir, oral tenofovir/emtricitabine or vaginal tenofovir gel in the VOICE study (MTN 003).* Paper presented at the 20th Conference on Retroviruses and Opportunistic Infections, Atlanta.

Martin, D. (1990). *Tongues of Fire: The Explosion of Protestantism in Latin America.* Oxford: Blackwell.

337

Maticka-Tyndale, E. (1992). Social Construction of HIV Transmission and Prevention among Heterosexual Young Adults. *Social Problems, 39*(3), 238-252.

Mayer, P. & Mayer, I. (1974). *Townsmen or Tribesmen: Conservatism and the Process of Urbanization in a South African City*. Cape Town: Oxford University Press.

Mbeki, T. (2002). Casto Hlongwane, Caravans, Cats, Geese, Foot & Mouth and Statistics: HIV/AIDS and the Struggle for the Humanisation of the African. Retrieved 23/3/2014, from http://www.virusmyth.com/aids/hiv/ancdoc.htm.

McCloskey, M. (1983). Naive Theories of Motion. In D. Gentner & A. Stevens (Eds.), *Mental Models*. New Jersey: Lawrence Erlbaum.

McNeill, F. (2009a). 'Condoms Cause AIDS': Poison, Prevention and Denial in Venda. Johannesburg: Department of Sociology, Anthropology & Development Studies, University of Johannesburg.

McNeill, F. (2009b). Venda: Magic? Talking about Treatment. In M. Crew (Ed.), *Magic: AIDS Review 2009*. Pretoria: Centre for the Study of AIDS, University of Pretoria.

McNeill, F. & Niehaus, I. (2009). Introduction. In M. Crewe (Ed.), *Magic: AIDS Review 2009*. Pretoria: Centre for the Study of AIDS, University of Pretoria.

Melville, H. (1972). *Moby-Dick*. Harmondsworth: Penguin.

Metropolitan. (2009a). Live the Future. Retrieved 12/10/2012, from www.livethefuture.co.za/b_the_future/b_the_future.

Metropolitan. (2009b). Pamphlet 'B the Future cellbook on HIV and AIDS'.

Metropolitian. (2012). Company Overview. Retrieved 25/1/2012, from http://www.metropolitan.co.za/index.php/metropolitan-holder/about-us/overview.html.

Ministry for Cooperative Government and Traditional Affairs. (2011). Service Delivery Challenges Immense but Past Achievements Lay a Solid Foundation for New Councils. Retrieved 27/11/2011, from http://www.cogta.gov.za.

Moodie, D. & Ndatshe, W. V. (1994). *Going for Gold: Men, Mines and Migration*. Johannesburg: Wits University Press.

Mpe, P. (2001). *Welcome to Our Hillbrow*. Pietermaritzburg: University of Natal Press.

Nattrass, N. (2007). *Mortal Combat: AIDS Denialism and the Struggle for Antiretrovirals in South Africa*. Durban: UKZN Press.

Nattrass, N. (2012). *The AIDS Conspiracy: Science Fights Back*. Johannesburg: Wits University Press.

Nguyen, V.-K. (2010). *The Republic of Therapy: Triage and Sovereignty in West Africa's Time of AIDS*. Durham, NC: Duke University Press.

Nicholson, Z. (2011). Etv ordered to pull 'miracle' ads, *IOL News*. Retrieved from http://www.iol.co.za.

Niehaus, I. (2009). Bushbuckridge: Beyond Treatment. In M. Crewe (Ed.), *Magic: AIDS Review 2009*. Pretoria: Centre for the Study of AIDS, University of Pretoria.

Niehaus, I. & Jonsson, G. (2005). Dr. Wouter Basson, Americans and Wild Beasts: Men's Conspiracy Theories of HIV/AIDS in the South African Lowveld. *Medical Anthropology, 24*, 179-208.

Nzioka, C. (1996). Lay Perceptions of Risk of Hiv Infection and the Social Construction of Safer Sex: Some Experiences from Kenya. *AIDS Care, 8*(5), 565-580.

Paroz, R. A. ([1961] 1988). *Southern Sotho-English Dictionary*. Morija, Lesotho: Morija Sesuto Book Deposit.

Parran, T. (1937). *Shadow on the Land: Syphilis*. New York: Reynal & Hitchcock.

Peltzer, K., Preez, N. F., Ramlagan, S. & Fomundam, H. (2008). Use of Traditional Complementary and Alternative Medicine for HIV Patients in KwaZulu-Natal, South Africa. *BMC Public Health, 8*(255). doi: doi:10.1186/1471-2458-8-255.

Peltzer, K. & Promtussananon, S. (2005). HIV/AIDS Knowledge and Sexual Behaviour among Junior Secondary School Students in South Africa. *Journal of Social Science, 1*(1), 1-8.

Piot, P. (2008). *AIDS: Exceptionalism Revisited*. London: London School of Economics and Political Science.

Reynolds Whyte, S. (2009). Health Identities and Subjectivities: The Ethnographic Challenge. *Medical Anthropology Quarterly, 23*(1), 6-15.

Robins, S. (2004). 'Long Live Zackie, Long Live': AIDS Activism, Science and Citizenship after Apartheid. *Journal of Southern African Studies, 30*(3), 651-672.

Rödlach, A. (2006). *Witches, Westerners, and HIV: AIDS & Cultures of Blame in Africa*. Walnut Creek, CA: Left Coast Press.

Rogers, E. M. (2003). *Diffusion of Innovation* (5 ed.). New York: The Free Press.

Rosenbrock, R., Dubois-Arberb, F., Moersc, M., Pinelld, P., Schaeffere, D. & Setbonf, M. (2000). The Normalization of AIDS in Western European Countries. *Social Science & Medicine, 50*(11), 1607-1629.

Saethre, E. & Stadler, J. (2009). A Tale of Two 'Cultures': HIV Risk Narratives in South Africa. *Medical Anthropology, 28*(2), 268-284.

SAnews. (2011). 100 million fake cigarettes destroyed. Retrieved 16/8/2013, from http://oldsanews.gcis.gov.za/rss/11/11020414451001.

Schneider, H. (2002). On the Fault-line: The Politics of AIDS Policy in Contemporary South Africa. *African Studies, 61*(1), 145-167.

Schneider, H. & Fassin, D. (2002). Denial and Defiance: A Socio-political Analysis of AIDS in South Africa. *AIDS, 16* (Supplement 4), S45-S51.

Sidibe/UNAIDS, M. (2011). *UNAIDS Report 2011*. Geneva.

Society for Family Health. (ND). Condom Packet Insert: 'Lovers Plus: Cross over to real style'.

South African National AIDS Council (SANAC). (2013). World AIDS Day – Call to Action. Retrieved 1/12/2013, from http://www.sanac.org.za.

South African Press Service (SAPA). (2012). Eskom: Soweto debt stands at R3.3bn, *Business Report*. Retrieved from www.iol.co.za.

Squire, C. (2007). *HIV in South Africa: Talking about the Big Thing*. London: Routledge.

Stadler, J. (2003a). Rumor, Gossip and Blaime: Implications for HIV/AIDS Prevention in the South African Lowveld. *AIDS Education and Prevention, 15*(4), 357-368.

Stadler, J. (2003b). The Young, the Rich and the Beautiful: Secrecy, Suspicion and Discourse of AIDS in the South African Lowveld. *African Journal of AIDS Research, 2*(2), 127-139.

Statistics South Africa. (2004). Census 2001: Primary Tables South Africa. Pretoria: Statistics South Africa.

Statistics South Africa. (2012a). Census 2011: Census in Brief. Pretoria: Statistics South Africa.

Statistics South Africa. (2012b). Census 2011: Statistical Release P0301.4. Pretoria: Statistics South Africa.

Steinberg, J. (2008). *Three Letter Plague: A Young Man's Journey through a Great Epidemic*. Johannesburg: Jonathan Ball.

Stevens, M., Weiner, R., Mapolisa, S. & Dickinson, D. (2005). Management Responses to HIV/AIDS in South African Workplaces: A Baseline Survey. *South African Journal of Economic and Management Science,* 8(3), 287-299.

Stillwaggon, E. (2005). *AIDS and the Ecology of Poverty*. Oxford: Oxford University Press.

Sundkler, B. (1961). *Bantu Prophets in South Africa*. London: Oxford University Press.

Thom, A. (2009). The Curious Tale of the Vitamin Seller. In K. Cullinan & A. Thom (Eds.), *The Virus, Vitamins & Vegetables: The South African HIV/AIDS Mystery*. Johannesburg: Jacana Media.

Thomas, L., Schmid, B., Gwele, M., Ngubo, R. & Cochrane, J. (2006). *Let Us Embrace: The Role and Significance of an Integrated Faith-Based Initiative for HIV and AIDS:* Ahrap.

Thomas, S. & Quinn, S. (1991). The Tuskegee Syphilis Study, 1932 to 1972: Implications for HIV Education and AIDS Risk Education Programmes in the Black Community. *American Journal of Public Health, 81*(11), 1498-1505.

Tomaselli, K. (2011). Sham Reasoning and Pseudo-Science: Myths and Mediatisation of HIV/AIDS in South Africa. In K. Tomaselli & C. Chasi (Eds.), *Development and Public Health Communication*. Cape Town: Pearson.

Treichler, P. (1999). *How to Have a Theory in an Epidemic: Cultural Chronicles of AIDS*. Durham: Duke University Press.

Turner, V. (1981). *The Drums of Affliction: A Study of Religious Processes among the Ndembu of Zambia*. Ithaca, New York: Cornell University Press.

University of Natal Medical School. (2013). The Medical School History. Retrieved 8/3/2013, from http://scnc.ukzn.ac.za/doc/EDU/UnivColl/Medical_School.pdf.

US Department of Health and Human Sciences. (2006). *Your Guide to Lowering Your Blood Pressure with DASH*.

Vaughan, M. (1991). *Curing their Ills: Colonial Power and African Illness*. Cambridge: Polity.

Vernazza, P., Hirschel, B., Bernasconi, E. & Flepp, M. (2008). HIV-positive Individuals Not Suffering from Any Other STD and Adhering to an Effective Antiretroviral Treatement Do Not Transmit HIV Sexually. *Bulletin des Medecens Suisses, 89*(5).

Weiss, R. (1994). *Learning from Strangers: The Art and Method of Qualitative Interview Studies*. New York: The Free Press.

Whyte, W. (1989). Advancing Scientific Knowledge through Participatory Action Research. *Sociological Forum, 4*(3), 367-385.

Willis, P. (1978). *Learning to Labour: How Working Class Kids Get Working Class Jobs*. Westmead: Saxon House.

Wogan, P. (2004). Deep Hanging Out: Reflections on Fieldwork and Multisourced Ethnography. *Identities: Global Studies in Culture and Power, 11*, 129-139.

Yamba, B. (1997). Cosmologies in Turmoil: Witchfinding and AIDS in Chiawa, Zambia. *Africa, 67*(2), 200-223.

Zola, I. K. (1966). Culture and Symptoms – An Analysis of Patients' Presenting Complaints. *American Sociological Review, 31*(5), 615-630.

Endnotes

Introduction

1 Dickinson (2002); (Dickinson, 2003).

2 Dickinson (2004); Dickinson and Innes (2004); Dickinson and Stevens (2005) and Stevens, Weiner, Mapolisa, and Dickinson (2005).

3 The 1ˢᵗ Wits HIV/AIDS in the Workplace Research Symposium, June 2004, Wits Business School, Johannesburg, co-chaired with Marion Stevens and the 2ⁿᵈ Wits HIV/AIDS in the Workplace Research Symposium, May 2008, Wits Business School, Johannesburg, co-chaired with Courtney Sprague.

4 A project that ended in tears, see Cairns, Dickinson, and Orr (2006).

5 Prior to this, antiretroviral drugs were only available privately (and effectively only for the 15 or so per cent of the population who had medical aid), through a handful of NGOs and, from 2002, for the employees of some of South Africa's largest companies.

6 South African Business Coalition on HIV/AIDS (Sabcoha) Second Private Sector Conference on HIV and AIDS, November 2008. South African HIV Clinicians Society, February 2009. Colloquium for Social Entrepreneurs, February 2009. Sabcoha's Satellite Programme to the Fourth SA AIDS Conference, Durban, April 2009. Third Annual Workshop on Advanced Clinical Care (AWACC) – AIDS (Durban), October 2009. International Federation of Chemical, Energy, Mine and General Workers' Unions (ICEM) HIV/AIDS Sub-Saharan Regional Workshop, November 2009.

7 Dickinson (2008b).

8 To whom I am grateful for his willingness to share his knowledge and his warmth. I can only apologise that no publication emerged from the information that he provided. You can find him at www.facebook.com/mmsibeko.

9 By this time, the late 2000s, Mbeki's denialism had largely disappeared from the scene.

10 South Africa used, and continues to use, racial categories as a demographic variable. Under Apartheid four racial categories were legislated, African, Coloured, Indian and White. The racial hierarchy saw the creation of separate townships for Africans, Coloureds and Indians. This book focuses on African townships. The primary historical purpose of townships was to house industrial and domestic labour adjacent to White towns and cities. Africans constitute some 80 per cent of South Africa's population and, in a society that remains deeply divided along racial categories, many townships remain racially homogeneous. While this inquiry is based within African township populations, it should not be assumed that alternative accounts of HIV/AIDS are restricted to either this racial category or geographical location.

11 Dickinson (2009).

12 In addition to the African peer educators, one White peer educator actively participated in the project. I have excluded this data from the analysis.

13 Dickinson (2005).

14 South African National AIDS Council (SANAC) (2013).

15 Gauteng and the Free State are two of South Africa's nine provinces. Gauteng, the smallest, is heavily urbanised and accounts for more than 30 per cent of the country's GDP. The Free State is a largely rural province that borders the southern boundaries of Gauteng.

16 South African townships are complex and changing places and not all residents can or should be regarded as constituting a subordinate population. However, as an approximation, categorising the populations of African townships in South Africa as a subordinate population is valid.

Chapter 1: More than one kind of AIDS

1 A few months earlier, I had written a short opinion piece that I had opened with the observation that AIDS is rarely cited as the cause of death at funerals. 'I live in a country where it has become normal to bury men and women in their thirties. At least it is so at township funerals. At the cemetery while the women, standing to one side, sing hymns, the men labour in relays to fill the grave. We work shoulder to shoulder, but we do not share what we are thinking: that this person died of AIDS.' (Dickinson, 2008a). Later in the piece, I outlined how one peer educator had recounted to me the difficulty of talking about AIDS at the funeral of a relative. He had explained the intense conflict within his family as to the cause of death. Three options were in play: AIDS, tuberculosis (TB) or witchcraft (of which the deceased's wife was being accused). The peer educator reported how, after exhaustive efforts to convince the family to pronounce the cause of death as AIDS, he had only got agreement to say his brother had died of TB. As his account had unfolded, I was hoping that he would tell me that he had broken the silence, but later saw the significance of what he had achieved. In the face of competing explanations of AIDS, the easiest thing would have been to say nothing and keep the peace. This account of the peer educator's funeral speech is also recounted in Dickinson (2009).

2 The Gospel and not the Country & Western version.

3 Jonathan Stadler (2003a, p. 358).

4 A state of affairs that is punctuated by periodic concerns that this knowledge is slipping, or in some way insufficient, and that further education efforts are necessary, see for example John (2012).

5 Such surveys consist of questionnaires in which respondents are asked to answer questions designed to assess their knowledge, attitudes and perceptions of HIV/AIDS (or other topic of concern). Typically, the questions are in a 'closed response' format where respondents choose from a set of possible answers (i.e. multichoice-type questions) or say whether a statement about HIV/AIDS is 'true', 'false' or they 'don't know'. Attitudes and perceptions about HIV/AIDS and people living with the disease take similar formats, with the options being a scale of agreement. Such formats allow for the quick collection of clear data points. They do not allow for nuances, doubts or deception.

6 Peltzer and Promtussananon (2005, p. 358).

7 The Metropolitan Company is one of the top three insurance groups in southern Africa. It operates in more than half a dozen African countries and its Head Office is in Cape Town. Its products include life assurance, retirement annuities, medical scheme administration, managed health care, asset management services and collective

investment schemes. Its large client base and business focus on (privately provided) social protection products, including health care, have lead it to support an extensive Corporate Social Responsibility (CSR) programme, which includes a strong emphasis on HIV/AIDS. The company's CSR initiatives are linked to its corporate slogan of 'Together We Can' and a belief that, 'Our brand positioning remains true to our unwavering core ideology of being people and community focused'. Metropolitian (2012).

8 The idea of the cellbook was that information on HIV/AIDS could be downloaded onto a cell phone (without the use of internet connectivity) and take advantage of the wide cell phone penetration in South Africa.

9 Metropolitan (2009b).

10 Metropolitan (2009a).

11 Kleinman (1988).

12 Helman (1978).

13 Helman (1978, p. 132).

14 Zola (1966).

15 The only reference in literature that I have located on *nyoko* is John Gay's (1993) *Disease in Lesotho: Perceptions and Prevalence*. Gay translates *nyoko* as 'bile' and describes it as a condition without a Western counterpart. His account then starts to wobble because he never clearly grasps the emic understanding of *nyoko*. Gay rightly suggests that *nyoko* 'relates to a general malaise … and corresponding discontent and low spirits' (1993, p. 74) and that the diversity of symptoms suggests that *nyoko* is an explanation for unspecific health concerns which may or may not have objective validity. This has some truth; a self-diagnosis of *nyoko* can, in the township, be simply saying you are feeling off colour or, alternatively it can be used as an acceptable foil if you don't want to discuss your actual illness. But what is overlooked in the report is that there is a well-developed understanding of the cause, symptoms and treatment of *nyoko* within African communities.

16 Other ways to remove *nyoko* include: induced vomiting (*ho kapa*) using warm water usually laced with either vinegar or salt; using laxatives either bought over the counter or prescribed by traditional healers as medicine to clean the blood (*moriana ho hlatswa madi*); and by steaming.

17 Church prophets generally stick to steaming, while traditional healers typically use all methods, other than over-the-counter laxatives.

18 Kleinman (1980).

19 This division is of course political; biomedicine has emerged over the last hundred years as the dominant healing model in South Africa and claimed professional status, whereas a range of other healing systems have been relegated to folk status via legislative and other restrictions.

20 Kleinman (1980).

21 L. Thomas, Schmid, Gwele, Ngubo, and Cochrane (2006, p. 53).

22 Typically, they are opposed by an alliance of medical professionals, the state and large employers using legal, economic and reputational attacks. Though this is not a one-way street, popular media in South Africa gives coverage to errors made by medical practitioners and the resulting harm to individuals.

23 Peltzer, Preez, Ramlagan, and Fomundam (2008).

24 Horton (1971).

25 Horton (1971, p. 261).

26 Haram (1991).

27 Nzioka (1996).

28 Macdonald (1996).
29 Liddell, Barrett, and Bydawell (2005).
30 Fassin and Schneider (2003).
31 L. Thomas et al. (2006).
32 McNeill and Niehaus (2009); Rödlach (2006) and Steinberg (2008).
33 Last (1981).
34 African Initiated Churches (with the 'I' in the abbreviation 'AIC' flexibly used to stand for Initiated, Indigenous and Independent) are varied and widespread in Africa. Their key features are African leadership and membership (in frequent historical contrast to missionary-introduced 'mainline' Christian denomination) and various syncretisation of orthodox (European/North American) Christianity and traditional African beliefs. The South African 2001 Census estimated that 31.8 per cent of the population were affiliated to AICs, just behind the 32.6 per cent affiliated to mainline churches and well ahead of the 5.9 per cent affiliated to Pentecostal churches (Statistics South Africa, 2004). The question of religious affiliation was not asked in the 2011 Census.
35 Heald (2006).
36 Unlike Christian and traditional African theories of AIDS, the racial explanation does not offer any alternative cure, its role is, therefore, limited to a preventive role.
37 It is possibly only by chance that the major South African folk theories of AIDS have significant bio-moral aspects. Such bio-moral components of folk theories of AIDS may not be necessary. Alternative healing systems, such as Ayuvedic medicine (the presence of which in South Africa is largely confined to the Indian population and is absent in African townships), which can be located in the folk sector of Kleinman's schema, have only a minimal moral explanation of health and sickness (Lalbahadur, 2013).
38 Allopathic medicine is, of course, far from free of bio-moral influences. It is especially strong in the public health sector with the stigmatisation of unhealthy behaviour such as excessive drinking, smoking and being overweight.
39 Illich (1974).
40 Vaughan (1991).
41 There is now doubt as to how accurate the syphilis diagnoses were (Vaughan, 1991, p. Chapter 6).
42 Vaughan (1991), Chapter 6: Syphilis and Sexuality: The Limits of Colonial Medical Power.
43 Vaughan (1991, p. 133).
44 Jordanova (1995, p. 368).
45 Fee (1988).
46 Parran (1937).
47 Fee (1988, p. 136). Emphasis in the original.
48 As Fee (1988) points out, public health officials deliberately undermined the centrality of sexual transmission in their educational campaigns to reduce stigmatisation in order to facilitate discussion, testing and treatment.
49 Fee (1988, p. 142).
50 Treichler (1999).
51 A lack of access to prevention services has also been put forward as an explanation of the epidemic, but in the case of adult-to-adult transmission this has worn thin as South Africa has been flooded with free condoms. Other forms of prevention, such as faithfulness or abstinence, cannot of course be provided as a 'service'. Though this does not prevent such an argument been trotted out in rote communications, see for example Bathabile Dlamini, South Africa's Minister of Social Development (2011). The emergence

of treatment as prevention (through lowering the viral load of infected individuals, reducing the chance of them infecting others) may lead to a resurgence of the argument of a lack of prevention access, though this will now be synonymous with treatment.

52　Stillwaggon (2005).

53　Gilbert (2012).

54　The major exception here is of course the American Presidential Fund for HIV/AIDS which, in response to religious lobbies in the US, positively promoted prevention campaigns that focused on abstinence and faithfulness and downplayed or omitted condom messages.

55　Dickinson (2009).

56　Kunda and Tomaselli (2010, p. 110).

57　Both prevention-as-treatment and circumcision have been promoted as responses to the epidemic for at least a decade, but only gained traction in recent years.

58　Sidibe/UNAIDS (2011, p. 5).

Chapter 2: Hunting myths, finding theories

1　Eliade (1964).

2　Malinowsk (1984).

3　For example, surveys conducted by Health & Development Africa for Johns Hopkins Health and Education in South Africa (2009) in four South African provinces asked a range of questions to between 750 and 870 people in order to understand the 'local dynamics' of the AIDS epidemic. The 'misconceptions about condoms' that are reported in these studies (Health & Development Africa, 2009a, 2009b, 2009c, 2009d) include that 'condoms may contain worms' and that 'you should always check the expiry date before using a condom'. Getting people to check the expiry date on a condom shouldn't prove too hard to rectify with conventional education methods. Convincing people that there aren't worms in condoms (that cause HIV) is likely to be a more complex process. Yet the reports make no attempt to distinguish between what is a belief embedded in racial perceptions of the world and (a small number of) people not appreciating that condoms, like food, have expiry dates.

4　But in line with the common linguistic use of the term myth, this misunderstanding over the efficacy of two condoms is frequently termed an AIDS myth, for example, the information pack of Lovers Plus condoms, marketed by the Society for Family Health (SFH), has a section on 'Common myths and facts about condoms'. These include not needing to use a condom with your regular partner, not needing to use a condom if other contraception is being used, and that using two condoms is better than one (Society for Family Health, ND).

5　Though some AIDS myths may draw upon myths of origin for support. For example, some Christian explanations of AIDS as a punishment from God for sin draw on the Creation narrative, human sinfulness and prophecy of the Last Days, in addition to a wide range of specific Bible verses.

6　In the literature that deals with alternative explanations of AIDS, different terminology is used. Thus, for example, Goldstein (2004) uses the term 'AIDS legends' for what I describe as AIDS myths.

7　Piot (2008).

8　Irwin, Millen, and Fallows (2003).

9　Farmer (2003, p. xviii).

10　Not because of the 'so-called' prefix, here Farmer is correctly pointing to all beliefs being in a constant process of adaptation, rather than frozen in some past configuration.

11   Levine and Siegel (1992).

12   Lowy and Ross (1994, p. 481).

13   Epstein (1997).

14   Goldstein (2004).

15   Mackenzie (2011).

16   Researchers looking at some of this range of AIDS explanations include: Ashforth
     (2005) on witchcraft in South Africa; Rödlach (2006), Robins (2004) and Stadler
     (2003a) on witchcraft and racial conspiracy beliefs as mechanisms for blaming others
     in Zimbabwe and South Africa; Fassin (2007) and Fassin and Schneider (2003) on
     racial conspiracy beliefs emerging from South Africa's Apartheid past; Ingstad (1990)
     and Heald (2002) on AIDS as a traditional disease in Botswana; and (Liddell et al.,
     2005) working across the three core components of traditional beliefs in sub-Saharan
     Africa.

17   Green (1994).

18   Hunter (2010).

19   Steinberg (2008).

20   Niehaus and Jonsson (2005).

21   Jonathan Stadler (2003b).

22   McNeill (2009b).

23   Niehaus (2009, p. 31)

24   Steinberg (2008).

25   Fassin (2007).

26   Studies that include a physical check on what is said can, at least, establish the scale of
     the problem. Thus, in reporting the failure of the VOICE HIV drug-based prevention
     study, it was established that while 90 per cent of the study's participants reported
     adherence to the drugs, chemical tests for the drugs in their blood/vaginal fluids
     showed adherence rates of under 30 per cent (Marrazzo et al., 2013).

27   Seventy-five per cent of the peer educators were men, a figure that needs to be
     compared with the workforce of Digco which, not untypically for a mining company,
     is 89 per cent male overall. On average they had been employed by Digco for
     11.9 years (ranging from 1 to 28 years). Their home languages indicate a range of
     ethnicities reflective of the townships around Digco. The predominant home language
     was isiZulu (17 peer educators). Additionally, four spoke Sesotho at home, two
     isiXhosa, two Sepedi, two Xitsonga and one siSwati.

28   Over 300 recordings were submitted in English, Afrikaans, isiXhosa, isiZulu, Sepedi
     and Sesotho. These were translated and transcribed into English. The majority of
     reports were on AIDS myths that had been encountered within peer environments.

29   The idea of stories to counter myths did not come out of nowhere; I had observed
     such a process spontaneously developed during a peer educator meeting in my 2006
     research into peer educator informal activity. Subsequently, I had run a number of
     workshops with peer educators which replicated the process of generating 'myth-
     busting stories' in a structured way. The Digco research extended this by running it
     over a nine-month project held together by a number of workshops and a range of
     data-collecting methods, see Dickinson (2011).

30   Nevertheless, by virtue of their peer educator status, while they may be close to their
     peers, they are also distinct as a result of their peer educator status. As peer educators
     they are on the battle lines of the epidemic and what they report must always be read
     with this in mind. Given that peer educators' biomedical knowledge will, inevitably,
     be incomplete, they may not know what is, defined against scientific consensus,
     a myth. This is further complicated by changes in the biomedical consensus. My
     interest in HIV/AIDS myths, and the possibility of peer educators responding with

stories, was sparked during participatory observation research with a group of peer
educators in 2006 when I was struck by how they responded to reports of a new (to
them) AIDS myth – that because antiretroviral drugs put HIV to 'sleep', HIV-positive
people taking treatment did not need to use condoms (Dickinson, 2011). That HIV-
positive people should use condoms even if on antiretroviral drugs was considered an
important health promotion message at the time, see Crepaz, Hart, and Marks (2004).
In 2008, medical advice that HIV-positive individuals should not have unprotected
sex was reversed (Vernazza, Hirschel, Bernasconi, & Flepp, 2008). An HIV-positive
person with a comprehensively suppressed viral load would not, it was concluded,
in the absence of other STIs, infect a sexual partner. Indeed, apart from challenges
such as the case of HIV-positive women whose viral load in vaginal secretions may
intermittently surge to levels capable of infecting sexual partners (Cu-Uvin et al.,
2010), the value of treatment in lowering viral loads is now credited as a factor in
lower incidences rates in South Africa (Sidibe/UNAIDS, 2011). Yesterday's AIDS
myths that need to be dispelled can become today's AIDS facts that need to be
disseminated.

31 This was one of a minority of recordings made by peer educators who directly
recorded peers talking about HIV/AIDS. Most submitted recordings were of the peer
educators themselves recounting what they had heard.

32 Semen, in Sesotho and Nguni languages and ethno-physiology, is classified as a form
of blood.

33 In this I used an adapted version of Kleinman's (1980) division of explanatory models
of illness into three areas: professional, folk and popular (which I replace with lay).
There remained a small number of AIDS myths that I have been unable to link to
these folk and lay theories. This may be because I failed to see how these particular
AIDS myths support one or more of the listed core ideas at the heart of each of these
theories, because there are core ideas that I failed to identify, or because these were
flighted suggestions or idle supposition that got caught up in the net of the research
project. If so, and they really are 'stumps' not linked to any core idea, they are unlikely
to thrive and may never be heard of again.

34 This organisation of folk and lay theories of AIDS draws inspiration from Imre
Lakatos' (1978) outline of how rival scientific research programmes compete.
Lakatos argues that each scientific programme seeking to explain a field or area has
a 'core idea' that lies at its heart. Protagonists of these core ideas generate 'auxiliary
hypotheses' which explain and predict phenomena in the field of study. As well as
reflecting the power of the underlying idea (and of course the strength and funding
of the scientific teams committed to particular programmes), auxiliary hypotheses
also protect the core idea from attack; as long as the belt of auxiliary hypotheses have
vigour, the scientific programmes of which they are a part retain adherents who will
generate new hypotheses based on the core idea. Lakatos was, however, modelling
competition between different *scientific* theories that share common principles of
method, evidence and falsification. We should not, therefore, directly compare the
model of competing scientific research programmes with the competition of rival
explanations of AIDS. Thus, while an analogy is useful, we need to recognise that
these rival theories of AIDS exist in different paradigms of thought. Usually, they do
not even share common methods for evaluating the auxiliary hypotheses that surround
their different core ideas.

35 Farmer (1994).

36 Epstein (1997).

37 Heald (2006).

38 Horton (1971).

39 In which Afro-Americans were enrolled in a scientific experiment documenting the progression of untreated syphilis. Participants were not offered effective antibiotic treatment when this became available in the 1940s and active measures were taken to prevent this being provided through other channels. The experiment was only closed, after being brought to public attention, in the 1970s (S. Thomas & Quinn, 1991).

40 Niehaus and Jonsson (2005).

41 The Truth and Reconciliation Commission, set up by an Act of Parliament and chaired by Archbishop Desmond Tutu, aimed to identify and rectify human rights violations conducted under Apartheid.

42 Schneider and Fassin (2002).

43 Mackenzie (2011).

44 The appearance of Indian doctors in these accounts is based on Indians' relatively superior position within the Apartheid racial hierarchy and the social (and physical) distances between Indian and African populations in South Africa.

45 Liddell et al. (2005, p. 694).

46 Douglas ([1966] 2006).

47 In interviews, peer educations were divided over whether cleansing after an abortion or miscarriage could be adequately achieved 'in the hospital' (i.e. D&C or 'womb scrape') or whether traditional purification rites (use of herbal medicines and rituals) were necessary. In keeping with the moral underpinning of pollution theory, an abortion was seen as more dangerous than a miscarriage.

48 Fassin (2007).

49 This case took place prior to the research period. It had been heard directly by the interviewed peer educator in a *shebeen* (township pub or bar). When the peer educator had threatened to call the police, the man relating the myth had made a getaway.

50 Cohen (2002).

51 Ashforth (2005); Macdonald (1996); Rödlach (2006); Robins (2004); Stadler (2003a).

52 Ashforth (2002).

53 An additional myth linked to religious belief was that 'You don't have to wear a condom if you trust in God'. This presents a tension between the two main ideas at the heart of this folk theory: God's power and the need to obey God's laws. Other than in the case of a discordant couple, this myth lies on the fault line of these two core ideas, since faith that you won't be infected is set against what would be regarded typically within this paradigm as breaking God's law by engaging in sex outside marriage (and assumed sexual safety). This myth was recorded on one occasion and reported to have been heard by three out of nine peer educators in a vox pop count. This can be compared to, for example, the AIDS myth that God can cure AIDS, which had seven recordings and eight out of 16 peer educators having heard it in a vox pop count.

54 Maticka-Tyndale (1992, p. 245).

55 Apart from eliminating the possibility that the virus can pass through an intact mucous membrane, friction theory is otherwise in line with scientific understanding of HIV transmission, particularly the heightened risks of infection when ulcerative STIs are present or there is damage to the vagina as a result of rape or dry-sex practices.

56 See Niehaus (2009, p. 26) for a separate observation of this belief and Mpe (2001, p. 4) for a fictional account.

57 Clearly, early in the response to AIDS there were rival scientific research programmes competing against each other. Now, excluding AIDS denialists, while competing research programmes continue, these dispute detail rather than fundamental principles of the disease.

58 Digco (2009, p. 25).

59 Yamba (1997, p. 200).
60 Yamba (1997, p. 216).
61 The question of whether HIV-positive individuals need to wear condoms or not is critical here. Not having to wear them makes antiretroviral drug therapy, the closest Western medicine has to a cure, much more attractive.
62 Other than beliefs that a cure is available for Whites/people overseas. This is, however, a minority variation, with the myth primarily concerned with Whites infecting Blacks.
63 Ashforth (2002).
64 Rödlach (2006).
65 Bayer (1999); Niehaus and Jonsson (2005, p. 179).
66 Thus, for example, even if we can agree on a mutually acceptable mechanism, showing that the 'worms' in condoms aren't HIV, that doesn't disprove other possible mechanisms, such as injections by White doctors, by which HIV is being used genocidally. Nor does it mean that condoms are going to be used (but White doctors avoided) since condoms may be opposed as the result of auxiliary theories of other core ideas, such as traditional ideas for the need for blood/semen to be exchanged between people and the dangers of one's own blood/semen being reabsorbed if a condom is worn. And this is even before we get to other objections to condom use, such as reducing pleasure or the value of fertility.

Chapter 3: Managing a mosaic of beliefs

1 Bayer (1999).
2 Parran (1937).
3 Bayer (1999, p. 1042).
4 Bayer (1991); Bayer (1999); Cock, Mbori-Ngacha, and Marum (2002); Lazzarini (2001).
5 Bayer (1999).
6 Rosenbrock et al. (2000, p. 1607). What exactly these innovations in prevention are is not spelt out, suggesting that optimism over the response to HIV/AIDS overtook reality.
7 Cock et al. (2002).
8 The prominent exception, regarding alternative explanations to that of mainstream medical science, was the confrontation between the South African health professionals and human rights HIV/AIDS activists on the one side, and President Thabo Mbeki and a small number of AIDS dissidents on the other. Even here, however, open defiance of the AIDS establishment was that of a dissident elite, not a popular belief, see Chapter 10.
9 Heald (2006, p. 34).
10 At this opening stage in the project there were 32 African peer educators participating. Thirteen 'strongly agreed' with the statement that 'My ancestors can protect me from danger', eight 'agreed', two said they had 'no strong view', two 'disagreed' and seven 'disagreed strongly'. It was a striking bimodal distribution, with views split on either side of the question of ancestral benevolence.
11 That is not to say that everybody chose to speak in open forum on all issues. Informal discussions during breaks or giving peer educators lifts back to their homes after the workshops, along with the final individual interviews, saw peer educators adding their own views on topics that had been discussed, but for one reason or another they had not spoken up. Sometimes these reasons were mundane, the point had already been made or time was short. On other occasions their public silence was for more significant reasons, such as their viewpoint being based on experiences they didn't want to be public knowledge.

12 Twenty-six peer educators had come to the workshop, but not all were able to stay for the whole workshop, due to work or domestic commitments, a problem that affected all the workshops.

13 One of the peer educators volunteered that she had suffered from an offensive vaginal discharge that the clinic had been unable to cure but a traditional healer had been able to clear up. The implication was that the problem must have been sent by a witch, since it was treatable only by traditional means.

14 A percentage that rose only slightly in the privacy of the research interviews, in which 5 out of 23 peer educators believed in witches' ability to send HIV/AIDS.

15 Here the peer educator is linking traditional healers to involvement in harming people, an accusation that most if not all healers would deny. The situation is, however, complex. At what point does a traditional healer's assistance of a client cross the boundary into witchcraft? Traditional healers are asked to help clients woo potential lovers, to keep current lovers faithful, and to bring lost lovers back by prescribing traditional remedies. All this can be characterised by healers as *ho thusa batho* (to help people), but helping one person may well be at the expense of others (on the assumption that the healer can indeed project power in this way). This overlap between helping and hurting occurs even before we get to those healers who may be less scrupulous over what they are willing to do for paying clients.

16 One thing that the entire group was, however, united on was that as peer educators they should not be talking about witches with their peers. They were now comfortable enough with one another and with me to have this discussion, but talk about witches wasn't to go beyond the workshop. They didn't want to even consider my suggestion of working on a story to counter the myth that witches could send AIDS. Believers and disbelievers in witches alike made the same argument; talking about witches and AIDS would drive people to traditional healers since these are the people who can protect you from witchcraft. And traditional healers were a key opponent they faced as peer educators, notwithstanding the fact that the majority of them reported consulting a traditional healer in the last five years.

17 Dickinson (2011).

18 In South Africa such a criticism is, almost inevitably, overlaid with a racial analysis: Whites are paid to come in as experts, Blacks in general and Africans in particular remain in low-skilled, low-paid jobs. I, the project leader, was White; they, the peer educators, were almost exclusively Africans.

19 A shorthand expression for the research funds that I was using to pay for my costs: transport, research assistance, transcriptions and so on. Digco provided a venue, lunch and teas and, of course, bore the cost of the peer educators being 'paraded' (the term in mining companies for workers being taken off their normal duties) for the workshops.

20 An unprotected strike in South African labour law, often wrong, described as 'illegal', means that striking workers can be dismissed. In this instance, all the peer educators were reinstated. Whether my diplomatic advocacy on their behalf (and in the interests of the project's continuity) influenced this decision, I don't know.

21 This was helped by them making a 'special' report for me during each recording period. This was in part to make sure that every peer educator had at least one recording to hand in each workshop, but the topics were also selected to help me better understand each peer educator and their beliefs. The topics were: why they had become a peer educator; and their views on traditional healers, race and gender issues.

22 Demonstrating the value of maintaining confidences was achieved by, among other things, always making sure that, when I introduced material that individuals had

submitted in their recordings, that they were not identified. An innovation, which I started midway through the projects also assisted in setting the project's values. I started to give 'commendations' to peer educators for particular attributes in their submitted recordings. This was done by means of listing their names on a Powerpoint slide during the workshops. The categories of commendation were: for responding to myths by telling stories (i.e. the ultimate practical objective of the project), for research innovation (i.e. they had been innovative in collecting or following up on AIDS myths), for developing their own thinking (about myths and HIV/AIDS), for having energy (in collecting AIDS myths), for being frank and honest (about their beliefs), and for participating. The last commendation meant that all peer educators were included in the list of those commended since I was anxious that this public naming did not also imply any shaming by omission. In fact, my introduction of these commendations was extremely popular and helped reinforce some of the values that I wanted the project's participants to embrace.

23 This was particularly interesting because we had discussed this practice during one of the workshops and the peer educator now felt it important that I hear her firsthand account. She believed that her problem, which she identified as *makgome*, had arisen from a failure to cleanse after the death of a boyfriend and that this had resulted in the death of her next partner. She had then seen a traditional healer who had identified her problem and prescribed, among other ritual treatments, sleeping with a stranger. The peer educators pointed out that finding an opportunity to do this had not been hard. She firmly believed that what she had done was the reason why her current partner was still alive. She was also happy to tell me, since some versions of these cleansing practices see the problem being transmitted to the unwitting sexual partner, that she had seen the man she had slept with several years later and could report he was alive and well.

24 Cornwell (1984).

25 The peer educators' level of education ranged from nine years of schooling to post-school diplomas. Of the 23 interviewed peer educators, just over half had completed school (12 years of schooling). All but three had received an initial peer educator training course which varied between 3 and 14 days (average 4.8 days). Initial peer educator training in Digco has, for a number of years, been a three-day course, based on a 174-page manual, run by a service provider and assessed against a South African Qualifications Authority Unit Standard (SAQA 8555: Contributing to Information Distribution Regarding HIV/AIDS in the Workplace). Twelve peer educators received refresher training, which they estimated varied between one and five days per year, organised on an *ad hoc* basis by Digco industrial nurses. On average, at the time of interviews, each peer educator had received a total of 11.5 days of training on HIV/AIDS, though this varied widely between zero, for two peer educators (in one case because the individual had only recently become a peer educator and in the other because of clashes with vocational training obligations), and 64 days, for one peer educator. The amount of knowledge gained from less formal education sources was much harder to quantify, as was the degree to which peer educators were proactive in attempting to further their understanding of HIV/AIDS, though both these factors clearly varied widely between individuals.

26 The peer educators often enjoyed providing a detailed description of how, as a result of an accident, blood could be transferred if a first-aider had an open cut on his or her hands.

27 The limited bio-medical grasp of the peer educators also illustrates the wider point of how the combined health education efforts in South Africa have made little impact on how most people regard HIV/AIDS. This group was, after all, receptive to these public

health messages and recipients of additional inputs as a result of their membership of Digco's peer educator programme.

28 Dickinson (2009).

29 Issues regarding condoms include: moral and religious mores, restrictions on sexual pleasure and intimacy, as well as questions over their efficacy.

30 Twenty-one out of the 23 reported attending church at least twice a month.

31 Such as the Roman Catholic and Zion Christian Church (ZCC).

32 This process, and the calculations made around it by the peer educator, illustrate how traditional beliefs serve to maintain social cohesion within extended families. The performance of traditional rituals within families, and the obligation to attend them, ensure regular gatherings around at least one point of agreement – that the rituals need to be performed if there is not to be disharmony within the family.

33 The Universal Church of the Kingdom of God: a Pentecostal-type church in South Africa, originating in Brazil, blends prosperity, theology and miracle healing into its services.

34 I excluded from 'other problems' relatively trivial concerns, such as soiled bedding in the case of having sex with a menstruating woman.

35 Care was taken to ensure that pollution beliefs were not conflated with the medical model of infection, for example clarifying that the discussion was dealing with the danger of menstrual blood outside the issue whether the women was HIV positive or had another STI.

36 Using the McNemar Test, the difference between HIV/AIDS and other problems is statistically significant (P value ranging from 0.0001 to 0.0027), indicating statistical significance for the identified pattern among this small sample of peer educators. Statistical analysis kindly provided by Michael Greyling.

37 Digco (2009, p. 24).

38 One of the peer educators suggested sex as the transmission route, and explained the dangers of contact between humans and animals though pollution beliefs: that any sexual mixing, including between different races, was inherently dangerous.

39 In an attempt to impose some order on this data, I constructed four different profiles against which to measure the compatibility of the peer educators' beliefs with a medically based peer education programme such as Digco's.

The first was a 'hard science compatibility' profile that would maintain a purely rational scientific view of the world, which very few people other than staunchly atheist scientists hold. For those holding such a belief, there would be no agreement with any of these alternative beliefs. They would fit intellectually within a peer educator programme, but might be faulted on human empathy (and they would certainly not be seen as peers by others in Digco or their communities). Not surprisingly, no peer educator matches this profile.

The second was a 'psychosocial support' profile that allowed for belief in the value of traditional healers, church prophets, prayer and ancestors outside curing HIV/AIDS or protecting a person from HIV infection. Such a position might not be very different from what we could expect of professional health practitioners who, while basing their professional work on scientific medicine, would also promote psychosocial support from sources important to the patient. Peer educators with this perspective would be able to work alongside health professionals with minimal differences over appropriate communication and action regarding HIV/AIDS. (The compatibility between peer educators fitting these profiles and sharing the same views of HIV/AIDS education with medical professionals assumes, of course, that medical professionals fit the criteria that have just been suggested; holding beliefs based on scientific medicine, but agreeing to the value of psychosocial support from sources important to the patient. What has emerged from characters appearing in the more detailed case-study chapters of this book is that at least some medical professionals in South Africa do not comply with that profile. In this regard they are, in some areas of belief, closer to some of the peer educators in Digco. In these situations practitioner and peer educator share common ground and can work together, though not on a basis that would be approved by medical scientists or those who place their faith in medical scientists). However, still no peer educator from the 23 fitted this profile (though, if the profile was expanded to include a belief in witches, excluding the ability to send HIV, a view many health professionals would balk at, one peer educator would match this profile).

The third profile was a 'united front on AIDS' profile that further expands acceptable beliefs, and accepts any view that does not make a claim over the cause, prevention or a cure for HIV/AIDS that is incompatible with scientific understanding. Such a position would be uncomfortable for health professionals, since it tolerates witches and traditional pollution beliefs, but if it was agreed to disagree on these issues (including when they intruded into medical conditions), then peer educators and medical professionals could work alongside each other over AIDS. Eleven out of the 23 peer educators, or just under 50 per cent, would meet this wide compatibility profile.

The fourth category, which included the remaining 12 peer educators, held one or more beliefs over HIV/AIDS that are heretical to the medical model.

40   A total of 25 beliefs deviated from the third 'united front on AIDS' profile (see previous footnote). Five peer educators believed that witches could send HIV/AIDS, four that prayer could cure or prevent HIV/AIDS, three that AIDS was being used to kills Africans, three that sex with an uncleansed woman who had had an abortion could result in HIV/AIDS, three that ancestors could protect somebody from HIV/AIDS, two that sex with a woman who had not cleansed after the death of her spouse could result in HIV/AIDS, two that traditional healers have a cure for HIV/AIDS, two that sex with a menstruating woman could result in HIV/AIDS, and one that a church prophet could cure HIV/AIDS.

41   Even though two peer educators privately continued to believe that it was possible that HIV/AIDS could be cured by traditional healers.

42   The Zion Christian Church (ZCC) to which the peer educator belonged.

43   Niehaus (2009).

44   Rödlach (2006).

45   Steinberg (2008, p. 131).

46   Rogers (2003).

Chapter 4: AIDS backchat

1   This is true even when there is face-to-face contact between expert and lay recipients. The context of such encounters, whether it be in the consultation room or on company wellness day, provides enough clues for people to know that it's not appropriate to suggest, seriously, that God can cure AIDS, even if that is what they believe.

2   At least those who adhere to a purely scientific account of illness. As we see at various points in this book, nurses, for example, not infrequently believe in alternative healing cosmologies while working within the Western medical system.

3   Heald (2002, p. 3).

4   Traditional African understandings of body fluids typically see blood and semen as different forms of the same bodily fluid (e.g. *madi* in Sesotho indicates both blood and

semen).

5 This belief has a number of implications. One common one is, for example, the need for the ritualistic cleansing of blood after your spouse dies if pollution, resulting from the decay of what has become a shared blood, is to be avoided. Such pollution can result in traditional diseases which may be misdiagnosed as AIDS.

6 Nobuya Inagaki (2007) outlines three models of communication aimed at bringing about behavioural change. First, a 'modernisation paradigm' that is top-down, relies on mass communication, and assumes the superiority of its messages. Second, a 'diffusion model', which is also top-down and assumes the superiority of its messages, but focuses on the importance of interpersonal communication. The most well-known proponent of the diffusion model is Evert Rogers, whose diffusion of innovation model is vertical in nature, with change agents or experts who conceive or develop new innovations and who are 'usually professionals with a university degree in a technical field' at the top of a communication channel that utilises lay promoters of innovation or peer educators (Rogers, 2003, p. 28). Third, Inagaki lists a 'participatory model', which aims to be horizontal and interpersonal, and seeks not to provide knowledge or solutions but to generate these as the result of discourse. The value of drawing on people's knowledge of their own situation, through participatory development appraisal, is now widely recognised (Chambers, 1994).

    The diffusion and participation models of communication both envisage a role for peer education: the diffusion model incorporates them within a vertical process of message delivery, the participatory model places them within a horizontal process of knowledge generation. In the diffusion model, information flows down; in the participatory model, the information generated should flow up.

7 A focus on the social determinants of health would give room for a participatory model since grassroots discussions can provide useful information on how social conditions and cultural values constrain or support different behaviours. On this basis, peer educators might well be considered, though other methods, such as focus groups, are usually used to extract this information.

8 Frankham (1998, p. 11).

9 Albeit one that is often threatened by the competing pressures for production, typically personified in the form of a supervisor who may not be happy to see HIV/AIDS discussed in a time that could otherwise be used to meet production targets.

10 See Dickinson (2007).

11 Twenty-seven of the 28 Digco peer educators reported going to church at least twice a month. Several were lay preachers and one ran his own church.

12 This was one of the clear, though unanticipated, successes of the action research project in Digco.

13 Though this depends on the peer educator's relationship with a health professional who is able to provide the required information.

14 Myth 33, Box 4, Chapter 2.

15 Earlier in this book I critiqued a survey that caught out respondents with a question on the risks of HIV transmission from kissing. I was here myself caught in the complexities that this presents.

16 See McNeill (2009a), who makes this point in the case of community peer educators in Venda.

17 The peer educators generally portrayed men, rather than women, as being attracted to other sexual partners than their spouse.

18 Low-Beer and Stoneburner (2003).

19 Officially renamed the Thomas Titus Nkobi Memorial Park, but the new name is

rarely used.

20 The humour stems from the play on words regarding the political formation of the Triple Alliance (ANC, the COSATU trade union federation and the South African Communist Party) and its alliance with SANCO (South African National Civics Organisation), which was christened 'Three plus One' in the township politics of the 1990s.

21 See the description of the lay friction theory of HIV transmission in Chapter 2.

22 He also pointed out that men have to be careful with their preference for tight sex, in line with his friction theory of HIV infection.

Chapter 5: The kasi

1 The Census data splits the township of Bohlokong into the four contiguous sections of: Old Location, Thorisong, Vuka and Bohlokong. I have merged these into one figure and name representing the local geography and understanding of town and township. The data excludes the previously Coloured township of Bakenpark, which lies over the R26 highway from Bohlokong. Bakenpark has a population of some 2 000 people, of which 54 per cent are Coloured and 45 per cent African. Including this population into either the town or the township would lower the percentage of Bohlokong which is African and the percentage of Bethlehem which is White. All data is taken from Frith (2013).

2 Townships are divided into sections. In larger townships these are officially demarcated and each section has a set of house numbers (house numbers linked to a particular street are not used). Smaller townships have only one set of house numbers for all houses and sections are less formally demarcated.

3 The term 'garden boy', still widely used, refers to a man of any age working as a domestic gardener. Like the term 'kitchen girl' for a domestic worker/maid, the terms carry the legacies of racial domination referring to Black domestic workers as children. Rebecca Malope's song *My Mother was a Kitchen Girl* subverts these terms in a sugary celebration of Black servants' resilience and commitment to their children's future. An adapted version, sung by workers during protests, cuts the sugar out, 'My mother was a kitchen girl, my father was a garden boy/That's why I'm a *Komunista'* (Communist).

4 The *Daily Sun* is South African's biggest circulation newspaper. It is a sensational tabloid paper, notorious for its tall stories, that focuses on the concerns of township residents. The *Sowetan* is a serious tabloid newspaper that, prior to the arrival of the *Daily Sun,* was the most commonly read township newspaper.

5 Duncan (2013, p. 27).

6 As outlined in the Introduction, Potlakong and Butleng are fictitious townships.

7 The quart bottle, the most common size of beer bottle in South Africa, is, in contrast to US or UK measurements, 750 ml.

8 The Reconstruction and Development Programme (RDP), South Africa's first post-1994 economic policy, included low-cost houses subsidised by the government. The RDP programme was superseded in 1996, but the name has stuck to the small, four-roomed houses that, despite being built in their millions, have failed to keep pace with demand.

9 The African Bank, a relative newcomer to South Africa's financial sector, is the largest provider of unsecured loans in the country. These loans are made without collateral. They are, however, given to those in employment, who must sign garnishee or direct debit orders that deduct monthly repayments. Loan applications are quickly processed. Loans are relatively small (up to R180 000). Repayments are between 2

and 2.4 times the original loan, depending on the repayment period, but additional charges, including compulsory loan insurance, increase the total costs. The bank targets the lower-income market that is otherwise badly serviced by the more established banks. It claims that with its loans, 'You don't have to wait for life to start, you can enjoy the lifestyle you want now ...' (African Bank, 2013).

10 Pampers is a trade name of Procter & Gamble; however, it is used as a generic term for disposable nappies.

11 In January 2012, the time of this account.

12 *Spaza* shops are small independently run township stores selling a small range of basic items.

13 There are local Sekasi names for each coin and note in circulation. *Ponto* goes back to 1961 when the rand, as a new currency, was initially pegged at R2 to a British pound (the currency that had previously been legal tender in South Africa). The Sesotho transliteration of the English pound has stuck with R2, initially a note, and from the 1990s a coin.

14 Extra large cans of 440 ml.

15 The term is drawn from Peter Wogan (2004), though originally used by Clifford Geertz.

16 Reynolds Whyte (2009).

17 Gausset (2001).

18 As can their breakdown, such as the weakening of traditionally prescribed sexual relationships.

19 Saethre and Stadler (2009).

20 They end up serving the role of tourist destinations, destinations for school trips and conference venues.

21 One of the major telecommunications companies in South Africa providing cellular telephone and internet services.

22 Television soap operas.

23 Both these teams, which are constantly in competition to top the 'log' (football league) are based in Soweto and have by far the largest following of the domestic teams.

24 South African Press Service (SAPA) (2012).

25 Statistics South Africa (2012b); Ministry for Cooperative Government and Traditional Affairs (2011).

26 The slogan was used by the ANC in the first democratic elections of 1994.

27 Most visibly in the explosion of xenophobic riots that occurred across South Africa in May 2008 when more than 60 people were killed. Xenophobic tensions and violence are, however, endemic in townships and foreign-owned shops are almost invariably looted during disturbances.

28 Notably the strike at the Marikana mine in August/September 2012 which saw 34 people die in a confrontation with police on 16 August, and other 'wildcat' strikes across the mining industry in late 2012.

29 Pick n Pay is a South African mid-level supermarket chain; U$ave is the low-income brand of the Shoprite retail group.

30 Despite the widespread practice of selling 'loose draw', it has, since the introduction of the Tobacco Products Control Amendment Act of 2008, been illegal, with all tobacco products having to be sold in packets printed with health warnings.

31 Although social relationships are changing within African society, it is still common that a child remains within, and has the surname of, the mother's family until formal marriage arrangements, including the payment of *lobola* (bride wealth), have been completed.

32 The fictitious, historically White town, with which Butleng is linked.

33 Sekasi like Fanagalo is a *lingua franca* made up of different languages. However, while Fanagalo, used extensively on South African mines, was formalised as a language of command, Sekasi has emerged from an uncontrolled, and ongoing, process within townships. There are wide variations in Sekasi based on geography and also the relative dominance of particular languages among speakers. See Appendix 1 for more on Sekasi.

Chapter 6: The precarious life of Bafana Radebe

1 The University of Natal Medical School (now the University of KwaZulu-Natal) in Durban was established in 1951 for Black (African, Coloured and Indian) students within what was otherwise a university for Whites. For two decades it was the only tertiary education institution focused on training Black medical students in South Africa. It first admitted White undergraduate students in 1995 (University of Natal Medical School, 2013).

2 R500 or five hundred rand (the South African currency unit) was worth approximately US$60 at the time. This sum, in Sekasi 'Five Clipper', is a considerable amount of money. The old-age state pension was a little over R1,000 a month at the time.

3 In Sesotho the third person singular pronoun does not distinguish gender – *yena* refers to him or her.

4 Miliary or disseminated tuberculosis (TB) is characterised by widespread disease lesions throughout the body. These give the appearance on X-ray pictures of millet seeds, hence the name of this form of TB.

5 The sick role involves an ill person being given or taking permission to be absolved of normal responsibilities and duties and to be afforded special privileges and favours, such as Bafana being able to legitimately reject any food that he disliked or request any that took his fancy.

6 CD4 tests provide a measure of how strong a person's immune system is. Monitoring this allows the commencement of antiretroviral drugs before the immune system is too compromised and the individual succumbs to opportunistic infections that will require extensive, costly medical intervention. Left too late, as is commonly the case, such interventions may not be effective and the patient may die before it is possible to commence antiretroviral therapy.

7 Under Apartheid policies of separate development, ten ethnically based 'homelands' were created, often as a patchwork of discontinuous territories, frequently referred to derogatorily as Bantustans. Four of these became nominally independent states but remained dependent on South Africa and were not recognised internationally. They were absorbed back into South Africa following the 1994 transition to democracy.

8 The self-governing, but not independent, homeland for ethnic Basotho was established in 1974 and comprised some 650 square kilometres. It is now part of the Free State and home to some 300 000 people.

9 Since independence in 1980, Zimbabwe.

10 The Rand is the strip of land running east-west through Johannesburg and is the site of extensive mining activity in the past and is now largely industrialised and/or urbanised. On either side of Johannesburg, the East and West Rand form large urban centres. The East Rand now forms the Ekurhuleni Metropolitan Municipality, but the term East Rand remains in common use.

11 Of South Africa's nine official African languages, four, isiZulu, siSwati, isiXhosa and isiNdebele, form the Nguni language group and are, largely, mutually intelligible. The

Sesotho group of languages, again largely mutually intelligible, consists of Sesotho (sometimes called Southern Sotho), Sepedi (Northern Sotho) and Setswana. See Appendix 1 for more on South Africa's languages.

12 Paroz ([1961] 1988).

13 In fact a series of three parliamentary Acts, promulgated in 1950, 1957 and 1966 (with numerous amendments), that determined, on the basis of race, where people could live or run businesses in the urban areas. It was repealed in 1991.

14 Meaning, in this context, that she had passed her final-year school exams.

15 Hunter (2010).

16 The Ekurhuleni Metropolitan Municipality was created in 1999 from the merger of the seven towns and their associated townships that had previously been separate municipal entities.

17 Alternatively, Northern Sotho (*Sesotho sa Leboa*), one of South Africa's nine official African languages. It forms part of the Sesotho language group and is spoken by some four million people, primarily in Limpopo, Gauteng and Mpumalanga provinces; see Appendix 1.

18 The Zion Christian Church (or ZCC), established in 1924, is one of the largest African-initiated churches in southern Africa. There are two main divisions within the church, both with their headquarters in South Africa's Limpopo Province. Like many Apostolic or Zionist churches, the ZCC promotes faith-healing through the laying on of hands, the use of blessed water, the drinking of tea and coffee brewed and blessed by a church member, and the wearing of blessed cords or cloth.

19 The complaint that patients with sexually transmitted infections are not treated with respect in government health facilities is common. In additional to the often poor levels of care and respect in clinics and hospitals, gender and moral factors are at play. Nurses typically represent a higher social strata in the townships and are frequently strongly religious; those coming in for treatment of sexually transmitted infections are seen as both immoral and irresponsible and unnecessarily adding to their workload.

20 An international insurance company with its headquarters in South Africa, with 14 million clients worldwide.

21 Apostolic and Pentecostal churches accounted for some 38 per cent of the population in the 2001 National Census. Both forms of churches appear to be growing, particularly among township residents.

22 'Throwing the bones' is a common form of divination practised by many African traditional healers. It involves casting a bag of small objects (traditionally animal bones) which represent characters and forces. The alignment of the objects, when thrown out onto a mat, is used to probe the patient's condition, in particular his or her relationship with other people, including their ancestors. There are a host of other divination techniques that are used; the absence of these in Bafana's consultations indicates a focus on the physical symptoms that Bafana presented, rather than an exploration of their underlying causes. As we see in this narrative, Bafana is using this absent diagnostic event to suggest that it wasn't witchcraft; a good healer would have sensed if this was the case and proceeded to investigate.

23 As the biggest circulation daily paper in South Africa, the *Daily Sun* provides often sensational coverage of issues relevant to township residents, including witchcraft. While an important source of information, Bafana recognises the limited credibility of any individual *Daily Sun* story when put under scrutiny.

24 Fassin (2007, p. 230).

25 As a measure of an individual's immune system strength, a CD4 count of 200 (cells/ mm^3) is cause for alarm. The CD4 count of a healthy individual ranges between 500

and 1 000 cells/mm³.

26 A 'please call me' is a free SMS message with which the sender can request somebody who has airtime or a phone contract to ring them back (and pay for the call).

27 South Africa allocates a unique 13-digit identity (ID) number to citizens and permanent residents, which is used extensively in bureaucratic and commercial processes.

28 Commissioners of Oaths are required to stamp document copies in South Africa before they will be accepted by bureaucracies or companies.

29 Jonny Clegg. 2002. 'Impi.' In: *The Best of Juluka/Savuka* (CD). The song is a pro-Zulu account of the 1879 battle of Isandlwana during the Anglo-Zulu War.

30 In South Africa *madam* refers to wives who would be in charge of one or more domestic servants. Given South Africa's past, this inevitably meant White women in charge of Black servants. Depending on context, the title can be respectful, sarcastic or derogatory.

31 These condoms, branded as 'Choice' in an attempt to increase their consumer appeal, are free and widely distributed in South Africa.

32 All tuberculosis results from strains of the *mycobacterium bacillus* infecting the body. By far the most common site of infection is the lungs (pulmonary tuberculosis), but any part of the body can be infected, resulting in different conditions. The severity of any infection will depend on factors, including the health of the individual (and the strength of their immune system) and the degree to which the *bacillus* variety has acquired drug resistance.

33 Bafana's observation is sound. In large part to aggressive campaigns to combat syphilis and other STIs, in the hope that this would reduce HIV infections, prevalence among pregnant women attending public health care facilities, measured by the *South African National Antenatal Sentinel HIV & Syphilis Prevalence Surveys*, has dropped from 11.2 per cent in 1997 to 1.6 per cent in 2011 (Department of Health, 2011, p. 58).

34 See Chapter 2.

35 The part of Pentecostal church services (in particular) in which congregants go forward to ask God for help, confess sins or acknowledge a commitment to God; see Chapter 9 for more details.

36 Willis (1978).

37 Willis (1978, p. 41).

Chapter 7: The certainties of Paseka Radebe

1 Such reclaiming of property into the man's family when the wife dies is not uncommon though the presence of children, bearing the dead man's surname, usually mitigates this.

2 The term applies only to degrees of cousinship without states of removal. Any removal ends the *bana ba motho* link, with the generational difference changing the nature of the relationship. Thus, for example, a first-cousin-once-removed would be regarded as an aunt or uncle and would stand in a very different status to each other compared to the 'sibling'-type relationship between *bana ba motho*.

3 Weddings are less significant in this role, though they play an important part in transferring women between families, a process symbolised through the payment of *lebola* (bride wealth) and the two-stage ceremony, usually over a weekend, starting at the bride's *habo* (family home) and moving to the groom's *habo*.

4 In the original Sesotho-Sekasi: "*Now ke paiya revenge. E ne e le nako ya ka hore, ha ke re, yena o se a painelwa o utlwa bohloko ... [Di]ntho tse nkutlwisitseng bohloko... now tshwantse nna ke mo utlwele bohloko. At the same time, ke jumpe speed ke lo mo safe.*"

5 I use the term 'love' in a straightforward and practical way. Love is shown by care: caring for somebody, when it is unpleasant, burdensome, time-consuming or costly in any way, demonstrates love.

6 This latter sacrifice makes no sense in terms of high blood pressures, since dietary recommendations, such as the Dietary Approaches to Stop Hypertension (DASH), recommend the use of spices as an alternative to salt (US Department of Health and Human Sciences, 2006). The high salt content of popular pre-prepared synthesised spice-mixes in South Africa, such as the Aromat brand, whose name is synonymous with real spice, may account for this common belief in spices being bad for health.

7 Cleansing refers to the belief in removing polluting substances from the body.

8 See Chapter 1 for an account of the ethnoecological disease *nyoko*. Additionally to this role as a cleansing agent, some of these over-the counter patent medicines can be used, in large dosages, as an abortifacient.

9 The normal range for blood pressure is 90-119/60-79 [systolic or arterial pressure/ diastolic or veinal pressure]. Hypertension is classified as 140/90 or higher.

10 This is contestable; Dr Sibonyani needed to justify his R200 consultation fee. Fiddling with the dosage of the hypertension-lowering drugs would be one justification. Getting the right dosage for an individual is a process of trial and error. The problem here is that three people were simultaneously adjusting the dosage: the clinic nurse, private doctor and patient. Ultimate control lay in Paseka's hands, only she knew how many pills she was really taking. Dr Sibonyani could also justify his role and his fee by prescribing an additional drug with possible benefits.

11 A common household cleaning soap, generally used for scrubbing and washing clothes.

12 Steaming is widely practised by church prophets as well as by traditional healers and, of course, more mainstream spa treatments.

13 Apostolic/Zionist churches generally have both a *moruti* or preacher and *baprofeta* or prophets. The *moruti* heads the church and addresses the congregation, while the prophets conduct the processes of divination and healing.

14 Turner (1981).

15 In addition to questions of belief and relief, her work as a healer had been a source of income, which was not the case with church membership, but with most church activities on the weekends she had been freed up and was able to find employment as a domestic worker.

16 Paseka explain, *Dipilisi tsa sepetlele di mo thusitse but ntho e neng e mo booster haholo e leng hore nna ke mo thusitse ka yona ke di motoho wa diherbs o ne ke mo rekela ona.* (The pills from the hospital helped him, but the thing which boosted him a lot was that which I helped him with, the fortified *pap* which I bought for him.)

17 Nor that, linguistically, she slipped partly into Sekasi with '*diherbs*'.

18 Initiation schools, in which young men (and sometimes young women) are secluded from society for a period of time remain widespread in South Africa. A key and highly controversial feature is the traditional circumcision of men. There is a wide variation on how 'going to the mountain' takes place (a common euphemism for attending circumcision school across South Africa). However, it is far from universal among Africans. It is not practised by all ethnic groups within the African population and it is viewed as a remnant of backwardness by many educated sections of the township, particularly those attending Pentecostal churches. Even here, however, circumcision is frequently seen as important for men and is conducted through hospital or clinic-based procedures. Although public attention is often focused on the circumcision component of the school, and particularly the not infrequent maiming and deaths

that result from poorly run schools, these institutions are more than traditional ways of circumcising men. They also provide a rite of passage into manhood, form a key component of a traditional African worldview, and establish bonded groups of *mathaka* (age-mates) and networks.

Chapter 8: The struggles of Grace Dlamini

1 The South African name for 'Blu-Tack' or 'Sticky Fix'.

2 Service delivery protest is the generic term used to describe the increasingly frequent township disturbances in post-Apartheid South Africa. These disturbances usually result from a multiplicity of frustrations, prominent among these being the lack of services, poor services or slow implementation of services such as water, electricity, roads and sewerage.

3 Previously part of the Transvaal and now the most northern of South Africa's nine provinces.

4 The Pedi or Bapedi classificatory group consists of a range of related ethnic groups, predominantly in the north of South Africa, that speak a number of dialects of Sepedi or Northern Sotho.

5 The largest classificatory ethnic group in South Africa, speaking isiZulu and concentrated in the KwaZulu-Natal Province, which borders the Indian Ocean on the east coast of the country.

6 Located, as can be assumed, in the north-west of South Africa and bordering Botswana. Approximately half of the Gross Provincial Product comes from mining activities, which include platinum, gold and diamonds.

7 *Simba* is the generic Sekasi loan word for potato crisps, taken from a common brand of crisps.

8 A South African brand of cider particularly popular among women.

9 Stories of similar treatment are not uncommon from the early years of the epidemic. With no effective treatment and resources limited, there was widespread shunning of those diagnosed as HIV positive even among medical professionals.

10 A brand of milk powder manufactured by Nestlé and popular in South Africa.

11 The provision of antiretroviral drugs in the public sector was delayed by the Mbeki government (see for example, Geffen, 2010). Chapter 10 discussed some of the background to this state resistance to treatment provision.

12 The roll-out of antiretroviral drugs initially started with a small number of key sites, near large population centres.

13 *Toyi-toying* refers specifically to the dancing employed during protest marches in South Africa. More generally it can reference any form of protest or resistance.

14 See Chapter 2 for a description of ancestral belief and its linkage to HIV/AIDS.

15 Revelation, Chapter 2, Verses 20–23.

16 Sundkler (1961, p. 266). Italics in the original.

17 The standard public health message at the time, which has since been modified for people on antiretroviral therapy and undetectable viral loads.

18 Nguyen (2010).

19 The three-letter acronym PWA, despite being incomplete and technically incorrect, has stuck. Attempts to establish the more complete and more accurate PLWHA (Person Living with HIV/AIDS) have not been successful.

20 Of 18 May 2011.

21 SAnews (2011).

Chapter 9: The salvation of Neo Pakwe

1   In Sekasi, the card suit of Diamonds is called 'Dice', while Clubs is 'Fly'. Hearts and Spades are the same.

2   The qualifying 'feela' (only) is important here in suggesting that it was a minor ailment. *Sefuba* without a qualification could refer to any chest infection – that it was TB would be clarified as *sefuba sa TB*. In formal Sesotho, TB is *lefuba*, though this term is rarely used outside translated information sheets on TB.

3   John, Chapter 1, Verse 29.

4   Martin (1990).

5   Hunter (2010); Mayer and Mayer (1974); Moodie and Ndatshe (1994).

6   Such as *mashoba* (fly whisks made from the tails of cows, which are symbols of traditional authority).

7   The Living Waters Church made an effort to welcome Africans from other countries residing in Butleng. On occasion they would be encouraged to give short prayers in other African languages, such as Shona.

8   The church encourages its members, whether men or women, to progress in practical ways. This means escaping poverty, even if only to *zama* (try through business) and earn a few rands selling *makwena* (fatcakes or dumplings) to neighbours. The promise, held out in the services, is much more than a few rands. But this will not come all at once. After *makwena,* the next step might be to open a *spaza* shop or sew clothes. The church runs a small credit scheme that operates entirely without collateral other than reputation and doesn't account in any formal way for repayment. Church members explain their plan and, if approved, the money is handed over. The repayment is via the *boshome* (tenth, i.e. tithing) of their income that church members are encouraged to give. If the business is successful, their contribution to the church will increase. It was, however, stressed that it is prayer that was critical in ensuring that these endeavours succeed and attention was paid in Bible classes as to how one should pray.

9   The same mixture of prayer and practicality applied to getting a job as well as in making business enterprises succeed. This was more applicable to the youth of the church. *Moruti* Mofokeng's key advice was for them to respect themselves by paying attention to their personal appearance and by dressing as smartly as they could. While God looks at the heart, *Moruti* Mofokeng explained, such an attitude shows the person is making an effort and truly does want to do something to better him- or herself. And if this happens in the eyes of God then, no doubt, it will also be the case in the eyes of others who have to select from the vast pool of unemployed youth.

10   See Chapter 1.

11   While the widespread belief in witchcraft within African township society is rooted in traditional beliefs, the Bible does refer to witches, notably the Witch of Endor (Samuel 1, Chapter 28, Verses 3–25).

12   *Bontate*: the senior men. There are women who carried out this role in the Holy Spirit Church but they were few and far between. Women can take up senior positions, if they are called by God to do so, but as *Moruti* Mofokeng pointed out without any embarrassment, the Bible says that women are weak, so while some women would have the spirit for this it was not likely to be many.

13   When I discussed the role of church leaders in healing with some of the *bontate*, a key concern was that any person who took on this role in mediating between a *mokopi* (supplicant) and *Modimo* (God) must be secure in his or her own faith. It was also possible for people to imitate this power without having the Holy Spirit within them. The book of Jude predicts that impostors will infiltrate the church in the Last Days.

The Living Waters Church elders argued that such men, acting as pastors, could use *maslamosa* (magic) to cure people. That was, of course, something from Satan, not God; the *bana by lefifi* (children of darkness) would walk among the *bana ba lesedi* (children of light). Nothing should be taken at face value.

14 More sceptical visitors cited this thrust, which many preachers utilise when laying on hands, as a trick used to demonstrate apparent power. Some church members reported tussles during these altar calls, especially with visiting preachers. If they didn't feel the Spirit overcoming them, they would not cooperate with the preacher's attempts to get them to go over backwards. Such disagreements were visible during altar calls, but so were many cases where *bakopi* (supplicants) were clearly overcome and would have been hurt without the stewards there to break their fall. At times the emotional atmosphere in the church could be intense and powerful during altar calls.

15 The distinction between preacher and evangelist is not absolute. Some preachers are known for their evangelistic ability, that is to convert people to Christianity, and this would be put to use within specific events such as 'revival missions'.

16 The older Sesotho translation of the Bible (*Bibele e Hlalelang,* First Edition, South African orthography, 1961, based on a 1907 translation) is still much more widely used than the newer translation (*Bibele: Phetolelo e Ntjha,* First Edition, 1989) in Butleng's churches.

17 It lists *feba* and *boka* (arguably translated as adultery and fornication) as well as translating debauchery as *bootswa* (which has strong connotations of prostitution).

18 McNeill and Niehaus (2009).

19 The allies of health promotion, such as Sister Maurine mediating her medical role as nurse with the bio-moral understanding of the Butleng churches, operate largely below the radar of public health scrutiny. Their messages are adapted and transformed to suit local cultural formations, without official approval.

20 Squire (2007).

21 Squire (2007, p. 158).

22 Or further, for example, misunderstanding an 'undetectable viral load' as HIV being cured.

23 This is not so different from how other cosmologies of cure within the South African plural health care systems operate. Each seeks, for want of a better word, to 'brand' themselves as being able to assist. In a competitive environment this is necessary; you must attract adherents. Once drawn in, the real work of healing can proceed, though the problem of 'patient' loyalty and adherence to treatment remains.

We can attempt to evaluate the strengths and weaknesses of each system's promotion and practice, but since this would need to cover, *inter alia*, the scope of authority claimed, access, costs, the efficacy of treatment, the quality of care, empathy experienced, and the psychological as well as physiological dimensions involved in these treatment practices, such calculations are all but impossible – other than pointing out a range of strengths and weaknesses for each healing system. In any case, isolating one component of healing, such as its efficacy to correct physiological dysfunction, is a scientific exercise that is not reflective of health-seeking behaviour. The continued existence of plural health care systems indicates that, from users' perspectives, these tallies of strengths and weaknesses fail to point exclusively to one or other of the contending options.

Over HIV/AIDS, the ability of alternative health systems to claim therapeutic parity with Western medicine has been noted. Western science doesn't have a cure and what it does offer requires strict adherence and is attended by risks and side-effects. As with Neo's sister, Holekane, following an HIV diagnosis there is a period of patient training, a test of commitment, before treatment will be commenced. Once this begins, regular checks must be made to monitor the treatment's effectiveness. Despite this, those adhering to their drug regimes are subject to inexplicably fluctuating CD4 counts and the side-effects that the drugs bring.

24 Passed on to a witch, the supplicant's problem would be apparently responded to by an ancestor visiting them in a dream. Once the *mosebetsi* (celebration to honour the ancestors) was held and the situation subsequently improved, it would be the ancestors that would be thanked, not God, for their help, even though God had been the true benefactor.

25 In Sesotho, some of this is short-cut by the verb *belaela,* which connotes the ideas of suspicion and doubt.

26 Accidents are also out of the control of those using minibus taxis. Car safety belts are not worn in minibus taxis and, in townships, even for private cars these are seen as an accessory only appropriate for long journeys. My insistence on wearing seatbelts in my car has on several occasions been opposed on the grounds that it would mark us out as not being from the township (and therefore a target for crime). Pointing out the obvious, that my white skin gives the game away belt or no belt, exposes that it is really my passengers' embarrassment at wearing a seatbelt in opposition to the township norm that is the issue. When I insist, using the joking formula, '*Ke molao kahare koloi ya ka hore batho ba tswanetse ho apara mabanta'* (It's the law in my car that people must wear [seat]belts), and we belt up, it is not uncommon that I have to assist first-time passengers on the use of this unfamiliar safety device.

27 And a largely uncatalogued herbal pharmacopoeia.

28 An alternative way in which Neo stood her ground against *setso* was to ask whether it was in the Bible. In this way she dismissed traditional rituals around funerals, such as the careful ordering of male relatives of the deceased throwing earth into the grave and the shaving of the heads of the bereaved family. There was, she contended, no justification for these practices to be found. Once on a roll, she would continue her offensive against *setso. Jwala* (alcohol), which played a central part within traditional rituals, was in her view the supercharger of sin and the cause of suffering. So *setso* was promoting sinful behaviour and leading people into misery. Finally, if there was a need to be more direct over the harm caused by *setso,* she cited polygamy and widow inheritance practices as affronts to God's laws and the cause of HIV infection.

Chapter 10: An elite dispute

1 Melville (1972, p. 261). Italics in the original.

2 Schneider (2002, p. 153).

3 Geffen (2010, p. 2).

4 Mbeki (2002).

5 Gevisser (2007, p. 736).

6 Though others ascribe authorship differently. For example, Keyan Tomaselli (2011, p. 30) cites the authorship of *Castro Hlongwane* to Peter Mokaba.

7 In addition to scientists, the document references various institutional sources, such as the World Bank and World Health Organisation.

8 Even if some of the arguments made in the document are not themselves good science. For example, the document argues that the HIV virus had never been isolated or analysed and that 'nobody knows what it looks like'. Without this information, the document argues that HIV as a cause of death is simply speculation.

9 Mbeki (2002, pp. 54-55).

10 Mbeki (2002, p. 16). The argument is later buttressed with reference to the UNDP's approach to health in India (Mbeki, 2002, p. 68).

11 Anthony Butler (2005).

12 Gevisser (2007, p. 750).

13 Mbeki (2002, p. 8). Emphasis in the original.

14 For example, Fourie and Meyer (2010); Kalichman (2009); Nattrass (2007) and (2012).

15 Though Nattrass (2007) and others would reluctantly find themselves in agreement with Mbeki's social determinant of health argument.

16 A point made by Fourie and Meyer (2010) even though it contradicts the thrust of their arguments over Mbeki's role in the epidemic.

17 Caution over what impact political leadership has had within the AIDS epidemic should not be used to mitigate judgement on Mbeki's record in holding back the state's response to HIV/AIDS, notably over antiretroviral drug provision.

18 This professional twitchiness over what the population is believed to believe and its apparent gullibility is also illustrated by the outrage provoked by the then Vice-President Jacob Zuma's courtroom revelation that he had taken a shower after having sex with an HIV-positive woman. The ensuring commentary rarefied his post-coital activity from the practical act of washing sexual fluids from his penis, which would reduce the chance of infection, if only marginally, to the allegation that he held mystical beliefs in the power of showering to retrospectively prevent HIV infection. Having unprotected sex with an HIV-positive partner is not a smart thing to do, but then ridiculing Zuma for the little he could do after the event is not smart either. Of course, if the commentators who condemned Zuma for his showering actually knew much about the lives of township residents, then they might not have been so indignant about the harm his courtroom statement would do. Very few township residents have showers and wash in a *waskom* (washing bowl).

19 Kalichman (2009, p. 25).

20 Into which Kalichman has no hesitation in placing Duesberg, given his earlier work on cancer-causing genes.

21 Kalichman (2009, p. 150).

22 Steinberg (2008, p. 153).

23 The document also reports that they assumed he was a rapist because of his race. The section of the document relating to Casto Hlongwane reads as follows: 'More recently than everything we have said about racism and AIDS, what we have recounted above was illustrated in an ugly racist incident that took place at a Caravan Park near Port Edward in southern KwaZulu-Natal at the end of December 2001. A group of White school children decided to have an end-of-year party at this Caravan Park. Among them was one Black boy, Castro Hlongwane, 17, their schoolmate. Because he is Black, the owners of the Park ordered him to leave, despite the fact that he was properly booked in together with his White friends. One of the witnesses to this incident, Amy Godfrey, said this was "pure racism like I have never seen in my life".

Relevant to our story, *The Sunday Times* of January 6, 2002, reported: '*Schoolmate Ryan Templar, 18, said he was told by (Park owner) Theresa Smit that Hlongwane had AIDS and would rape other campers.*' The unsophisticated Theresa Smit expressed openly a conviction and belief that many other sophisticated 'Theresa Smits' hold, but would never express in public, *because they are mature practitioners of the deceits of the sophisticated.* Nevertheless, they do everything they can to demand the implementation of policies and programmes based on the conviction and belief that, *because he is Black, "Hlongwane has AIDS and will rape other campers!"* When they are caught red-handed in their immersion in racism, they readily respond that their accusers seek to silence them by "playing the race card!"

Thus does the victim of racism get transformed into a racist, while the racist escapes scot-free by the transformation of the perpetrator into a victim! In spite of the spectacular advances in science, miracles are still part of our daily lives!

(NB: the Hlongwane incident and Foot & Mouth Disease have provided us the title to this dissertation.)' (Mbeki, 2002, p. 58). Emphasis in the original.

24 The one reference to religion in the document is in Chapter 2, referring metaphorically to the book of Genesis, which expresses the hope that the authors will be able to 'separate the light from the darkness with regard to the issue of AIDS' even though they do not have the power of the Creator (Mbeki, 2002, p. 9).

25 Cullinan and Thom (2009, p. xii).

26 Fourie and Meyer (2010).

27 Though even here we have to accept that the cosmologies, from which folk theories of AIDS arise, pre-date AIDS's arrival as well as Mbeki's interventions. We also have to recognise the doubt created by denialism does not support, in any direct way, many of these theories.

28 Thom (2009).

29 Nicholson (2011).

30 eNCA (2013).

31 Before Hercules and Iolaus worked out that if they cauterised each bloody stump of the Hydra's decapitated heads they would not regenerate.

Chapter 11: Agency from below

1 Nattrass (2007, p. 184).

2 The Treatment Action Campaign is aware of this. It has attempted to link courtroom cases with community mobilisation. The campaign to develop a cadre of AIDS activists in working class, often African communities was bold and ambitious. Zackie Achmat (2003, p. xvii) has explained, 'the TAC believes that it is an individual's responsibility to study ethics, science, law, politics and economics, medicine and history. This is the duty of every HIV/AIDS activist, whether HIV positive or negative, literate or illiterate, and it is the key to stopping the epidemic.' However, McNeill and Niehaus (2009, p. 115) have persuasively argued that equating treatment literacy with a commitment to biomedical models is mistaken.

3 Fee (1988, p. 121).

4 Their character differs enormously and it is difficult to calibrate the degree to which their situations are the result of circumstance dealt to them and how much is the outcome of choices they have made within these circumstances.

5 People use various sources of information and inspiration to imagine these different kinds of AIDS. Some information and inspiration may have trickled down from high-profile AIDS dissidents. As outlined in Chapter 10, a 'strong thesis' that they have taken on, verbatim, the dissident views expressed by Mbeki or other prominent denialists lacks credibility. It may be that the 'weak thesis' that Mbeki's doubt gave people more leeway to work with alternatives to that of medical science has some credibility. Nevertheless, it is clear that the admixture of their beliefs contains much that comes from within their own social environments and not a little that they have individually formulated.

6 Goffman (1974).

7 Though that does not mean, as Goffman outlines, that both parties understand a frame in the same way. 'Fabrications' involve the keying of a situation by one party in a way that is credible, but not correct, for another party. Scams and other frauds are examples of such fabrications in which the dupe is lured into a framing of the

situation that is, in fact, false.

8 She also felt that her cousin's belief that Bafana's AIDS was caused by an evil spirit was undermining her attempts to mobilise practical help for him.

9 At least when 'on duty'. Sister Maurine, who spoke at the Bulteng World AIDS Day (Chapter 9) event, provides a good example of how nurses (and peer educators) may well be juggling different systems of belief themselves.

10 De Certeau (1984).

11 Integrated into this is a degree of trust for experts who work, usually for a fee, on our behalf to provide advice on how to proceed.

12 Something that also needs to be taken into account in understanding the treatment odysseys often undertaken in response to HIV infection.

13 That were only kept at bay when the aunt was 'born again' and slept with a Bible under her pillow.

14 Ashforth (2002, p. 13).

15 See Chapter 10 for a brief account.

16 Especially within the age- and gender-demarcated groupings that inevitably form themselves on these occasions.

17 Gausset (2001, p. 512).

18 Kempton (1987, p. 223).

19 A point that he illustrates by outlining how spouses continue to hold different theories of how their (shared) thermostat works, with their different ways of achieving the same desired objective being a source of ongoing domestic tension.

20 Michael McCloskey (1983, p. 318) reaches the same conclusion with university physics students finding that 'many ... emerge from a physics course with their impetus theories [a theory of motion similar to that held in the pre-Newtonian 14th century] largely intact'.

21 Holland and Quinn (1987). Collins and Gentner (1987, p. 284) make the same point in a study of how educated Americans understood evaporation. Often they utilised a number of 'component models' to explain different phenomena associated with evaporation, to create a 'pastiche model'.

22 Rather, like the wider South African social welfare system, and the men working away from Butleng, Western medicine was important to but distant from Neo; something in the background that is taken for granted on a day-to-day basis.

23 A noun that originates from the mythological event.

24 Arthur Klienman *et al.* have highlighted the difference between patients' understanding of illness and the medical practitioners' focus on disease. They argue that at its extreme, 'this [scientific disease] orientation, so successful in generating technological interventions, leads to a veterinary practice of medicine.' Kleinman, Eisenberg, and Good (1978, p. 252).

Appendix 1: The unwritten language of the kasi

1 Statistics South Africa (2012a).

2 Though the census does not take into account the degree to which these languages are spoken across South Africa's international borders.

3 I take issue with the idea of 'rural areas', at least in some dimensions, in Chapter 5.

4 Unless, perhaps, you happen to be in China or maybe Latin America.

5 So, if you try to learn, say, Sesotho, you will struggle to find even basic educational resources, current material or skilled tutors (isiZulu and, to an extent, isiXhosa are better provided for in this respect, but it's a relative advantage only).

6 Or, reflecting the lack of any fixed orthography, Sekasie.

7 Paroz ([1961] 1988).
8 Doke and Mofokeng (1957).
9 Itself already heavily influenced by other languages.
10 On the South African platinum belt this has played out with the use of Fanagalo (or Fanakalo), the formal *lingua franca* of the mining industry that was banished (at least officially) with democracy as demeaning, under pressure from the National Union of Mineworkers (NUM). Twenty years later, insurgent mineworkers have re-appropriated Fanagalo, effectively a version of Sekasi, for themselves, leaving the now establishment NUM with English, which its officials share with mine management.

Appendix 3: Methodology
1 Dickinson (2009).
2 See Whyte (1989) for a description of participatory action research.
3 Weiss (1994, p. 119).

Index